Introduction to Geographic Information Systems in Public Health

Alan L. Melnick, MD, MPH

Director
Joint Residency in Family Medicine/Preventive Medicine
Oregon Health Sciences University
Portland, Oregon

Health Officer,
Clackamas County, Oregon

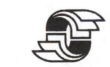

AN ASPEN PUBLICATION®
Aspen Publishers, Inc.
Gaithersburg, Maryland
2002

Library of Congress Cataloging-in-Publication Data

Melnick, Alan L.
Introduction to geographic information systems in public health/Alan L. Melnick
p. cm.
Includes bibliographical references and index.
ISBN 0-8342-1878-X
1. Public health—Data processing. 2. Geographic information systems. 1. Title.

RA566.M435 2002
614.4'0285—dc21
2001056635

Cover map has been reprinted from www.cdc.gov/nchs/data/atmapall.pdf (January 2002),
National Center for Health Statistics.

Orders: (800) 638-8437
Customer Service: (800) 234-1660

About Aspen Publishers • For more than 40 years, Aspen has been a leading professional publisher in a variety
of disciplines. Aspen's vast information resources are available in both print and electronic formats. We are
committed to providing the highest quality information available in the most appropriate format for our
customers. Visit Aspen's Internet site for more information resources, directories, articles, and a searchable
version of Aspen's full catalog, including the most recent publications: **www.aspenpublishers.com**
Aspen Publishers, Inc. • The hallmark of quality in publishing
Member of the worldwide Wolters Kluwer group

Editorial Services: Megg Mueller Schulte
Library of Congress Catalog Card Number: 2001056635
ISBN: 0-8342-1878-X

Printed in the United States of America

1 2 3 4 5

To my wife Kelly, for your patience, for giving me time to write, for your love, and for inspiring me to do the right things.

To my son Martin, for giving me the time to write, for your love and support, and for teaching me how to teach.

"Place absorbs our earliest notice and attention, it bestows on us our original awareness; and our critical powers spring up from the study of it and the growth of experience inside it. From the dawn of man's imagination, place has enshrined the spirit; as soon as man stopped wandering and stood still and looked about him, he found a god in that place; and from then on, that was where the god abided and spoke from if ever he spoke."

–Eudora Welty, *"Place in Fiction"*

Table of Contents

Foreword

Historically, public health has often provided the proof that it's a whole lot easier to collect data than to put it to any good use. The result—an unfortunate reputation for an action-oriented discipline that strives to have data driven decisions. Yet, even today, almost every health department can point in most any direction at accessible data that in theory could inform programs and policy makers, but in practice do not.

The underlying problem is that it's always been simpler to gather data than to analyze it. Analysis requires the synthesis and integration of many bits of data into recognizable patterns and relationships. The ability to translate data into useful, understandable information—critical to our effective functioning—is the basis of the scientific discipline of epidemiology. But our epidemiologic tools have not been equally up to the task for all kinds of data. And in practice, geographic information has always been the runt of the litter, largely unexploited because of the inadequacy of our existing epidemiologic tools to usefully manipulate and modify it.

Why has geographic information been a particular problem? One of the biggest issues has been our inability to display it. There's just no getting around the fact that a picture has always been the most effective way to synthesize data and translate it into information. Perhaps from an evolutionary standpoint, we've been subjected to a lot more selection pressure to develop visual skills to integrate information and recognize patterns than to develop analytic skills to assess a data base. Whatever the explanation, most of us can look at a table of graph coordinates all day and not see patterns that are immediately obvious once those same data are plotted on a scattergram. Fortunately, most traditional public health data are scalar and can be expressed in one dimension. Complex interrelationships between variables can be relatively easily translated into simple two dimensional pictures—figures and graphs—that can be used to simplify analysis and effectively transmit findings visually. Unfortunately, geographic information is already two dimensional and contextual. As such, it has been more difficult to abstract, manipulate, combine with other information, and depict.

Although a very good carpenter can make beautiful things with simple, old tools, most of the rest of us can't. Instead, we need the right tool to complete complex tasks. While we've conducted rudimentary analyses of geographic information for many years using primitive tools, geographic information systems (GIS) is that new, right tool that now allows us to see more clearly and explain more easily the relationship of geographic data to other issues and concerns, and to create the pictures we need to understand and translate geographic data into public health information.

So, read a GIS instruction manual, fire up the computer, and start churning out brilliant analyses.

If only it were that easy. Knowing how to operate a tool is only a small part of knowing how to use it. Instead, most of us really learn how to use a tool by seeing what others have done with it. That's what Dr. Melnick offers in this book, explaining not only the basics of GIS, but also providing a comprehensive range of examples of what public health researchers have done with it. In the process he gives all of us a better sense of how this tool can be used.

New technologies always have their advocates, and for more than a few years now, GIS zealots have tried to make us believe all manner of wondrous things about this one. The truth of the matter, though, is that as you wend your way through this book, the story that unfolds is one of a new potential being realized. GIS is being used to provide important new insights into infectious disease control, the bedrock of public health, and into environmental health, perhaps the

xii INTRODUCTION TO GEOGRAPHIC INFORMATION SYSTEMS IN PUBLIC HEALTH

most obvious application of this technology. But the story doesn't end there. The arrival of GIS is broadly nurturing the growth of the modern age of public health. Elegant work based on this technology is pushing back the frontiers in chronic disease control, injury prevention, maternal and child health, substance abuse, and delivery of health care services. GIS is fostering the growing importance of community as a locus of action and mobilization. And GIS is speeding our move away from outdated, single-focus surveillance systems that serve only one categorical program to a system approach where data from a variety of sources can be manipulated and integrated to serve many needs.

Putting data to good use is a stepwise process. Historically we've done well in the data collection process but have faltered in converting these data to information, particularly for geographic data. As shown in this book, GIS now better enables this next step to science-driven policy. And this is good news, because in a world of increasingly complex, interconnected issues, it seems at least possible that problems defined by place may have simpler, more satisfactory solutions than many of the other health issues confronting us today. At a minimum, a better understanding of place and its relation to other variables will permit a more reasoned community-based approach to the development of effective interventions. This book teaches how GIS can help, but in the context of a tool that we need to learn to use rather than a technology that will provide our salvation. In fact, looking at what others have done with GIS offers the best evidence that it's in the brain and not in the computer that most of the really hard work still needs to be done.

Dr. David Fleming
Deputy Director
Centers for Disease Control and Prevention

Preface

From the beginning, the use of information has been an essential component of public health practice. Public health practitioners have used epidemiology, the core science underlying public health, to analyze information on the distribution of health and disease within populations. On the basis of their analyses, health officials have implemented programs designed to control disease outbreaks, to prevent future occurrences, and to protect the public. An indication of the pivotal role of information management in public health practice is that all master's degree programs in public health require completion of core courses in epidemiology and biostatistics.

Over the past decade, rapid changes in technology and information management have begun to create quite a revolution in public health practice. Some of the changes have been quantitative, in that the newer tools promise to speed up traditional tasks. Other changes, however, have been qualitative, in that they promise to change fundamentally the way we practice public health. Much more data from many more sources are available compared to a decade ago. Available data include data not traditional to public health, such as transportation data, hospitalization data, and law enforcement data. Besides being available, the data are also much more accessible. State and local government officials no longer have a monopoly on access to data. Using a personal computer with an Internet connection at home or at a library, anyone can quickly access a variety of data sets maintained by commercial vendors as well as state and local governments.

In addition to data, technological tools to use the data have become easier to obtain. Powerful personal computers, rapid Internet connections, and sophisticated software have become available at home, libraries, and schools. In the health care arena, patients now have access to the same technological tools and data as their physicians, and the relationships between physicians and patients are changing. Patients are beginning to take a much more active role in their care. Likewise, community access to the new technologies will forever change the relationship between public health officials and their constituents. Communities will take a much more active role in population health improvement.

Public health officials can view these new relationships as threats or as opportunities to public health practice, and probably both are true. The use of one of the most exciting technological developments, geographic information systems (GIS), as described in this book, provides the most tangible examples of these threats and opportunities. On one hand, GIS technology has the capacity to bring community health assessment and improvement down to the neighborhood level. With this new technology, data could become much more meaningful to neighborhood residents and non–public health professionals, providing public health officials with an opportunity to engage their constituents and partners in meaningful conversations and projects around public health improvement. On the other hand, these new technological tools provide a setup for abuse. For example, violations of confidentiality and misinterpretation of results by people without appropriate training could have disastrous consequences.

Although communities will have access to the same tools, data, and technologic resources as public health officials, these health officials should still have many important roles to play. Potential roles include building Internet-based GIS, mobilizing community partnerships, serving as resources, ensuring confidentiality, inserting (and teaching) science, and ultimately facilitating community health improvement. Many of these new roles will require leadership skills in communication and collaboration. Clearly, public health officials will not be able to leave these new roles to technicians. Consequently, the typical public health administrator of the twenty-first century will need a basic understanding of the new technologies, including GIS. Unfortunately, real and perceived barriers, such as poor data quality, lack of training in information technology, and costs have prevented public health students and practitioners from making optimal use of these new technologies.

This book is written for those people—public health students and public health officials, including managers—who want to know how GIS technology can enhance their performance and the performance of their agencies. Although it includes technical information, the book does not require an understanding of computer science. Knowledge of basic concepts of epidemiology, biostatistics, and information management, commonly obtained through survey courses, review courses, and practical experience, should suffice. Each chapter builds on the information of previous chapters.

The first three chapters provide a background of the basic technological aspects of geographic information systems. Chapter 1 explores the history of the use of geographic analysis in public health. In an example from the mid-nineteenth century, the chapter discusses valuable lessons learned that can help public health officials avoid one of the pitfalls of modern geographic analyses: the tendency to draw cause-and-effect conclusions based on ecologic data.

Chapter 2 begins with a definition of GIS, including their functional components. The remainder of Chapter 2 describes how to obtain the different types of data available for use in GIS, including data not traditionally used by public health practitioners.

Once the data are incorporated into the GIS, the mapmaking process can begin. Chapter 3 discusses how to make maps, including different types of map displays. In addition, Chapter 3 explains how students and practitioners can use GIS technology to analyze the data, including some simple statistical analyses.

Chapters 4 through 8 discuss how GIS technology can enhance public health practice by illustrating several different applications. Chapter 4 examines the uses of GIS technology in environmental health. It begins by providing examples of how the technology can help us understand the risks of disease related to environmental exposures and how the technology can help public health officials target public health interventions based on these risks. The second half of Chapter 4 explores how GIS technology can help us understand issues around environmental equity: whether and how environmental hazards differentially affect the health status of low-income and minority populations.

Chapter 5 is devoted to the use of GIS technology in communicable-disease control and prevention. It discusses how the technology can summarize the complex relationships between communicable-disease pathogens, associated disease vectors and reservoirs, the environment, and human populations. This way, GIS technology can help us better understand the causes of these diseases as well as better target our interventions. In addition, Chapter 5 examines how GIS technology can assist health departments in allocating their resources effectively by targeting services such as immunizations and directly observed therapy for tuberculosis to areas with the greatest need.

Chapter 6 explores how GIS technology can help public health officials use injury data available from non–public health agencies, such as law enforcement agencies and transportation departments, to increase their understanding of the etiology of injuries and prevent future occurrences. Examples in Chapter 6 include injuries related to motor vehicles, earthquakes, and fires. The last part of Chapter 6 examines how GIS technology can be helpful in targeting efforts aimed at reducing intentional injuries such as homicides.

Chapter 7 discusses the role of GIS technology in helping public health practitioners respond to the challenge of chronic disease in their communities. The chapter begins by exploring the use of GIS technology in targeting communities for relevant health education and health promotion messages. Many communities are concerned about the association between chronic disease, especially cancer, and local environmental hazards, yet differences in rates of chronic disease have many additional determinants, such as the behavioral, genetic, and socioeconomic characteristics of underlying populations. Chapter 7 discusses the role of GIS technology as a tool for evaluating many of these potential risk factors and displaying the results of a complex analysis to community residents in an understandable format.

Chapter 8 examines how public health practitioners can use GIS technology for community health assessment and improvement. The chapter begins by illustrating the flexibility of the technology to define communities in many different ways and the ability of the technology to incorporate many different kinds of data. Chapter 8 then explores how GIS technology can help in many aspects of community health assessment and improvement by:

- Evaluating access to health care.
- Identifying and locating multiple services that could be better coordinated and integrated.
- Encouraging community participation.
- Facilitating program evaluation at the neighborhood level.
- Moving from a needs-based approach to an assets-based approach by mapping community resources in addition to community needs.

As with any new technology, GIS use has caveats. Chapter 9 will describe the limitations of this new technology, such as data availability, data quality, trained workforce, and costs, and its pitfalls, such as community definitions, confidentiality, and misinterpretation of results. For each identified limitation and pitfall, Chapter 9 discusses the role of public health managers in ensuring the appropriate use of GIS.

Before a local health department or other agency invests in a GIS application, it should determine whether it really needs the application or whether less expensive alternatives might suffice. Chapter 10 explores issues that health agencies should consider before making the decision to invest in GIS. The chapter then provides basic information for the public health manager on how to get started using GIS, including hardware, software, and Internet essentials.

Finally, Chapter 11 explores how GIS fit into theories of public health management and practice by examining the use of GIS technology in facilitating what public health does and how public health performs its functions. In addition, Chapter 11 explores how GIS technology can enhance several of the newest public health practice tools, such as As-sessment Protocol for Excellence in Public Health (APEXPH) and its latest version, Mobilizing for Action through Planning and Partnerships (MAPP). Chapter 11 concludes by suggesting a national public health research agenda aimed at identifying new public health GIS applications and addressing barriers to their successful implementation.

Although modern GIS technology, including software and powerful personal computers, has been available for at least a decade, most public health agencies have not yet incorporated it into their routine practice. Reasons surely include the skills and resources necessary for developing GIS applications. To uninitiated public health professionals, these requirements may appear needlessly complex and overwhelming. The organization and content of this book are designed to stimulate interest in GIS technology by making it easy to understand and by demonstrating to students and health officials how they can use the technology to improve their practice. We hope this book will inspire public health professionals to begin using and sharing this wonderful technology with their communities.

Acknowledgments

Kalen Conerly, Acquisitions Editor, created the idea of this book, and her enthusiasm, commitment, and support helped me turn this idea into a reality.

I would also like to express my gratitude to Judith Hayes, Tuality Hospital (Hillsboro, Oregon) Medical Librarian, who provided assistance for my literature searches, and to Megg Mueller Schulte, Associate Editor, who supported the final preparation of the manuscript.

CHAPTER 1

Introduction

The mission of public health is to fulfill "society's interest in assuring conditions in which persons can be healthy."[1(p.7)] To carry out this mission, the public health system relies on three components: the public health workforce; the employers of this workforce, including local, state, and federal organizations, governmental and private; and the information and communication systems used by these organizations in collecting and disseminating accurate data.[2] Revolutionary developments in the last component, information technology, promise to change the way public health is practiced.

Historically, our public health information (surveillance) system, based in our local, state, and federal governments, has collected and tabulated data on illness, disabilities, causes of death, injuries, behavioral and environmental risk factors, health costs, and other health issues.[1] For several reasons, health consumers and health planners have rarely used these health data. First, the data have not been timely. For example, up to two years can elapse before states release vital statistics data. Then, the data arrive in hard-copy form, containing limited analysis at the county level. Such hard-copy data are not amenable to further analysis, so local planners must ask the responsible state agency to make specific data runs, requiring additional time and staff support.[3] Second, many different agencies at the local, state, and federal levels collect and maintain health-related data in different formats in different locations, making the data less accessible for consumers, health planners, and local health departments. Third, data analyzed and reported at the county level and above are not useful for assessing the health of diverse communities within large or even medium-sized counties. Such macrolevel data fail to capture the unique essential characteristics of the individual communities, leaving little opportunity for local public health professionals to seek dialogue and strengthen relationships with populations within their counties.

To solve these problems, the public health system must make health data timely, accessible, and accurate.[2] We must link our various data systems, public and private, at federal, state, and local levels.[2] Additionally, data must be available, accessible, analyzable, and understandable at geographic levels smaller than counties, such as neighborhoods, enabling public health practitioners to engage diverse communities in a partnership to improve community health.[3] Recent advances in information technology, including hardware and software, culminating in modern geographic information systems (GIS), have made such solutions possible.[4] For several reasons, GIS may be the answer.

First, data collected by many agencies, public and private, health related and non–health related, usually include information on geography, such as residence address. While many public health program managers may have a good sense of the geography of health conditions, they may not be familiar with other relevant but less traditional health-related issues such as age of housing stock, home addresses of clinic patients, public transit routes, or locations of senior centers.[4] Using geography, GIS can link and integrate such multiple data sets rapidly and accurately.[5] Additionally, the process of linking these data sets encourages data-sharing partnerships between local health departments and other entities of local and state governments and the community.[5]

Second, by portraying the analysis on a map, GIS technology gives communities an easily understandable visual picture of community health. An ancient Chinese proverb, "A picture is worth more than 10,000 words," applies to GIS. Epidemiologists often present analyses in formats comprehensible only to other epidemiologists at best. GIS presents these analyses in an attention-capturing way that program managers, policy makers, community partners, and others can digest and believe.[4] Third, GIS allow public health practitioners and their partners to analyze and display data at the subcounty, community level, such as neighborhoods. As we will discuss in Chapter 8, maps at this level are especially useful in developing partnerships with community groups and stimulating community action to improve public health.[3,5]

Fourth, as GIS technology evolves, it promises to make public health information as accessible as a desktop computer.[5] Web-based versions are beginning to allow public health departments to present data and maps on the Internet, so that anyone with access to a library can analyze and display information on the health of the community.[3]

Despite its promise, the incorporation of GIS data, methods, and software into public health management and practice is just beginning.[5] Knowledge of this technology will become increasingly important for the successful public health manager of the twenty-first century. Objective 23–3 of *Healthy People 2010* is to "increase the proportion of all major National, State and local health data systems that use geocoding to promote nationwide use of geographic information systems at all levels."[2(pp.23-10)] The *Healthy People 2010* report adds that the capacity to achieve national health goals is related to the ability to target strategies to geographic areas.[2]

Considering the growing importance of GIS for public health practice, practicing and future public health practitioners must have a basic understanding of the uses and limitations of this technology. The purpose of this textbook is to introduce practitioners and graduate students in public health to GIS. We will begin by exploring the history of geographic analysis.

HISTORICAL USES OF GEOGRAPHIC INFORMATION IN PUBLIC HEALTH

Of the three core epidemiologic variables of time, place, and person, place has always been the most difficult and time consuming to analyze and depict.[4] Over 150 years ago, early public health professionals learned that maps could solve this problem.[6] In 1840, Robert Cowan used a map to show the relationship between fever and overcrowding in Glasgow. He attributed increased mortality to "excessive immigration without any corresponding increase in housing" and to the "steady decline in the proportion of the wealthy middle class."[6,7] In 1843, also in Glasgow, Robert Perry described a sixfold difference in the prevalence of fever in different neighborhoods. He showed the extent of the 1843 typhus epidemic by individually identifying affected households on a map.

In 1854, as every good epidemiologist knows, London was in the throes of a cholera epidemic. John Snow, considered one of the fathers of modern epidemiology, plotted the geographic distribution of cholera deaths in London, demonstrating the association between these deaths and contaminated water supplies (see Figure 1–1).[8] In doing so, he forever linked the new science of epidemiology with the use of geographic information to reveal relationships between environment and disease.[4] By the 1960s and 1970s, Melvyn Howe was using maps to show the geographic variation in all-cause and specific-cause mortality in London and Glasgow.[6,9,10] For example, he described a two- to threefold geographic variation in mortality from ischemic heart disease in adjacent city wards.[6]

The use of computers for geographical analyses and display began in the 1960s,[11,12] with GIS developing as a multidisciplinary field of study in the 1970s.[12] The disciplines underlying modern GIS include cartography, urban planning, and computer database management.[12] Over the past three decades, several factors contributed to the accelerated development of GIS. Computers became smaller, faster, more accessible, and less expensive. Software became easier to use. Landscape and census data became available in digital format, allowing linkage of health-related data sets to a geographic map.[12]

Long before the development of computer technology, the conclusions drawn from the London cholera epidemic revealed one of the pitfalls of modern geographic analyses. As Aesop noted in 500 B.C., "Appearances often are deceiving."[4] Most geographic analyses assessing whether there is an association between geography and health outcome will find one. Usually, however, outcomes such as cholera will cluster geographically because of underlying population characteristics, not because of the geography itself. In the hands of people inexperienced in basic epidemiologic principles, the temptation will be to leap too quickly to inferences about why the geographic clustering is occurring—to use a map as proof of one's own favored hypothesis. The investigation of the 1854 cholera example provides a good example.

John Snow's investigation of cholera deaths in the Golden Square neighborhood of London was one of three contemporaneous studies.[13] The Cholera Inquiry Committee of the vestry of the Parish of St. James, Westminster, conducted the second investigation, and England's General Board of Health conducted the third. All three investigations performed a geographic analysis using epidemic dot maps of cholera deaths. Although Snow and the Cholera Inquiry Committee correctly concluded that the contaminated Broad Street pump was the source of the epidemic, the General Board of Health reached a very different conclusion.[13] Even though it published the most complete and detailed map, the England General Board of Health concluded that deadly nocturnal vapors emanating from the Thames River caused the epidemic.[13]

The Board of Health's erroneous conclusion provides a basic lesson in ecologic fallacy for modern-day public health professionals. Although the Board of Health developed a general hypothesis that airborne vapors caused the epidemic,

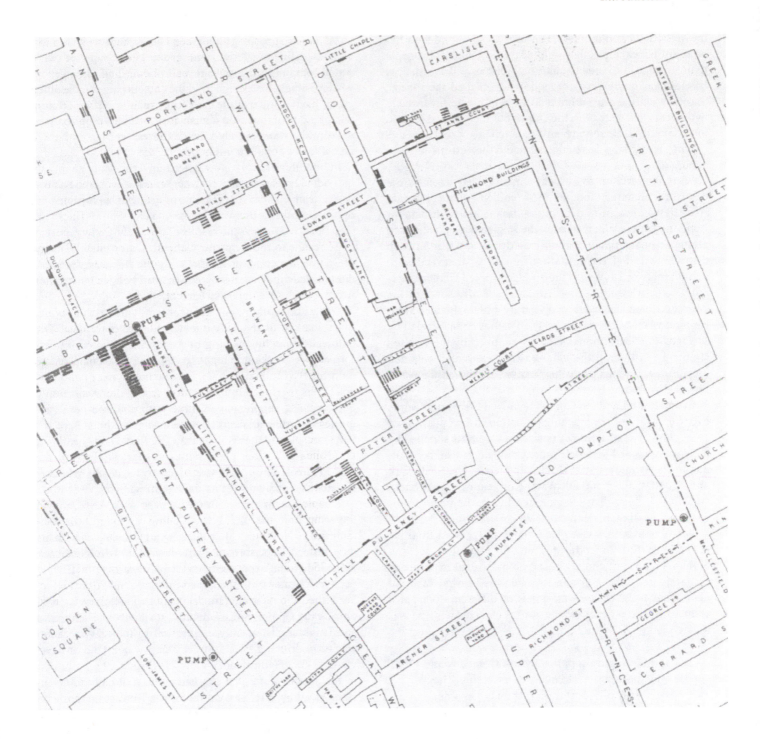

Figure 1–1 Map 1

they relied only on individual cases that supported their hypothesis. For example, they ignored cases of cholera in people living outside the Golden Square outbreak as well as instances of Golden Square residents who had escaped the illness. Snow, in contrast, used his map to help create his testable hypothesis that water was the culprit but then looked beyond his ecologic map, relying on two studies—a retrospective cohort study and a case-control study—to test his hypothesis.[14]

Snow had reason to suspect contaminated water as the culprit for cholera before the 1854 Golden Square outbreak. In earlier studies, he had looked at cholera mortality data for London districts, obtained from the Registrar-General, based on the company that was supplying drinking water for each district. Table 1–1 shows cholera mortality for several London districts in 1849 with their water supply.[8] Cholera mortality rates were higher in districts, generally south of the Thames River, that were supplied by water obtained from Battersea Fields, a location on the Thames contaminated by sewage.[8] One exception was water supplied by the Chelsea Company. Although the Chelsea Company also obtained contaminated water from the Thames, it filtered the water before distributing it.[8]

In 1852, the Lambeth Company moved their water works to an area free of sewage contamination.[8] In an analysis of 1853 cholera deaths, Snow showed that districts supplied by the Southwark and Vauxhall Water Company had higher cholera mortality rates than districts supplied by the Southwark and Vauxhall and Lambeth Water Companies.[14] Even more significant, three districts supplied by the Lambeth Company had no cholera deaths that year[8,14] (see Table 1–2).

With his hypothesis in place, Snow progressed from his ecologic analysis to studies testing this hypothesis, looking at the incidence of cholera based on individual exposure to contaminated water supplies. As he noted in his Table VI (see Table 1–2), because the pipes of different companies went down every street,[8] many houses received a mixed water supply:

> A few houses are supplied by one Company and a few by the other. . . . In many cases, a single house has a supply different from that on either side. . . . Each company supplies both rich and poor. . . . There is no difference either in the condition or occupation of the persons receiving the water of the different Companies.[8(p.75)]

Snow designed an experiment on the "grandest scale,"[8(p.75)] a retrospective cohort study:

"No fewer than three hundred thousand people of both sexes, of every age and occupation, and of every rank and station, from gentlefolks down to the very poor, were divided into two groups without their choice, and, in most cases, without their knowledge; one group being supplied with water containing the sewage of London, and, amongst it, whatever might have come from the cholera patients, the other group having water quite free from such impurity. To turn this grand experiment to account, all that was required was to learn the water supply to each individual house where a fatal attack of cholera might occur."[8(p.75)]

In his cohort study, Snow determined the water supply to individual houses in districts where mixing occurred and the deaths from cholera for residents of each house. As noted by Snow and others, this was no easy task.[14] Snow's Table IX (see Table 1–3) shows the results of the study. Snow reported these results to the Registrar General. Unfortunately, many of Snow's contemporaries, including the Registrar General, did not share his conclusion and instead believed that water was merely a "predisposing" factor.[14(p.S8)]

While still working on his cohort study in South London, Snow learned of the 1854 Golden Square outbreak.[15] The outbreak began the evening of August 31.[8] Snow first performed his geographic analysis, making a dot map of the outbreak[8,15] (see Figure 1–1). He obtained a list of all cholera deaths registered in that district during the week ending September 2, supplemented these with house-to-house inquiries regarding all deaths between August 31 and September 2, and plotted these on his map. He found that "nearly all the deaths had taken place within a short distance of the [Broad Street] pump. . . . There were only ten deaths in houses situated decidedly nearer to another street pump."[8(p.39)]

This was surprising to Snow because when he examined the water from the Broad Street pump, he found little contamination. However, Snow did not end his analysis with his map. Instead, he performed a case-control study, looking back at the individual exposure of cases and controls (unafflicted people) to water from the Broad Street pump. For example, he learned about the cholera deaths of two victims who lived outside the Golden Square district, residents of Hampstead and Brighton. Their only connection to the neighborhood was from drinking Broad Street pump water. One of these victims, the "Hampstead Widow," had such a high opinion of the pump's water that she had some sent daily to her in Hampstead by cart. She and her niece from Brighton, who also drank the water, died of cholera. No other Hampstead residents became ill.[15] Additionally, Snow discovered that cholera-infected children who lived near another pump passed by the Broad Street pump on their way to school and had been exposed to its water. Snow then looked at exposure to water for individual Golden Square residents who did not become ill. He discovered that 70 Golden Square brewery workers who lived in the district had a different water supply.[13,14] None of these workers died from cholera. Likewise, only 5 recorded cholera deaths occurred in a population of

Table 1–1 Water Supply and Cholera Mortality, London, 1849

District	Population in the Middle of 1849	Deaths from Cholera	Deaths by Cholera to 10,000 Inhabits	Annual Value of House and Shop Room to Each Person in £	Water Supply
Rotherhithe	17,208	352	205	4.238	Southwark and Vauxhall Water Works, Kent Water Works, and Tidal Ditches
St. Olave, Southwark	19,278	349	181	4.559	Southwark and Vauxhall
St. George, Southwark	50,900	836	164	3.518	Southwark and Vauxhall, Lambeth
Bermondsey	45,500	734	161	3.077	Southwark and Vauxhall
St. Saviour, Southwark	35,227	539	153	5.291	Southwark and Vauxhall
Newington	63,074	907	144	3.788	Southwark and Vauxhall, Lambeth
Lambeth	134,768	1,618	120	4.389	Southwark and Vauxhall, Lambeth
Wandsworth	48,446	484	100	4.839	Pump-wells, Southwark and Vauxhall, river Wandle
Camberwell	51,714	504	97	4.508	Southwark and Vauxhall, Lambeth
West London	28,829	429	96	7.454	New River
Bethnal Green	87,263	789	90	1.480	East London
Shoreditch	104,122	789	76	3.103	New River, East London
Greenwich	95,954	718	75	3.379	Kent
Poplar	44,103	313	71	7.360	East London
Westminster	64,109	437	68	4.189	Chelsea
Whitechapel	78,590	506	64	3.388	East London
St. Giles	54,062	285	53	5.635	New River
Stepney	106,988	501	47	3.319	East London
Chelsea	53,379	247	46	4.210	Chelsea
East London	43,495	182	45	4.823	New River
St. George's, East	47,334	199	42	4.753	East London
London City	55,816	207	38	17.676	New River
St. Martin	24,557	91	37	11.844	New River
Strand	44,254	156	35	7.374	New River
Holborn	46,134	161	35	5.883	New River
St. Luke	53,234	183	34	3.731	New River
Kensington (except Padding-ton)	110,491	260	33	5.070	West Middlesex, Chelsea, Grand Junction
Lewisham	32,299	96	30	4.824	Kent
Belgrave	37,918	105	28	8.875	Chelsea
Hackney	55,152	139	25	4.397	New River, East London
Islington	87,761	187	22	5.494	New River
St. Pancras	160,122	360	22	4.871	New River, Hampstead, West Middlesex
Clerkenwell	63,499	121	19	4.138	New River
Marylebone	153,960	261	17	7.586	West Middlesex
St. James, Westminster	36,426	57	16	12.669	Grand Junction, New River
Paddington	41,267	35	8	9.349	Grand Junction
Hampstead	11,572	9	8	5.804	Hampstead, West Middlesex
Hanover Square & May Fair	33,196	26	8	16.754	Grand Junction
London	2,280,282	14,137	62	—	

Note: The districts are arranged in the order of their mortality from cholera.

Table 1–2 Cholera Deaths, 1853

Subdistricts	Population in 1851	Deaths from Cholera in 1853	Deaths by Cholera in Each 100,000 Living	Water Supply
St. Saviour, Southwark	19,709	45	227	
St. Olave	8,015	19	237	
St. John, Horsleydown	11,360	7	61	
St. James, Bermondsey	18,899	21	111	
St. Mary Magdalen	13,934	27	193	
Leather Market	15,295	23	153	Southwark and Vauxhall Water Company only
Rotherhithe*	17,805	20	112	
Wandsworth	9,611	3	31	
Battersea	10,560	11	104	
Putney	5,280	—	—	
Camberwell	17,742	9	50	
Peckham	19,444	7	36	
Christchurch, Southwark	16,022	7	43	
Kent Road	18,126	37	204	
Borough Road	15,862	26	163	
London Road	17,836	9	50	
Trinity, Newington	20,922	11	52	
St. Peter, Walworth	29,861	23	77	
St. Mary, Newington	14,033	5	35	Lambeth Water Company and Southwark and Vauxhall Company
Waterloo (1st part)	14,088	1	7	
Waterloo (2nd part)	18,348	7	38	
Lambeth Church (1st part)	18,409	9	48	
Lambeth Church (2nd part)	26,784	11	41	
Kennington (1st part)	24,261	12	49	
Kennington (2nd part)	18,848	6	31	
Brixton	14,610	2	13	
Clapham	16,290	10	61	
St. George, Camberwell	15,849	6	37	
Norwood	3,977	—	—	
Streatham	9,023	—	—	Lambeth Water Company only
Dulwich	1,632	—	—	
First 12 subdistricts	167,654	192	114	Southwark and Vauxhall
Next 16 subdistricts	301,149	182	60	Both companies
Last 3 subdistricts	14,632	—	—	Lambeth Company

*A part of Rotherhithe was supplied by the Kent Water company; but there was no cholera in this part.

535 inmates of a workhouse within the outbreak area. This workhouse had its own well.

Besides going beyond the map to look at individual exposure, Snow taught us to consider biologic plausibility in de- veloping our hypotheses about cause and effect. Unlike the England General Board of Health, Snow had a comprehen- sive understanding of how cholera caused disease. He un- derstood that cholera symptoms were due to fluid loss from

Table 1–3 Cholera Deaths per 10,000 Houses

	Number of Houses	Deaths from Cholera	Deaths in Each 10,000 Houses
Southwark and Vauxhall Company	40,046	1,263	315
Lambeth Company	26,107	98	37
Rest of London	256,423	1,422	59

a gastrointestinal illness and that gastrointestinal disease was more likely due to an oral exposure than to a respiratory exposure. He was willing to admit and test that person-to-person transmission of cholera was possible. Although he could find no evidence of contamination in the Broad Street pump water, he saw that a sewer was nearby and that the pump well penetrated gravel that served as drainage for nearby cesspools.[14] In contrast, the Board of Health, like its Victorian contemporaries, was anticontagionist and tended to attribute epidemic disease to vapors. Consequently, the board reached an erroneous conclusion because members did not bother to link their vapor theory with the biologic symptoms of cholera.[13]

Like Snow, experienced modern public health practitioners must use the science of epidemiology to identify associations between exposures and disease and to determine whether and how these associations are due to cause and effect. As the technology for geographic analyses becomes more available, more people without public health training, some in policy-making positions, may be tempted to make premature conclusions based on ecological data and to make false assumptions about the nature of associations between geography, exposure, and health.[4]

In the early days of geographic analyses, when public health practitioners mainly focused on communicable disease control, pushpins or dots drawn on maps usually proved effective in helping to analyze and control disease outbreaks. The modern public health practitioner, however, is responsible for analyzing and responding to more complex health issues in a rapidly changing, diverse environment. The social, environmental, and behavioral determinants of health have a strong geographic component. To work effectively with communities in improving health status, modern public health practitioners and their community partners will need easy, immediate access to accurate geographically based data.[16] New developments in GIS technology are making this possible.

As we have experienced with other revolutionary developments, GIS technology will change how we practice public health, especially how we think about data and organize our collection, use, and display of data.[12] Successful GIS applications will need maintenance and support, will have significant costs, and will require training for their users (see Chapters 9 and 10). To the uninitiated, these changes and requirements may appear needlessly complex and overwhelming. We designed this book to make GIS easy to understand and, by doing so, to stimulate interest and use. As wonderful as it is, however, GIS technology comes with some important caveats. Like the England General Board of Health, future policy makers may be tempted to make false and simplistic assumptions about complex conditions and health. The potential for misuse increases with the complexity of the analyses. The job of public health officials will be to reinsert the science and ensure that those attempting to draw conclusions from geographic analyses account for potential confounders and modifiers of any exposure/disease association. We hope that the lessons in this book will help future public health GIS users meet this challenge, fulfilling the promise of GIS technology.

CHAPTER   REVIEW

1. The public health system relies on three components: the public health workforce; the employers of this workforce, including local, state, and federal organizations, governmental and private; and the information and communication systems used by these organizations in collecting and disseminating accurate data.
2. For several reasons, health consumers and health planners have rarely used health-related data:

- Data have not been timely.
- Data arrive in hard-copy form, containing limited analysis at the county level.
- Many different agencies at the local, state, and federal levels collect and maintain health-related data in different formats in different locations, making the data less accessible.
- Data analyzed and reported at the county level and above are not useful for assessing the health of di-

verse communities within large or even medium-sized counties.

3. GIS technology can help consumers and health planners make better use of health-related data by
   - Linking and integrating multiple data sets rapidly and accurately
   - Portraying data analysis on a map, giving communities an easily understandable visual picture of community health
   - Allowing public health practitioners and their partners to analyze and display data at the sub-county, community level, such as neighborhoods
   - Making public health information as accessible as desktop computers in public libraries

4. Knowledge of GIS technology will become increasingly important for the successful public health manager of the twenty-first century. Objective 23–of *Healthy People 2010* is to "to promote nationwide use of geographic information systems at all levels."[2]

5. Epidemiologists have used maps to depict disease incidence for over 150 years. The use of computers for geographical analyses and display began in the 1960s,

with GIS developing as a multidisciplinary field of study in the 1970s.

6. Over the past three decades, development of GIS technology accelerated because
   - Computers became smaller, faster, more accessible, and less expensive.
   - Software became easier to use.
   - Landscape and census data became available in digital format.

7. Conclusions drawn from the 1854 London cholera epidemic revealed one of the pitfalls of modern geographic analyses: the tendency to draw cause-and-effect conclusions based on ecologic data. John Snow reached the correct conclusion because he used his map to generate a testable hypothesis. Then he went beyond the map, using case-control and cohort study designs to test his hypothesis.

8. Public health officials of the twenty-first century will have the responsibility to ensure that those attempting to draw conclusions from geographic analyses will use appropriate study designs that account for potential confounders and modifiers of any exposure-disease association.

REFERENCES

1. Committee for the Study of the Future of Public Health, Institute of Medicine, Division of Health Care Services. *The Future of Public Health*. Washington, DC: National Academy Press, 1988.

2. U.S. Department of Health and Human Services. *Healthy People 2010* (conference ed., 2 vols.). Washington, DC: 2000.

3. A. Melnick et al. "Clackamas County Department of Human Services Community Health Mapping Engine (CHiME) Geographic Information Systems Project." *Journal of Public Health Management and Practice* 5, no. 2 (1999): 64–69.

4. A.L. Melnick and D.W. Fleming. "Modern Geographic Information Systems: Promise and Pitfalls." *Journal of Public Health Management and Practice* 5, no. 2 (1999): viii–x.

5. W.A. Yasnoff and E.J. Sondik. "Geographic Information Systems (GIS) in Public Health Practice in the New Millennium." *Journal of Public Health Management and Practice* 5, no. 4 (1999): ix–xii.

6. A. Gordon and J. Womersley. "The Use of Mapping in Public Health and Planning Health Services." *Journal of Public Health Medicine* 19, no. 2 (1997): 139–147.

7. R. Cowan. *Vital Statistics of Glasgow Illustrating the Sanitary Condition of the Population*. Paper read before the Statistical Section of the British Association. September 21, 1840.

8. J. Snow, "On the Mode of Communication of Cholera," in *Snow on Cholera*, 2d ed. New York: Commonwealth Fund, 1936.

9. G.M. Howe, "London and Glasgow: A Comparative Study of Mortality Patterns." *International Geography* 11 (1972): 1214–1217.

10. G.M. Howe, ed. *A World Geography of Human Diseases*. London: Academic Press, 1977.

11. W.R. Tobbler. "Automation and Cartography." *Geographical Review* 49 (1959): 526–534.

12. K.C. Clarke et al. "On Epidemiology and Geographic Information Systems: A Review and Discussion of Future Directions." *Emerging Infectious Diseases* 2, no. 2 (1996): 85–92.

13. N. Paneth et al. "Public Health Then and Now. A Rivalry of Foulness: Official and Unofficial Investigations of the London Cholera Epidemic of 1854." *American Journal of Public Health* 88, no. 10 (1998): 1545–1553.

14. W. Winkelstein. "A New Perspective of John Snow's Communicable Disease Theory." *American Journal of Epidemiology* 142, no. 9, suppl. (1995): S3–S9.

15. H. Brody et al. "John Snow Revisited: Getting a Handle on the Broad Street Pump." *Pharos* (winter 1999): 2–8.

16. W.L. Roper and G.P. Mays. "GIS in Public Health Policy: A New Frontier for Improving Community Health." *Journal of Public Health Management and Practice* 5, no. 2 (1999): vi–vii.

CHAPTER 2

GIS Data Acquisition and Storage

DEFINITION OF GIS

What are geographic information systems? Many definitions exist, although GIS can probably be defined better by their functions than by what they are.[1] Blakemore, in 1986, defined GIS as "computer packages, which integrate the storage, manipulation, analysis, modeling and mapping of digital spatial information."[2(p.173),3] Burrough defined GIS as "powerful sets of tools for collecting, retrieving at will, transforming and displaying spatial data from the real world."[3,4(p.9)] Others have defined GIS as "database systems in which most of the data are spatially indexed, and upon which a set of procedures are operated in order to answer queries about spatial entities in the database."[3,5(p.13)] Another definition describes GIS as "computer systems that store and link nongraphic attributes or geographically-referenced data with graphic map features to allow a wide range of information processing and display operations, as well as map production, analysis and modeling."[3,6(p.8)] Recent definitions describe GIS as "automated systems for the capture, storage, retrieval, analysis and display of spatial data."[1,7] *Healthy People 2010* defines GIS as "powerful tools combining geography, data and computer mapping."[8(p.23-10)]

Common to all of these definitions are several integrated GIS functions. These functions include the capture and incorporation of data sets, the storage of data, the retrieval of data, the statistical manipulation of data, data analysis, data modeling, and the display of the data on maps.[1,3] These functions are no different from what John Snow performed by hand. To display data on a map, the data must have a spatial or geographical component, and a map must be available. John Snow and the Board of Health obtained the street addresses of cholera victims in London and plotted them on a

hand-drawn map. Modern GIS combine these functions electronically, using appropriate electronic data sets, digital (computer-stored) maps, and geographic software. For example, if laboratories and physicians were to report cholera cases electronically, including an address of each case, and if a digital map and geographic software were available, a modern-day John Snow could instantly map an epidemic. Because much of the data collected electronically today has some geographic reference, such as a street address, modern electronic GIS have the potential to revolutionize public health practice. With GIS, public health practitioners can instantly plot health-related issues, such as mortality and birthrates, at the neighborhood or even street level.[9] In addition, GIS are tools for understanding and displaying disease or disease risks related to environmental exposures or social demographic data.[10] For example, studies have used GIS to demonstrate the relationship between childhood lead-poisoning cases by census block with older housing stock.[11]

The five functional components of GIS we will describe are

1. Data acquisition and data verification
2. Data storage and database management
3. Data transformation and analysis
4. Data output and presentation
5. User interface

In this chapter, we will discuss data acquisition, verification, storage, management, and transformation. Chapter 3 will discuss data output and presentation, including mapmaking. Subsequent chapters will discuss analysis and user interface. Figure 2–1 is a schematic of the mapmaking process that we will discuss in these chapters.[12]

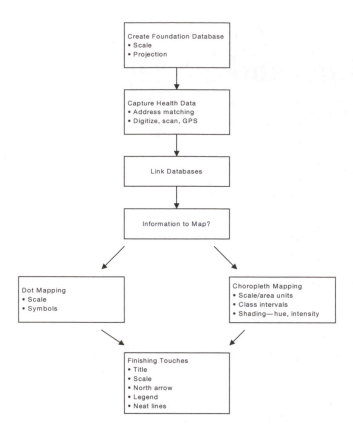

Figure 2–1 The mapping process

DATA ACQUISITION AND STORAGE: INCORPORATING SPATIAL DATABASES

To perform geographic analyses and make a map on a computer, GIS require a foundation of spatial (geographic) data. Spatial databases are contained in either a raster or a vector file format. Each has advantages and disadvantages, depending on the study.

Raster Format

The raster format (Figure 2–2) stores geographic data as images in a regular grid of cells.[13] The cells are generally the same size and usually square, although other types of polygons, such as rectangles, hexagons, and equilateral triangles, have been used.[3] Row and column numbers define the locations of each cell on the grid, or map. In raster format, cells (also called pixels) represent points, strings of connected cells represent lines, and aggregates of cells represent areas. Data scanned from maps, obtained from photographs, or obtained from space satellites are digitally stored in a raster format.[13]

The format assigns each cell a data value indicating the value of an attribute, such as land use type, within the cell. Through improved remote-sensing technology, images are available in infrared, thermal, radar, and other wavelengths at increasingly higher resolution. The raster format divides these images into cells, with the shades of each cell representing a value of a specific feature, or attribute. For example, shades of gray could indicate a specific type of land use within the area portrayed by the cell.[14] The accuracy of the raster data file is inversely proportional to the size of the cells: the smaller the cells, the greater the degree of resolution and the greater the accuracy. Some commercially available raster data files have resolution at the 1-foot level, although 5 to 10 m images are more common.[14]

With digital images incorporated into their GIS, investigators can identify and map environmental features, such as elevation, temperature, moisture content, and vegetation, which are associated with disease-transmitting insect populations.[15] Satellite data, secret during the Cold War, such as CORONA and Russian spy imagery, are now broadly available, even on the Internet. In the United States, the National Air Photo program plans to remap the United States every five years, at a scale of 1:12,000 with 1 m resolution, and to publish the images as CD-ROMs.[1] The National Aeronautics and Space Administration (NASA) developed LANDSAT, a program using U.S.–launched satellites, to produce images of the earth's surface. Through its Mission to Planet Earth and its Earth Observation System, NASA will provide vast amounts of data on the earth's geography and atmosphere. NASA then will make these data available on the Internet, distributed by a set of active archive centers.[1]

As an example of the use of raster-format data, a study of environmental risk factors for Lyme disease in Baltimore, Maryland, used six raster databases to create a grid map of Baltimore County[16] (see Chapter 5). The databases, maintained by the Baltimore County Department of Environmental Protection and Resource Management and the Department of Geography at Towson State University, had a resolution of 400 feet by 500 feet (121.9 m × 152.4 m). This resulted in a grid map of the county with 164,248 cells of that size. Like other raster databases, each cell had a value based on one or more attributes. In this study, these attributes included land use/land cover, forest distributions, soils, elevation geology, and watershed. A composite of a LANDSAT Thematic Mapper satellite image and planimetric maps of the urban portions of the county provided the land use/land cover data. (Planimetric maps are maps showing land features in a two-dimensional representation; they do not include topographical or relief data. Each thematic map displays a single attribute, or theme, such as soil types or vegetation cover.) The same LANDSAT image provided data on forest distribution. The U.S. Department of Agriculture provided soil data, and digitized Maryland Geological Survey maps

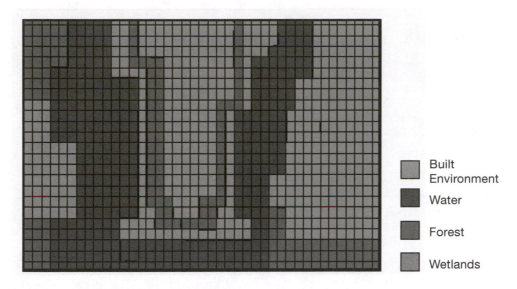

Built Environment

Water

Forest

Wetlands

Figure 2–2 The raster view of the world. The raster GIS references phenomena by grid cell location in a matrix. The grid cell is the smallest unit of resolution and may vary from centimeters to kilometers depending on the application.

supplied geology data, including rock formations. The digitized Baltimore City Department of Public Works watershed database supplied the geographic distributions of the 15 watersheds.

The raster format has several advantages. First, it is easy to obtain raster data from a digital photograph or satellite image. The database is simple and easy to handle in a computer.[3,17] It is also useful for studies based on environmental features easily scanned (with a computer scanner) from a map, such as vegetation cover. This format has several disadvantages, however. Each cell has a specific value for each attribute. If the resolution is low, cells can be quite large, leading to inaccuracies. On the other hand, a higher resolution requires a greater number of cells, increasing the size of the database (with concomitant computer storage requirements) and computer computational time. Although land use data based on images are easy to store in a raster database, linear and demographic data, such as street names and addresses, are not. Raster data are therefore less useful in community health applications that require analyses based on political boundaries and demographics.

Vector Format

Most public health GIS applications use a vector format or a combination of raster and vector formats. In a vector database, points, lines, and polygons represent geographic features[9] (see Figure 2–3). The computer stores these features as x and y coordinates based on latitude and longitude.

Points (e.g., location of alcohol-serving outlets) are objects on a map representing an exact location, with specific x and y coordinates. Lines, such as streets, are map objects that connect two or more points. Polygons are map objects consisting of lines enclosing specific areas, such as county boundaries or census tracts.[9] The vector format has several advantages over the raster format. While the raster format represents lines as a string of cells, the vector format, based on coordinates, can identify the exact middle of a line. While the raster format defines an area as a group of square cells, the vector format can define the exact boundaries of areas of any shape. This is particularly useful for community health applications, where political and social geographic boundaries, such as states, cities, counties, legislative districts, and neighborhoods, are essential. Disadvantages of the vector format include its complexity and size and the inability to easily store details of an image.[18] In addition, the vector format assumes that features are uniform within the polygon. Fortunately, modern GIS technology now has the ability to store and manipulate data in both formats. For example, GIS can convert satellite images into vector structures.

Creating a Foundation of Spatial Data

GIS require an accurate, geographic base map in digital format— raster, vector, or both.[19] This digital map contains data on the features that will contribute to the map, such as county boundaries, census tract and census block group

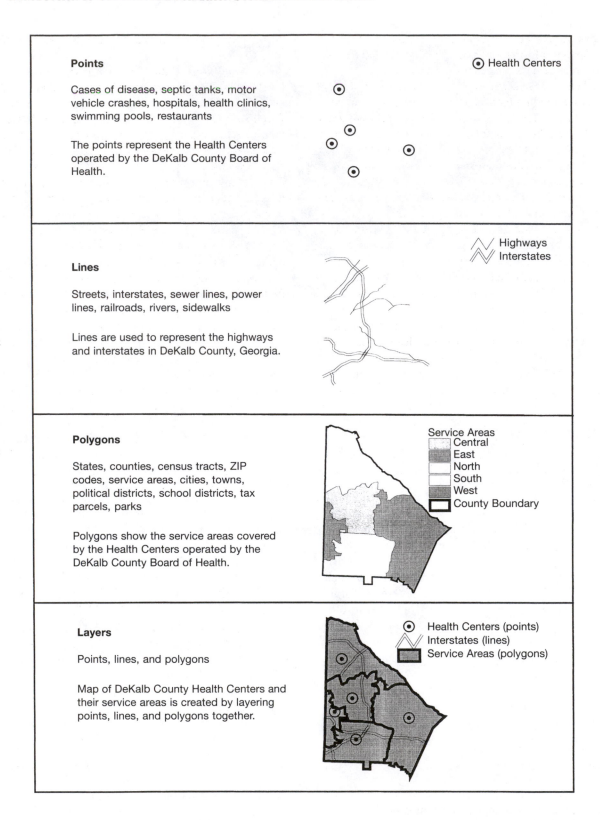

Points   ⊙ Health Centers

Cases of disease, septic tanks, motor vehicle crashes, hospitals, health clinics, swimming pools, restaurants

The points represent the Health Centers operated by the DeKalb County Board of Health.

Lines   Highways / Interstates

Streets, interstates, sewer lines, power lines, railroads, rivers, sidewalks

Lines are used to represent the highways and interstates in DeKalb County, Georgia.

Polygons

Service Areas
Central
East
North
South
West
County Boundary

States, counties, census tracts, ZIP codes, service areas, cities, towns, political districts, school districts, tax parcels, parks

Polygons show the service areas covered by the Health Centers operated by the DeKalb County Board of Health.

Layers

⊙ Health Centers (points)
Interstates (lines)
Service Areas (polygons)

Points, lines, and polygons

Map of DeKalb County Health Centers and their service areas is created by layering points, lines, and polygons together.

Figure 2–3 Points, lines, and polygons become multiple layers in a GIS

boundaries, streets, and environmental features such as rivers. This spatial information is the foundation for later adding health-related data for geographic analysis.

Public health GIS users can obtain spatial data from several sources, including local state and federal governmental agencies and commercial vendors.[19] With Executive Order 12906, "Coordinating Geographic Data Acquisition and Access: The National Spatial Data Infrastructure," President Clinton emphasized the importance of spatial data.[20] This order requires federal agencies to describe their spatial data, meet quality and compatibility standards for their data, and make their data accessible to the public.[18] Specifically, the order directs the Federal Geographic Data Committee (FGDC) to coordinate a national geospatial clearinghouse and encourages federal departments and agencies to join this committee. The order directs the FGDC to collaborate with state, local, and tribal governments in the development of the clearinghouse. As a result, each federal agency must document all new geospatial data that it collects or produces and make the documentation accessible to the clearinghouse. The agencies must follow data quality standards set by the FGDC. To increase efficiency, before collecting or producing any data, each agency must use the clearinghouse to determine whether any other agency has already collected the data in question. In addition, to encourage data sharing, each agency must first check with the clearinghouse to determine the feasibility of cooperating with other agencies to collect or produce the data.[20] Each agency must have a plan documenting how it will make its data accessible to the public.

The Geospatial Data Clearinghouse, sponsored by the FGDC, now allows agencies at all levels, federal, tribal, state, and local, government and private, to band together (in a decentralized way) to promote their available digital spatial data. The clearinghouse functions as a catalog service where various agencies can provide metadata. Metadata, data about data, described later in this chapter, include details on the data source, quality, timeliness, and reliability. After reviewing the metadata, potential users can access a data set that interests them. For small data sets, clearinghouse users can download the geospatial data in one or more formats. For larger data sets, unavailable through the Internet, the clearinghouse links users to on-line order forms. Map data products ordered this way are available on floppy disk and CD-ROM. Many geospatial data sets, in raster and vector format, are accessible through the clearinghouse, including environmental measurements from the U.S. Geological Service, the U.S. Environmental Protection Agency (EPA), and the National Oceanic and Atmospheric Administration (NOAA). For example, the EPA Spatial Data Library System (ESDLS) is a repository for the EPA's geospatial data holdings. EPA itself has a Geospatial Data Clearinghouse site that provides access to data down to the local level, identifying the location and characteristics of natural and manmade features and boundaries.[19] Exhibit 2–1 is a listing of available national sources of geospatial data with their Web addresses.[19]

Exhibit 2–1 Examples of On-Line Gateways to Geospatial and Attribute Data That Can Be Used in GIS

Bureau of the Census: www.census.gov
   TIGER Home Page: www.census.gov/tiger/tiger.html
CACI: www.demographics.com
Caliper Corporation: www.caliper.com
Centers for Disease Control and Prevention: www.cdc.gov
   WONDER System: http://wonder.cdc.gov
   National Center for Health Statistics: www.cdc.gov/nchswww
   Behavioral Risk Factor Surveillance System: www.cdc.gov/nccdphp/brfss
   STDs or AIDS Surveillance: www.cdc.gov/nchstp
Claritas: www.claritis.com
Dartmouth Atlas of Health Care in the United States: www.dartmouth.edu/~atlas/
Department of Health and Human Services: www.healthfinder.org
Environmental Protection Agency: www.epa.gov
   National GIS Program: www.epa.gov/ngspr
   EPA Envirofacts: www.epa.gov/enviro/index_java.html
Environmental Systems Research Institute: www.esri.com
Geographic Data Technology: www.geographic.com

Health Care Financing Administration: www.hcfa.gov/stats
Healthdemographics: www.healthdemographics.com
Health Resources and Services Administration: www.hrsa.dhhs.gov
International Association of Cancer Registries: www-dep.iarc.fr
   Cancer Registry Resources: www-dep.iarc.fr/resour/manuals.htm
MapInfo Corporation: www.mapinfo.com
National Association of Central Cancer Registries: www.naaccr.org
National Cancer Registrars Association: www.ncra-usa.org
National Oceanic and Atmospheric Administration Data: www.noaa.gov
National Program of Cancer Registries: www.cdc.gov/nccdphp/dcpc/npcr
National Institutes of Health: www.nih.gov
U.S. Geological Survey: Call: 1-800-USA-MAPS
   Main Home Page—www.usgs.gov
   EROS Data Center—http://edcwww.cr.usgs.gov

Many local health departments also have access to spatial data within their sister local government agencies. This source has several advantages. First, it tends to be low cost or even free. Other city or county agencies, especially land use and transportation agencies, often have staff that have expertise in the use of these databases and are willing to share these staff with public health departments. In addition, this kind of data partnership can be "contagious." Once local agencies begin working together on GIS projects, they discover the value of professional and data resource sharing in other areas.

The most commonly used spatial database is the U.S. Bureau of the Census's Topologically Integrated Geographic Encoding and Referencing (TIGER) files. The TIGER database is a result of a collaborative effort between the U.S. Geological Survey and the Bureau of the Census.[18] The creation of TIGER as a foundation database contributed to the development of modern GIS.[17] TIGER is a vector-format database representing physical features, including rivers, and governmental and statistical boundaries. Updated, easily obtainable versions of the TIGER geographic data files include detailed street and address range information, along with political and administrative boundaries such as counties, ZIP codes, census tracts, and census block groups.[12] The files exist in multiple partitions, such as counties or groups of counties, but they represent the entire U.S. space as a single seamless data set.

As defined by the U.S. Bureau of the Census, a census tract is a small, relatively permanent statistical subdivision of a county in a metropolitan area (MA) or a selected nonmetropolitan county. Census tract boundaries normally follow visible features, such as rivers, but may follow governmental unit boundaries and other nonvisible features. Although census tracts do not cross county lines, entities within counties, such as cities, may split them. Designed to be relatively homogeneous units with respect to population characteristics, economic status, and living conditions, census tracts usually contain between 1,000 and 8,000 inhabitants.

A census block is the smallest entity for which the Bureau of the Census collects and tabulates decennial census information. Census blocks are polygons bounded on all sides by visible and nonvisible features. A block group (BG) is a combination of census blocks that is a subdivision of a census tract or block numbering area (BNA). The BG, generally containing between 300 and 3,000 people, is the lowest level of geography for which the Bureau of the Census has tabulated sample data in the 1990 census. Figure 2–4 illustrates the relationship between counties, census tracts, block groups, and blocks.

An advantage to TIGER is that it allows the automated integration of census data for any geographic location within the United States. This enables users to perform analyses of socioeconomic factors easily for any geographic area. TIGER line files are available to order at the U.S. Bureau of the Census's TIGER home page, <www.census.gov/geo/www/tiger/index.html>.

While frequently updated TIGER files are easily available at low cost or even free, they are sometimes inaccurate. Especially in areas of rapid growth, new residences and streets may be missing, and street positional accuracy may need updating. Fortunately, updated geographic data files are available from commercial vendors, but they may be expensive.[9] For example, the Environmental Systems Research Institute (ESRI) provides a street map for the entire United States in one of its software products, ArcView GIS. Caliper Corporation provides spatial data, including U.S. streets and census tracts, in its Maptitude and U.S. Department of Housing and Urban Development (HUD) Community 2020 software products. Another company, Geographic Data Technology, Inc (GDT), provides geographic databases that include street, postal, and census information.[18]

SCALE AND PROJECTION

Two fundamental geographic characteristics that developers of GIS applications must consider are scale and projection.[12] Without the same scale and projection, different spatial databases cannot be viewed and mapped together. *Scale* refers to the ratio between the size of an object (or the length of a distance) on a map and the size of the object (or the actual distance) in the real world. On a map with a scale of 1:24,000, a distance of 1 cm is equivalent to a distance of 24,000 cm on the earth. Map scales do not necessarily have to use the same units. For example, some maps have scales such that 1 inch is equivalent to 1 mile. The smaller the scale, the larger the area displayed on a map. Maps of large areas, such as states or countries, use small scales ranging from 1:250,000 to 1:25,000,000, while maps of subcounty areas, such as towns or neighborhoods, typically use large scales of 1:100,000 or even larger. On the other hand, maps of large areas cannot display as much detail as maps of smaller geographic areas.

The earth is round and three-dimensional, while maps are flat.[9] Projection is the mathematical model that transforms three-dimensional features on the earth's curved surface to a two-dimensional map.[12] Locations on the earth's surface, as indicated by latitude and longitude coordinates, are unprojected data. To project from the earth's surface to a two-dimensional map, states within the United States use different coordinate systems. These coordinate systems are references used to display horizontal and vertical distances on a flat (planimetric) map. Depending on the projection used, some spatial relationships are lost during the transformation. For example, different projections cause different amounts of distortion in area measurements, area shapes, distances

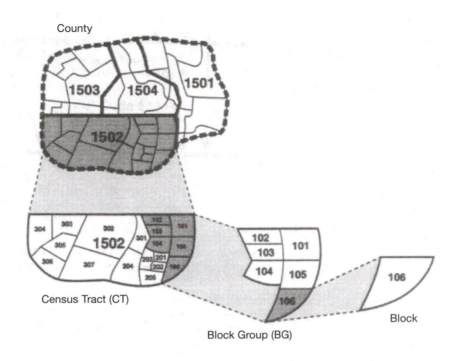

Figure 2–4 Relationship between counties, census tracts, block groups, and blocks

between points, or direction. The type of projection chosen depends on the geographic location, the commonly accepted map images used in a given area or region, and the type of analysis performed. To map areas accurately, the cartographer should select an *equal-area* projection; to measure distance accurately, an *equidistant* projection; and to preserve shape, a *conformal* projection.[9] For example, if the goal of a study were to measure distances from patient homes to the nearest clinic, an equidistant projection would make the most sense.

These considerations are much more important for maps of large areas than for maps of small communities because larger areas are more subject to distortion due to the curvature of the earth. However, even in small areas, spatial databases must use the same projection, or they will not link properly. For example, to simultaneously map a raster-based digital image with TIGER files, the two spatial databases must have the same scale and projection. Of course, even with the same scale and projection, most of these data sets will not line up perfectly. In such cases, GIS software can "rubber-sheet" (stretch) one database to fit the other.[12]

INCORPORATING ATTRIBUTE DATABASES

The next step in a GIS analysis is to obtain the attribute data and link them to the geographic database.[12] Attribute data relate to any public health issue of interest and can include disease information, such as reported cholera cases, social data, and environmental data. To map an attribute like cholera, the attribute data must link with the geospatial data. To do this, the attribute data set must include a geographic reference, such as a state, county, ZIP code, or street address. GIS can analyze any attribute database, such as birth data, that includes a field with a location. The level of geographic analysis depends on the specificity of location in the database. If the location field on an attribute database includes only residence by state, the GIS analysis can go no lower than the state level. To analyze birthrates by neighborhood, each record in the birth database must include a field with the mother's location by census block group or lower. Clearly, data sets including street addresses allow for the most detailed analysis. In addition, GIS can aggregate these data sets into larger areas, such as counties and states, permitting analysis at all levels.

Depending on the state and locality, many data sets are easily obtainable, such as vital statistics data (perinatal and mortality), health care expenditures, access to primary care, hospital discharge data, and behavioral risk factor data.[19] Public health practitioners will find that a large number of these health-related data sets meet the basic requirement of having an address field (see Tables 2–1 through 2–5). Some of them are "traditional" public health data familiar to most public health professionals and include things like vital statistics and reported communicable disease. The beauty of GIS technology is that it encourages the integration of many other data sets that will prove useful in improving community health. For example, because TIGER allows the automated integration of census data, public health professionals can easily incorporate population denominator data in calculating rates for many kinds of health-related issues.

DEMOGRAPHIC DATA

Electronic demographic data (Table 2–1) are critical in public health GIS applications for a couple of reasons.[19] First, for health planning, public health practitioners need information on the age, gender, race, and ethnic distribution of their community. Second, this information is essential for calculating incidence and prevalence of health-related conditions for diverse populations. In addition, age adjustment is impossible without denominator data. The "gold standard" of demographic data is the decennial census (1990 or 2000) and is available from the U.S. Bureau of the Census down to the census block-group level.[19] Sometimes, especially in rapidly growing areas, GIS users might prefer updated demographic data. Fortunately, reliable intercensus projections are available through commercial vendors.[21] One drawback to such commercial data sets is that, like updated geographic files, they can be expensive.

Table 2–1 Data for GIS-Based Community Health Planning: Geospatial, Demographic, Socioeconomics, Health Care Expenditures, Health Care Resources, and Access to Primary Care

Category (Examples)	Source	Data Set Name	Smallest Geographic Unit
Geospatial data for base maps (e.g., boundaries, streets, points)	U.S. Bureau of the Census U.S. Geological Survey National Oceanic and Atmospheric Administration U.S. Environmental Protection Agency	TIGER line files Geospatial Data Clearinghouse	Street
Demographic data (e.g., age, sex, race, and ethnic distribution)	U.S. Bureau of the Census	Decennial and Periodic Census	Census block
Socioeconomic data (e.g., educational level, poverty level, percent unemployed, age of housing, and number of workers by industry)	U.S. Bureau of the Census U.S. Bureau of Labor Statistics	Decennial and Periodic Census County Business Patterns	Census block group County
Health care expenditures data (e.g., number of persons on Medicaid, number of persons in Women, Infants, and Children Program, number of homeless persons, number of food stamp recipients)	Health Care Financing Administration	Estimates of National Health Expenditures Estimates of State Health Expenditures	National State
Health care resources and access to primary care data (e.g., number of primary care physicians, community and migrant health care centers, uninsured/ underinsured)	Health Resources and Services Administration	Area Resource File Physician Supply Estimates Nurse Supply Estimates National Health Provider Inventory National Home and Hospice Care Survey	County National National National National

SOCIOECONOMIC DATA

The U.S. Bureau of the Census provides useful socioeconomic data (Table 2–1) down to the block group level. Available socioeconomic variables include poverty, education level, and age of housing.[19] Housing age by block group is especially valuable in measuring the risk of childhood lead exposure because houses built before 1950 are more likely to contain lead-based paint.[9] Other useful available databases related to socioeconomic status include Food Stamp recipients, Medicaid recipients, and participants in the Women, Infants and Children (WIC) programs.[19]

VITAL STATISTICS DATA

Births

Births (Table 2–2) are reportable by law in every state. Many states and communities use birth data derived from these reports as measures of community and public health.[19] Birth reports, commonly known as birth certificates, include maternal residence address at the time of birth, making these reports available for geographic analysis (see Figure 2–5). Besides residence, data on birth certificates may include demographic data, such as maternal age, ethnicity, marital status, occupation, payment status (Medicaid, private insurance, or self-pay), and years of education. Additionally, birth reports usually contain several other useful measures. These include maternal smoking and drug use during pregnancy and birth outcomes (such as birth weight), gestational age, APGAR scores (an assessment of the newborn's color, pulse, respiration, tone, and response to stimuli), and congenital anomalies (birth defects). The birth report generally contains data on prenatal care, including the number of prenatal visits, the trimester that prenatal care began, and the adequacy of prenatal care. Many of the *Healthy People 2010* objectives, including adolescent pregnancy, prenatal care, rate of low birth weight, preterm birth, and prenatal substance abuse, rely on birth data.[8]

All states have participated in birth registration since 1933.[19] Many states are beginning to store birth data electronically, including data from earlier years. Conversion of these hard-copy reports to an electronic format allows for an automated time-trend analysis. Unfortunately, although most states have converted birth data into an electronic form, they have substituted county or ZIP code for full street address, prohibiting geographic analysis at the community level. Local health departments can solve this problem by entering the address data before they send the birth reports on to the state. Local health departments having access to such electronic birth records with a street address can use GIS to show measures such as prenatal care, prenatal substance abuse, and rate of low birth weight for neighborhoods within their jurisdictions. In addition, local health departments and their partners can use birth data to estimate future school enrollments and distribute government funding for education.[22] Other programs, such as the Healthy Start initiative, use infant mortality rates for cities to determine how to distribute public funds.[22]

Table 2–2 Data for GIS-Based Community Health Planning: Perinatal Indicators, Mortality, and Years of Potential Life Lost (YPLL)

Category	Source	Data Set Name	Smallest Geographic Unit
Perinatal indicators (e.g., total live births, teenage live births, prenatal care, low body weight live births, live births with mortality or birth defects)	National Center for Health Statistics	National Vital Statistics Program (Birth and Fetal Death Certificate)	County
	Centers for Disease Control and Prevention	Abortion services statistics	State
	State or local registries	Congenital malformation or birth defect registries	County, limited local
Mortality (e.g., leading causes of mortality by age and population subgroups)	National Center for Health Statistics	National Vital Statistics Program (Compressed Mortality File)	County
	State vital statistics	State vital statistics	Street
Years of potential life lost (YPLL)	State vital statistics	YPLL statistics (derived from age of death on death certificate)	County (subcounty analysis in some states)

U.S. STANDARD CERTIFICATE OF LIVE BIRTH

LOCAL FILE NO.   BIRTH NUMBER:

CHILD

1. CHILD'S NAME (First, Middle, Last, Suffix) | 2. TIME OF BIRTH | 3. SEX | 4. DATE OF BIRTH (Mo/Day/Yr)

5. FACILITY NAME (If not institution, give street and number) | 6. CITY, TOWN, OR LOCATION OF BIRTH | 7. COUNTY OF BIRTH

MOTHER

8a. MOTHER'S CURRENT LEGAL NAME (First, Middle, Last, Suffix) | 8b. DATE OF BIRTH (Mo/Day/Yr)

8c. MOTHER'S NAME PRIOR TO FIRST MARRIAGE (First, Middle, Last, Suffix) | 8d. BIRTHPLACE (State, Territory, or Foreign Country)

9a. RESIDENCE OF MOTHER-STATE | 9b. COUNTY | 9c. CITY, TOWN, OR LOCATION

9d. STREET AND NUMBER | 9e. APT. NO. | 9f. ZIP CODE | 9g. INSIDE CITY LIMITS? ☐ Yes ☐ No

FATHER

10a. FATHER'S CURRENT LEGAL NAME (First, Middle, Last, Suffix) | 10b. DATE OF BIRTH (Mo/Day/Yr) | 10c. BIRTHPLACE (State, Territory, or Foreign Country)

CERTIFIER

11. CERTIFIER'S NAME: _____
TITLE: ☐ MD ☐ DO ☐ HOSPITAL ADMIN. ☐ CNM/CM ☐ OTHER MIDWIFE
☐ OTHER (Specify)_____

12. DATE CERTIFIED ___/___/___ MM DD YYYY

13. DATE FILED BY REGISTRAR ___/___/___ MM DD YYYY

INFORMATION FOR ADMINISTRATIVE USE

MOTHER

14. MOTHER'S MAILING ADDRESS: ☐ Same as residence, or: State: City, Town, or Location:

Street & Number: Apartment No.:   Zip Code:

15. MOTHER MARRIED? (At birth, conception, or any time between) ☐ Yes ☐ No | 16. SOCIAL SECURITY NUMBER REQUESTED FOR CHILD? ☐ Yes ☐ No | 17. FACILITY ID. (NPI)

IF NO, HAS PATERNITY ACKNOWLEDGMENT BEEN SIGNED IN THE HOSPITAL? ☐ Yes ☐ No

18. MOTHER'S SOCIAL SECURITY NUMBER: | 19. FATHER'S SOCIAL SECURITY NUMBER:

INFORMATION FOR MEDICAL AND HEALTH PURPOSES ONLY

MOTHER

DRAFT 09/12/2001

20. MOTHER'S EDUCATION (Check the box that best describes the highest degree or level of school completed at the time of delivery)
☐ 8th grade or less
☐ 9th - 12th grade, no diploma
☐ High school graduate or GED completed
☐ Some college credit but no degree
☐ Associate degree (e.g., AA, AS)
☐ Bachelor's degree (e.g., BA, AB, BS)
☐ Master's degree (e.g., MA, MS, MEng, MEd, MSW, MBA)
☐ Doctorate (e.g., PhD, EdD) or Professional degree (e.g., MD, DDS, DVM, LLB, JD)

21. MOTHER OF HISPANIC ORIGIN? (Check the box that best describes whether the mother is Spanish/Hispanic/Latina. Check the "No" box if mother is not Spanish/Hispanic/Latina)
☐ No, not Spanish/Hispanic/Latina
☐ Yes, Mexican, Mexican American, Chicana
☐ Yes, Puerto Rican
☐ Yes, Cuban
☐ Yes, other Spanish/Hispanic/Latina
(Specify)_____

22. MOTHER'S RACE (Check one or more races to indicate what the mother considers herself to be)
☐ White
☐ Black or African American
☐ American Indian or Alaska Native (Name of the enrolled or principal tribe)_____
☐ Asian Indian
☐ Chinese
☐ Filipino
☐ Japanese
☐ Korean
☐ Vietnamese
☐ Other Asian (Specify)_____
☐ Native Hawaiian
☐ Guamanian or Chamorro
☐ Samoan
☐ Other Pacific Islander (Specify)_____
☐ Other (Specify)_____

FATHER

23. FATHER'S EDUCATION (Check the box that best describes the highest degree or level of school completed at the time of delivery)
☐ 8th grade or less
☐ 9th - 12th grade, no diploma
☐ High school graduate or GED completed
☐ Some college credit but no degree
☐ Associate degree (e.g., AA, AS)
☐ Bachelor's degree (e.g., BA, AB, BS)
☐ Master's degree (e.g., MA, MS, MEng, MEd, MSW, MBA)
☐ Doctorate (e.g., PhD, EdD) or Professional degree (e.g., MD, DDS, DVM, LLB, JD)

24. FATHER OF HISPANIC ORIGIN? (Check the box that best describes whether the father is Spanish/Hispanic/Latino. Check the "No" box if mother is not Spanish/Hispanic/Latino)
☐ No, not Spanish/Hispanic/Latino
☐ Yes, Mexican, Mexican American, Chicano
☐ Yes, Puerto Rican
☐ Yes, Cuban
☐ Yes, other Spanish/Hispanic/Latino
(Specify)_____

25. FATHER'S RACE (Check one or more races to indicate what the father considers himself to be)
☐ White
☐ Black or African American
☐ American Indian or Alaska Native (Name of the enrolled or principal tribe)_____
☐ Asian Indian
☐ Chinese
☐ Filipino
☐ Japanese
☐ Korean
☐ Vietnamese
☐ Other Asian (Specify)_____
☐ Native Hawaiian
☐ Guamanian or Chamorro
☐ Samoan
☐ Other Pacific Islander (Specify)_____
☐ Other (Specify)_____

Mother's Name _____

Mother's Medical Record No. _____

26. PLACE WHERE BIRTH OCCURRED (Check one)
☐ Hospital
☐ Freestanding birthing center
☐ Home Birth: Planned to deliver at home? ☐ Yes ☐ No
☐ Clinic/Doctor's office
☐ Other (Specify)_____

27. ATTENDANT'S NAME, TITLE, AND NPI
NAME: _____ NPI:_____
TITLE: ☐ MD ☐ DO ☐ CNM/CM ☐ OTHER MIDWIFE
☐ OTHER (Specify)_____

28. MOTHER TRANSFERRED FOR MATERNAL MEDICAL OR FETAL INDICATIONS FOR DELIVERY? ☐ Yes ☐ No
IF YES, ENTER NAME OF FACILITY MOTHER TRANSFERRED FROM:
_____

Figure 2–5 Sample birth certificate

Figure 2–5 continued

MOTHER

29a. DATE OF FIRST PRENATAL CARE VISIT
___/___/_____ □ No Prenatal Care
MM DD YYYY

29b. DATE OF LAST PRENATAL CARE VISIT
___/___/_____
MM DD YYYY

30. TOTAL NUMBER OF PRENATAL VISITS FOR THIS PREGNANCY
_____ (If none, enter "0".)

31. MOTHER'S HEIGHT _____ (feet/inches)

32. MOTHER'S PREPREGNANCY WEIGHT _____ (pounds)

33. MOTHER'S WEIGHT AT DELIVERY _____ (pounds)

34. DID MOTHER GET WIC FOOD FOR HERSELF DURING THIS PREGNANCY? □ Yes □ No

35. NUMBER OF PREVIOUS LIVE BIRTHS (Do not include this child)
35a. Now Living Number _____ □ None
35b. Now Dead Number _____ □ None

36. NUMBER OF OTHER PREGNANCY OUTCOMES (spontaneous or induced losses or ectopic pregnancies)
36a. Other Outcomes Number _____ □ None

37. CIGARETTE SMOKING BEFORE AND DURING PREGNANCY
For each time period, enter either the number of cigarettes or the number of packs of cigarettes smoked. IF NONE, ENTER "0".
Average number of cigarettes or packs of cigarettes smoked per day.

	# of cigarettes		# of packs
Three Months Before Pregnancy	_____	OR	_____
First Three Months of Pregnancy	_____	OR	_____
Second Three Months of Pregnancy	_____	OR	_____
Last Three Months of Pregnancy	_____	OR	_____

38. PRINCIPAL SOURCE OF PAYMENT FOR THIS DELIVERY
□ Private Insurance
□ Medicaid
□ Self-pay
□ Other (Specify) _____

35c. DATE OF LAST LIVE BIRTH ___/_____ MM YYYY

36b. DATE OF LAST OTHER PREGNANCY OUTCOME ___/_____ MM YYYY

39. DATE LAST NORMAL MENSES BEGAN ___/___/_____ MM DD YYYY

40. MOTHER'S MEDICAL RECORD NUMBER

MEDICAL AND HEALTH INFORMATION

DRAFT 09/12/2001

41. RISK FACTORS IN THIS PREGNANCY (Check all that apply)

Diabetes
□ Prepregnancy (Diagnosis prior to this pregnancy)
□ Gestational (Diagnosis in this pregnancy)

Hypertension
□ Prepregnancy (Chronic)
□ Gestational (PIH, preeclampsia, eclampsia)

□ Previous preterm birth

□ Other previous poor pregnancy outcome (Includes, perinatal death, small-for-gestational age/intrauterine growth restricted birth)

□ Vaginal bleeding during this pregnancy prior to the onset of labor

□ Pregnancy resulted from infert

□ Mother had a previous cesarean delivery If yes, how many _____

□ None of the above

42. INFECTIONS PRESENT AND/OR TREATED DURING THIS PREGNANCY (Check all that apply)
□ Gonorrhea
□ Syphilis
□ Herpes Simplex Virus (HSV)
□ Chlamydia
□ Hepatitis B
□ Hepatitis C
□ None of the above

43. OBSTETRIC PROCEDURES (Check all that apply)
□ Cervical cerclage
□ Tocolysis
External cephalic version:
□ Successful
□ Failed
□ None of the above

44. ONSET OF LABOR (Check all that apply)
□ Premature Rupture of the Membranes (prolonged, ≥12 hrs.)
□ Precipitous Labor (<3 hrs.)
□ Prolonged Labor (≥ 20 hrs.)
□ None of the above

45. CHARACTERISTICS OF LABOR AND DELIVERY (Check all that apply)
□ Induction of labor
□ Augmentation of labor
□ Non-vertex presentation
□ Steroids (glucocorticoids) for fetal lung maturation received by the mother prior to delivery
□ Antibiotics received by the mother during labor
□ Clinical chorioamnionitis diagnosed during labor or maternal temperature ≥38°C (100.4°F)
□ Moderate/heavy meconium staining of the amniotic fluid
□ Fetal intolerance of labor such that one or more of the following actions was taken: in-utero resuscitative measures, further fetal assessment, or operative delivery
□ Epidural or spinal anesthesia during labor
□ None of the above

46. METHOD OF DELIVERY
A. Was delivery with forceps attempted but unsuccessful? □ Yes □ No
B. Was delivery with vacuum extraction attempted but unsuccessful? □ Yes □ No
C. Fetal presentation at birth
□ Cephalic
□ Breech
□ Other
D. Final route and method of delivery (Check one)
□ Vaginal/Spontaneous
□ Vaginal/Forceps
□ Vaginal/Vacuum
□ Cesarean If cesarean, was a trial of labor attempted? □ Yes □ No

47. MATERNAL MORBIDITY (Check all that apply) (Complications associated with labor and delivery)
□ Maternal transfusion
□ Third or fourth degree perineal laceration
□ Ruptured uterus
□ Unplanned hysterectomy
□ Admission to intensive care unit
□ Unplanned operating room procedure following delivery
□ None of the above

NEWBORN INFORMATION

NEWBORN

Mother's Name _____
Mother's Medical Record No. _____

48. NEWBORN MEDICAL RECORD NUMBER:

49. BIRTHWEIGHT (grams preferred, specify unit) _____ □ grams □ lb/oz

50. OBSTETRIC ESTIMATE OF GESTATION: _____ (completed weeks)

51. APGAR SCORE:
Score at 5 minutes: _____
If 5 minute score is less than 6,
Score at 10 minutes: _____

52. PLURALITY - Single, Twin, Triplet, etc. (Specify) _____

53. IF NOT SINGLE BIRTH - Born First, Second, Third, etc. (Specify) _____

54. ABNORMAL CONDITIONS OF THE NEWBORN (Check all that apply)
□ Assisted ventilation required immediately following delivery
□ Assisted ventilation required for more than six hours
□ NICU admission
□ Newborn given surfactant replacement therapy
□ Antibiotics received by the newborn for suspected neonatal sepsis
□ Seizure or serious neurologic dysfunction
□ Significant birth injury (skeletal fracture(s), peripheral nerve injury, and/or soft tissue/solid organ hemorrhage which requires intervention)
□ None of the above

55. CONGENITAL ANOMALIES OF THE NEWBORN (Check all that apply)
□ Anencephaly
□ Meningomyelocele/Spina bifida
□ Cyanotic congenital heart disease
□ Congenital diaphragmatic hernia
□ Omphalocele
□ Gastroschisis
□ Limb reduction defect (excluding congenital amputation and dwarfing syndromes)
□ Cleft Lip with or without Cleft Palate
□ Cleft Palate alone
□ Down Syndrome
  □ Karyotype confirmed
  □ Karyotype pending
□ Suspected chromosomal disorder
  □ Karyotype confirmed
  □ Karyotype pending
□ Hypospadias
□ None of the anomalies listed above

56. WAS INFANT TRANSFERRED WITHIN 24 HOURS OF DELIVERY? □ Yes □ No
IF YES, NAME OF FACILITY INFANT TRANSFERRED TO: _____

57. IS INFANT LIVING AT TIME OF REPORT?
□ Yes □ No □ Infant transferred, status unknown

58. IS INFANT BEING BREASTFED? □ Yes □ No

Several problems with birth data antedated the development of GIS. These problems are a reflection of the reliability of self-reporting. For example, physicians filling out birth certificates may not accurately report maternal behaviors such as tobacco or drug use. Other unreliable information may include APGAR scores and gestational age.[19] Another limitation of birth data is that some congenital anomalies do not become apparent until several years after birth, making the birth data incomplete and unreliable for geographic analysis of birth defects. Some states and localities have created congenital malformation or birth defect registries to include these data, but most of these registries do not actively update or confirm their data, reducing their usefulness.[19]

Most states require reporting of fetal deaths after 20 weeks' gestation, but these data are less useful than birth data for geographic analysis.[19] A fetal death is a death *in utero* of a fetus that weighs 500 g or more, regardless of gestation. The reason these reports are less useful is that their accuracy is variable, depending on gestational age. Physicians are more likely to report deaths of fetuses older than 28 weeks' gestation because most of these fetuses weigh more than 500 g. Between 20 and 28 weeks, the reporting is less consistent and is very incomplete for fetuses younger than 20 weeks' gestation. Although abortions are reportable, the report generally does not include a street address, prohibiting geographic analysis below the county level.

Deaths

Mortality reporting (see Table 2–2) shares many strengths and limitations with birth reporting. Like births, deaths are reportable by law in every state. Many states and communities use mortality data derived from these reports as measures of community and public health.[19] For example, some states have adopted infant mortality and adolescent suicide rates as benchmarks to measure progress in reaching health objectives. Like birth data, many of the *Healthy People 2010* objectives, including those regarding cancer deaths, deaths from unintentional injuries, and homicide, rely on data obtained from death certificate reporting.[8]

As they have for births, states have required death reporting for many years, allowing for time-trend analysis. Death certificates include residence address at the time of death, making these reports available for geographic analysis (see Figure 2–6). Besides residence, death certificate data include some demographic information such as age, gender, and race. Unfortunately, the data lack other useful demographic variables such as occupation and socioeconomic status. Death certificate reports also contain immediate and underlying causes of death.

As with birth reporting, many states are beginning to store death data electronically, including data from earlier years.

However, the geographic information available in the mortality database shares its limitations with birth data. Although most states have converted death data into an electronic form, they have again substituted county or ZIP code for full street address, preventing geographic analysis at the community level. Local health departments can solve this problem the same way they can for birth data, by entering the address data before they send the death reports on to the state. For geographic analysis, even an accurate residence address may not be helpful. For example, for a study of the relationship between an environmental exposure and a specific cause of death, the residence address at the time of death may not be the residence at the time of the exposure of interest.[19] This is especially true for diseases with long latencies between exposure and illness, such as many cancers. For this reason, death data are more useful for studying conditions with short latencies before death, such as unintentional injuries, including traffic accidents, and intentional injuries, including suicides and homicides. Local health departments having access to such electronic death records can use GIS to show death rates by cause for neighborhoods within their jurisdictions.

At the national level, the National Center for Health Statistics (NCHS) provides the Compressed Mortality File (CMF) for public use. The CMF contains several variables, including state and county of residence, year of death, age group at death, race, sex, and underlying cause of death (four-digit International Classification of Disease [ICD] code).

Several death data limitations antedated the development of GIS. These problems are a reflection of the reliability of the person making the report. For example, either family members or funeral directors may report the demographic information listed on the death certificate. The accuracy of this report may reflect how well the reporter knows the deceased individual. One potential consequence is that the reported race of an individual may differ from birth to death.[19] Physicians, medical examiners, or coroners report the cause of death and may report inaccurately.

Years of Potential Life Lost

Years of potential life lost (YPLL), a measure of premature mortality, is derived from mortality data and can be included in a geographic analysis. To calculate YPLL, the first decision is to decide what age constitutes premature mortality. Most public health analyses have used 65 years as the cutoff point, although as life expectancy lengthens, studies are switching to 75 as the end point. Once the end point is set, the YPLL is equal to the age of death listed on the death certificate, if less than the end point, subtracted from the end point. Deaths occurring greater than or equal to the end point age count toward a YPLL of zero. For example, a death

DRAFT 07/10/2001

U.S. STANDARD CERTIFICATE OF DEATH

LOCAL FILE NO.   STATE FILE NO.

NAME OF DECEDENT
For use by physician or institution

To Be Completed/Verified By: FUNERAL DIRECTOR

1. DECEDENT'S LEGAL NAME (Include AKA's if any) (First, Middle, Last) | 2. SEX | 3. SOCIAL SECURITY NUMBER

4a. AGE-Last Birthday (Years) | 4b. UNDER 1 YEAR | Months | Days | 4c. UNDER 1 DAY | Hours | Minutes | 5. DATE OF BIRTH (Mo/Day/Yr) | 6. BIRTHPLACE (City and State or Foreign Country)

7a. RESIDENCE-STATE | 7b. COUNTY | 7c. CITY OR TOWN

7d. STREET AND NUMBER | 7e. APT. NO. | 7f. ZIP CODE | 7g. INSIDE CITY LIMITS? □ Yes □ No

8. EVER IN US ARMED FORCES? □ Yes □ No | 9. MARITAL STATUS AT TIME OF DEATH □ Married □ Married, but separated □ Widowed □ Divorced □ Never Married □ Unknown | 10. SURVIVING SPOUSE'S NAME (If wife, give name prior to first marriage)

11. FATHER'S NAME (First, Middle, Last) | 12. MOTHER'S NAME PRIOR TO FIRST MARRIAGE (First, Middle, Last)

13a. INFORMANT'S NAME | 13b. RELATIONSHIP TO DECEDENT | 13c. MAILING ADDRESS (Street and Number, City, State, Zip Code)

14. PLACE OF DEATH (Check only one: see instructions)

IF DEATH OCCURRED IN A HOSPITAL:
□ Inpatient □ Emergency Room/Outpatient □ Dead on Arrival

IF DEATH OCCURRED SOMEWHERE OTHER THAN A HOSPITAL:
□ Hospice facility □ Nursing home/Long term care fac □ Decedent's home □ Other (Specify):

15. FACILITY NAME (If not institution, give street & number) | 16. CITY, TOWN, AND ZIP CODE | 17. COUNTY OF DEATH

18. METHOD OF DISPOSITION: □ Burial □ Cremation □ Donation □ Entombment □ Removal from State □ Other (Specify): | 19. PLACE OF DISPOSITION (Name of cemetery, crematory, other place)

20. LOCATION-CITY, TOWN, AND STATE | 21. NAME AND COMPLETE ADDRESS OF FUNERAL FACILITY

22. SIGNATURE OF FUNERAL SERVICE LICENSEE OR OTHER AGENT | 23. LICENSE NUMBER (Of Licensee)

To Be Completed By: MEDICAL CERTIFIER

ITEMS 24-28 MUST BE COMPLETED BY PERSON WHO PRONOUNCES OR CERTIFIES DEATH | 24. DATE PRONOUNCED DEAD (Mo/Day/Yr) | 25. TIME PRONOUNCED DEAD

26. SIGNATURE OF PERSON PRONOUNCING DEATH (Only when applicable) | 27. LICENSE NUMBER | 28. DATE SIGNED (Mo/Day/Yr)

29. ACTUAL OR PRESUMED DATE OF DEATH (Mo/Day/Yr) (Spell Month) | 30. ACTUAL OR PRESUMED TIME OF DEATH | 31. WAS MEDICAL EXAMINER OR CORONER CONTACTED?

CAUSE OF DEATH (See instructions and examples)   Approximate interval: Onset to death

32. PART I. Enter the chain of events--diseases, injuries, or complications--that directly caused the death. DO NOT enter terminal events such as cardiac arrest, respiratory arrest, or ventricular fibrillation wit

IMMEDIATE CAUSE (Final disease or condition ---------> resulting in death)   a._____
Due to (or as a consequence of):

Sequentially list conditions, if any, leading to the cause listed on line a. Enter the UNDERLYING CAUSE (disease or injury that initiated the events resulting in death) LAST   b._____
Due to (or as a consequence of):

c._____
Due to (or as a consequence of):

d._____

PART II. Enter other significant conditions contributing to death but not resulting in the underlying cause given in PART I. | 33. WAS AN AUTOPSY PERFORMED? □ Yes □ No

34. WERE AUTOPSY FINDINGS AVAILABLE TO COMPLETE THE CAUSE OF DEATH? □ Yes □ No

35. DID TOBACCO USE CONTRIBUTE TO DEATH? □ Yes □ Probably □ No □ Unknown | 36. IF FEMALE: □ Not pregnant within past year □ Pregnant at time of death □ Not pregnant, but pregnant within 42 days of death □ Not pregnant, but pregnant 43 days to 1 year before death □ Unknown if pregnant within the past year | 37. MANNER OF DEATH □ Natural □ Homicide □ Accident □ Pending Investigation □ Suicide □ Could not be determined

38. DATE OF INJURY (Mo/Day/Yr) (Spell Month) | 39. TIME OF INJURY | 40. PLACE OF INJURY (e.g., Decedent's home; construction site; restaurant; wooded area) | 41. INJURY AT WORK? □ Yes □ No

42. LOCATION OF INJURY: State: City or Town: Street & Number: Apartment No.:   Zip Code:

43. DESCRIBE HOW INJURY OCCURRED: | 44. IF TRANSPORTATION INJURY, SPECIFY: □ Driver/Operator □ Passenger □ Pedestrian □ Other (Specify)

45. CERTIFIER (Check only one):
□ Certifying physician-To the best of my knowledge, death occurred due to the cause(s) and manner stated.
□ Pronouncing & Certifying physician-To the best of my knowledge, death occurred at the time, date, and place, and due to the cause(s) and manner stated.
□ Medical Examiner/Coroner-On the basis of examination, and/or investigation, in my opinion, death occurred at the time, date, and place, and due to the cause(s) and manner stated.

Signature of certifier:

46. NAME, ADDRESS, AND ZIP CODE OF PERSON COMPLETING CAUSE OF DEATH (Item 32)

47. TITLE OF CERTIFIER | 48. LICENSE NUMBER | 49. DATE CERTIFIED (Mo/Day/Yr) | 50. **FOR REGISTRAR ONLY**- DATE FILED (Mo/Day/Yr)

51. DECEDENT'S EDUCATION-Check the | 52. DECEDENT OF HISPANIC ORIGIN? Check the box that best | 53. DECEDENT'S RACE (Check one or more races to indicate what the

Figure 2–6 Sample certificate of death

at age 56 is equal to a YPLL75 of 19. Average YPLL is the average of the YPLL for all deaths in a community. Causes of death, such as homicide, that are common in young people contribute a larger amount to the average YPLL of a community. If a health department or community has access to electronic death report data, and if these data include an address field, the health department can use GIS to show the average YPLL for each community in its district.[19]

MORBIDITY DATA

Morbidity data include data on hospitalizations, ambulatory medical care, prevalence of disease, and other health indices (Table 2–3).

Hospitalization

Hospitalization rates, hospitalization causes, and other hospitalization data are important measures of community health for a couple of reasons. They are an indirect measure of the burden of specific diseases within a community and an indicator of health care costs.[19] If linked with death data, hospitalization data can show the relationship between intensive hospital care and death. For example, the data can portray the number and cost of nursing home patients with do-not-resuscitate orders who receive care in a hospital intensive care unit within six months of death.[19] Several of the *Healthy People 2010* objectives use cause-specific hospitalization as a measure of community health status. For example, heart failure hospitalization is a measure related to the goal

Table 2–3 Data for GIS-Based Community Health Planning: Hospitalization, Ambulatory Medical Care, and Estimated Prevalence of Disease

Category (Examples)	Source	Data Set Name	Smallest Geographic Unit
Hospitalization (e.g., leading causes of hospitalization by age and population subgroup)	National Center for Health Statistics	National Hospital Discharge Survey	Census regions
	Health Care Financing Administration	Medicare Statistical System	Varies (some data include ZIP code)
	Dartmouth Center for Clinical Evaluative Services	Dartmouth Atlas of Health Care	Hospital referral region
	State Medicaid Agency	State Medicaid Data	Varies with each state
Ambulatory medical care	National Center for Health Statistics	National Hospital Ambulatory Medical Care Survey	Four national regions
		National Ambulatory Medical Care Survey	Four national regions
Estimated prevalence of disease	Local Health Department	Reportable diseases (e.g., sexually transmitted diseases, childhood lead poisoning)	Street
	Centers for Disease Control and Prevention	National Notifiable Diseases Surveillance System	State
		AIDS Surveillance	
	National Center for Health Statistics	National Health Interview Survey	National
		National Health and Nutrition Examination Survey	
	National Institute of Health	Surveillance, Epidemiology, and End Results Program (SEER)	County
	State cancer registries	Cancer and tumor registries	County, ZIP code, limited street

of improving cardiovascular health through the early identification and treatment of heart attacks and prevention of recurrent cardiovascular events. Hospitalization for asthma relates to the goal of promoting respiratory health through better prevention, detection, treatment, and education. Hospitalization for ambulatory care–sensitive conditions is a measure related to the goal of improved health care access.[8]

At the national level, the National Hospital Discharge Survey provides a continuing sample survey of short-stay hospitals in the United States.[19] Short-stay hospitals have an average patient admission of less than 30 days. Newborn discharges and discharges from federal hospitals are not included in the database. The geographic report level is at the census region. In 1942, the U.S. Bureau of the Census established census regions as four groupings of states (Northeast, South, Midwest, and West). Obviously, this database is not useful for analysis of hospitalization causes and rates at the community level.

The Medicare Statistical System provides data useful in analyzing hospital and health care utilization. This database has information on program effectiveness, including enrollees' eligibility and the benefits they use, certification of institutional providers, and payments for services. The system has four files related to health insurance: service providers, hospital insurance claims, and supplementary medical insurance payment records. Although most of the information is at the state level, some ZIP code information is available.[19] Compared to Medicare, geographic analysis of Medicaid data presents a more difficult challenge.[19] Because Medicaid is a state program, availability of its hospitalization data is dependent on the specific state. Currently, analyzing Medicaid data requires obtaining permission from individual state Medicaid agencies and performing analysis one state at a time. Definitions used in the Medicaid database may differ from state to state, making state and regional comparison difficult.[19] On the other hand, Medicaid data that include an address can be quite helpful for investigation of hospitalization and other health care utilization and access by the Medicaid population at a local level.

Some states have established electronic hospital discharge records that may be useful at the local level. For example, Massachusetts has hospital discharge data tape files that aggregate cause of hospitalization by diagnosis-related groups (DRGs) by patient residence by ZIP code.[23] If hospitals would report their discharge data with a street address, local health departments could use GIS to show rates of hospitalization by cause by neighborhood.[19]

Figure 2–7 is a map, based on state Uniform Hospital Discharge Data Set files, showing pediatric hospitalization rates based on discharge diagnosis for asthma for the 69 hospital service areas (described later in the chapter) of northern New England.[24] The map displays these hospitalizations as a ratio of each service area's age- and sex-adjusted pediatric asthma discharge rate to the rate for the entire region. Any service area with a ratio of 1 has a rate equal to that for the region. The map shows that 17 service areas have pediatric asthma discharge rates at least 30 percent greater than the regional rate, including one area with a rate 300 percent greater than the regional rate. Seventeen other areas have rates at least 70 percent below the regional rate. These large variations are occurring across relatively racially homogeneous populations, in environments without substantial differences in air quality.

Like the 1854 Golden Square cholera outbreak investigation, such maps showing regional variation can be deceiving. Without further analysis, this ecological study could lead to the conclusion that there are differences in asthma illness rates across the service areas.[24] However, no study has ever documented such large variations in asthma prevalence between neighboring small areas.[24] Further analysis reveals other possible explanations. Rather than burden of illness, higher bed supply is a strong and independent predictor of hospital admission. Other possibilities include proximity and accessibility of hospitals for residents of an area. The closer the hospital, the more likely an admission due to the greater use of emergency rooms for routine acute care. Physician practice, including whether local physicians prescribe the most effective asthma medications, may be another independent predictor of hospitalization for pediatric asthma.[24] This example points out the benefits and limitations of geographic analysis of health care utilization. The maps help us raise some interesting questions and often point us in the right direction, but we must consider further epidemiologic analysis before developing conclusions.

Ambulatory (Outpatient) Data

Over the past two decades, in an attempt to reduce health care expenditures, our health care system shifted patient care from hospital settings to ambulatory settings. Consequently, for health planning, for evaluating use of health care resources, including preventive services, and for evaluating the burden of illness in a community, ambulatory health care utilization data have become increasingly important. Data included in ambulatory records include information on diseases that are not rapidly fatal, do not necessarily lead to hospitalization, and are not available in registries. For example, ambulatory data are useful in estimating the prevalence of hypertension in a community.

Besides revealing substantial regional variation in hospital resources, maps created from the Medicare Statistical System can reveal variation in the quantity and type of ambulatory health care utilization and physician workforce.[25]

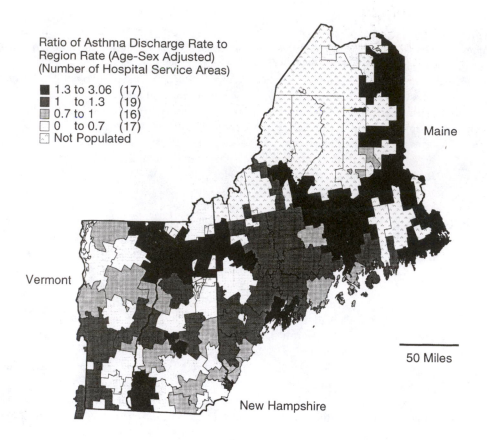

Figure 2–7 Pediatric asthma hospitalization (primary diagnosis ICD-9 493) for residents (age 0–17 years) of hospital service areas in northern New England, 1992–1996. *Source:* Data are from state departments of health Uniform Hospital Discharge Data Set files. Populations in hospital service areas exceed 10,000 person-years except for Colebrook, New Hampshire (discharge ratio 0.17), and Townsend, Vermont (discharge ratio 0). Average annual region rate is 1.47 discharges per 1,000.

The *Dartmouth Atlas of Health Care* provides an example of how GIS can use available Medicare data to analyze such geographic variation. The atlas based its geographic analysis on 3,436 hospital service areas (HSAs), health care markets where most Medicare beneficiaries receive inpatient care. These HSAs are grouped into 306 tertiary care regions, also known as hospital referral regions, based on hospitalization for major cardiovascular procedures.

Figure 2–8, a map from the atlas, shows considerable regional variation in breast cancer screening.[25] The U.S. Preventive Services Taskforce Guide to Clinical Preventive Services recommends screening mammograms at least every two years for all women aged 50 to 69 years.[26] The map clearly shows how well the American health care system is meeting this goal. In this case, the health care system failed to meet its goal in every region, although some regions performed better than others. Such information, if available at the local

level, could be useful in program planning and resource allocation, ultimately improving access to preventive services like mammography. Students and practitioners interested in obtaining a copy of the atlas can call the American Hospital Association at (800) 242–2626 or visit the Web site <www.dartmouth.edu/dms/cecs/>.

Another source of national level ambulatory data is the National Hospital Ambulatory Medical Care Survey. This survey, begun in 1992, is an ongoing annual national sample survey of patient visits to emergency rooms and outpatient departments in nonfederal, short-stay, or general hospitals.[19] Hospital staff complete record forms for a random sample of patient visits during a four-week period. The survey aggregates the data into four regions in the United States, so it is not available for local analysis. Similarly, the National Ambulatory Medical Care Survey is an ongoing national sample survey of outpatient medical visits. This survey also

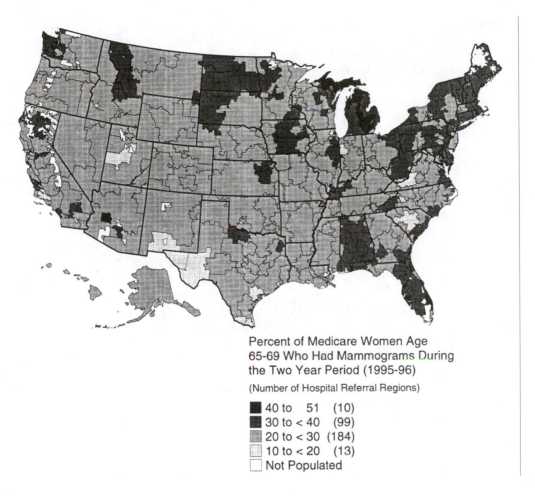

Percent of Medicare Women Age
65-69 Who Had Mammograms During
the Two Year Period (1995-96)

(Number of Hospital Referral Regions)

- ■ 40 to   51   (10)
- ▩ 30 to < 40   (99)
- ▤ 20 to < 30   (184)
- ▫ 10 to < 20   (13)
- ☐ Not Populated

Figure 2–8 Breast cancer screening rates in Medicare enrollees (age 65–69) by 306 hospital referral regions, 1995–1996. *Dartmouth Atlas of Health Care 1999.*

aggregates the data into four national regions and covers patient visits with non–federally employed physicians. Only actual outpatient physician office visits are included. The survey excludes telephone contacts, visits outside the office, and visits to hospital-based physicians. Also excluded are visits to anesthesiologists, pathologists, radiologists, and physicians involved in research, teaching, or administration.[19]

Limitations of Ambulatory Data

Although important as community morbidity measures, ambulatory data have substantial limitations preventing their broader use. Compared to inpatient data, ambulatory care data are much less likely to be stored in electronic form. Analyzing such hard-copy data requires the additional time and expense associated with coding and entering the data in a format compatible with GIS.[19] The definition of ambula-

tory care is broad, including emergency room visits, clinic visits, school health clinic visits, and visits by employees to their company health office. Because of this diversity, ambulatory records vary by quantity and quality of information. Even if physicians have converted their charting systems to an electronic medical record format, the availability of useful information in the data set can vary, depending on the software used. Billing systems, containing patient encounter data, are alternatives to electronic medical records for ambulatory care analysis. With billing systems, however, the quality of data can vary depending on the coding system. Epidemiologic analysis usually addresses a specific disease or outcome and requires disease-specific information. This is a problem with record coding using an administrative billing system based on disease groupings, such as DRGs. Compared to disease-specific systems, such as the International Classification of Diseases, 9th Revision (ICD-9) codes, systems based on lumping diseases into groups limit the value of the records for epidemiological analysis.[19]

Ambulatory data have several additional limitations. If a community has multiple practices, obtaining data sets from multiple offices is difficult. If physicians belong to a large group practice or health plan, proprietary policies may limit access to the data. In addition, patients' consent for release is required, even if personal indicators are not included with the data.[19] For studying rates, denominator data may be inaccurate or unavailable, especially if a subset of a community or region is the unit of analysis. Patients often travel out of their community or county for health care. Data based on records of health care providers within a county or community may underestimate the prevalence of disease because they exclude information on community residents who seek care elsewhere.

Disease Surveillance Data

Disease registries, created at the state and federal level, provide other sources for GIS analysis of disease patterns. State laws require physicians to report communicable diseases and other diseases with public health implications, such as lead poisoning. For example, reportable communicable diseases include

- Sexually transmitted diseases, such as syphilis, gonorrhea, and *chlamydia*
- Many diseases spread by the fecal-oral route, including (but not limited to) foodborne and waterborne diseases such as shigellosis, salmonellosis, *Escherichia coli* O157:H7, and hepatitis A
- Vaccine-preventable diseases, such as measles, rubella, and hepatitis B
- Airborne diseases with public health consequences, such as tuberculosis

Physicians and laboratories report these diseases to local health departments, who send a case report to the state and perform an investigation. Besides information on the disease, these reports include demographic information on the patient, including age, gender, and residence address. With these address data, local and state health departments can use GIS to map location of disease cases. If population data are available, health departments can also map reportable disease incidence rates and prevalence.

A geographic investigation conducted by Salt Lake County, Utah, provides an example of how a health department used reported hepatitis A data to map incidence rates by ZIP code[27] (see Figure 2–9). Health departments could use similar information to evaluate disease clusters. In addition, local health departments can develop maps adding information from other sources. For example, health departments could add data in location of childhood lead cases to information on housing age, creating maps that would show lead cases juxtaposed on older housing. As we will discuss in Chapter 4, these displays are useful for targeting lead-screening efforts.

As with other reportable communicable diseases, state and territorial health departments conduct surveillance for acquired immune deficiency syndrome (AIDS). Hospitals and physicians are generally required to report AIDS cases. In some states, HIV infection by name is also reportable. AIDS and HIV data are available at the state and, in some cases, county levels.

At the national level, the National Notifiable Diseases Surveillance System provides weekly provisional information on communicable-disease occurrence defined as notifiable by the Council of State and Territorial Epidemiologists (CSTE), with input from the Centers for Disease Control and Prevention (CDC).[19] The CSTE considers diseases notifiable if regular, frequent, and timely information regarding individual cases is necessary for the prevention and control of the disease.[28] As of January 1997, the CSTE and CDC designated 52 infectious diseases as notifiable at the national level (see Exhibit 2–2).

The CSTE and CDC periodically revise the list, depending on the public health impact of existing or new diseases. For example, they may add a disease to the list when a new pathogen emerges or may remove a disease when its incidence declines. The data come from voluntary reports from states and territories to the CDC. Because reporting is voluntary, the data set is not complete. All states generally report the internationally quarantinable diseases, such as cholera, plague, and yellow fever, in accordance with World Health Organization regulations. Data are available down to the state level, so they are not useful for community analysis. The system provides summary data annually.

Limitations of Disease Surveillance Data

Although local, state, and national communicable-disease data are helpful in analyzing disease burdens and trends, they underestimate the true incidence of disease. Patients with a severe clinical illness, such as rabies or plague, are more likely to see physicians, and physicians are more likely to recognize and report such severe disease. On the other hand, patients with clinically mild communicable diseases, such as salmonella, may not ever visit physicians or other health care providers. If they do visit physicians, the physicians may not recognize the disease as reportable, and even if they do, they may fail to report the disease. In addition, the availability of diagnostic resources, such as good laboratories, whether control measures are in effect (with concomitant public awareness of the disease), and the priorities of state and local public health officials responsible for disease surveil-

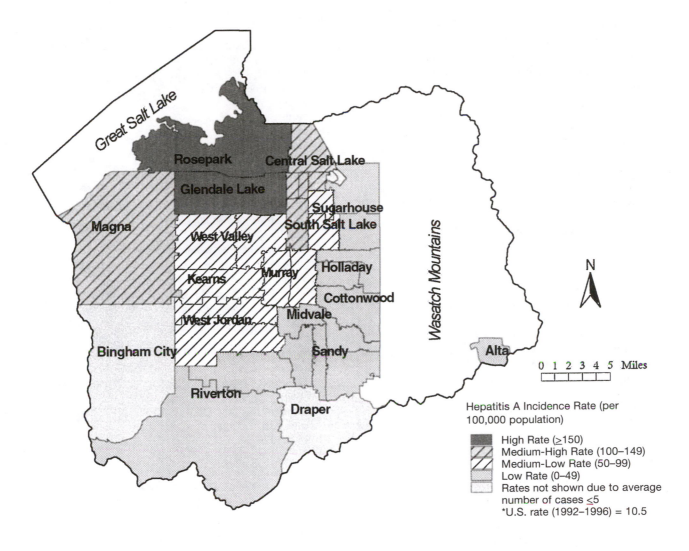

Figure 2–9 Incidence rates of hepatitis A by ZIP code area, Salt Lake County, Utah, 1992–1996

lance can further influence the likelihood that physicians will diagnose and report disease. Still other factors that can influence disease reporting up or down (independent of disease prevalence) include changes in case definitions, the introduction of new diagnostic tests, and the emergence of new diseases.

Communicable-Disease Prevention: Immunization Rates

Many states have established immunization registries to improve immunization rates of pre–school-aged children, especially children under two years of age. In these states, statutes require health care providers to report immuniza-

tions that they provide to young children. The reports usually include name, demographic information, and residence address. If street address data are included in the data set, public health practitioners can use GIS to study and report immunization rates for two-year-old children at the community level.[19] This information is extremely useful for targeting immunization outreach efforts.

Disease Incidence and Prevalence, Chronic Disease, and Risk Factors

Several other national data sets contain information on disease prevalence. The National Health Interview Survey

Exhibit 2–2 Nationally Notifiable Infectious Diseases, United States, 2000

Acquired immunodeficiency syndrome (AIDS)
Anthrax
Botulism
Brucellosis
Chancroid
Chlamydia trachomatis, genital infections
Cholera
Coccidiomycosis
Cryptosporidiosis
Cyclosporiasis
Diphtheria
Ehrlichiosis, human granulocytic
Ehrlichiosis, human monocytic
Encephalitis, California serogroup viral
Encephalitis, Eastern equine
Encephalitis, St. Louis
Encephalitis, Western equine
Escherichia coli O157:H7
Gonorrhea
Haemophilus influenzae, invasive disease
Hansen disease (leprosy)
Hantavirus pulmonary syndrome
Hemolytic uremic syndrome, postdiarrheal
Hepatitis A
Hepatitis B
Hepatitis C,/non-A, non-B
HIV infection, adult (≥ 13 years)
HIV infection, pediatric (< 13 years)
Listeriosis
Lyme disease
Malaria

Measles
Meningococcal disease
Mumps
Pertussis
Plague
Poliomyelitis, paralytic
Psittacosis
Q fever
Rabies, animal
Rabies, human
Rocky Mountain spotted fever
Rubella
Rubella, congenital syndrome
Salmonellosis
Shigellosis
Streptococcal disease, invasive, Group A
Streptococcus pneumoniae, drug resistant
Streptococcal toxic-shock syndrome
Syphilis
Syphilis, congenital
Tetanus
Toxic-shock syndrome
Trichinosis
Tuberculosis
Tularemia
Typhoid fever
Varicella (deaths only)

Note: Although varicella (chickenpox) is not a nationally notifiable disease, CSTE recommends reporting of cases of it via the National Notifiable Diseases Surveillance System (NNDSS).

(NHIS) collects data from household interviews on a continuous basis.[19] This information includes demographic characteristics, illnesses and injuries, disabilities, and health care utilization. The response rate has varied between 95 and 98 percent. Because it does not contain street addresses, this database is not useful for analysis of disease prevalence at the community level.

Another national data set includes the series of surveys performed by the National Center for Health Statistics (NCHS). The NCHS designed these surveys, the National Health and Nutrition Examination Surveys (NHANES), to estimate the prevalence of selected diseases and risk factors and to investigate reasons for trends in these diseases and risk factors. The surveys also contain information on the population distributions of several health measures.[19]

The purpose of the first survey, NHANES I, conducted in 1971–1974, was to measure the nutritional and health status of the U.S. public. The study population was civilian, noninstitutionalized persons between the ages of 1 and 74 who were living in the coterminous United States. The survey did not include Native Americans living on reservations. Measures included dietary intake, biochemical tests, physical measurements, and clinical assessments for nutritional deficiency.

NHANES II, conducted in 1976–1980, expanded the nutrition component. In this survey, the medical components included diabetes, kidney and liver function, allergy, and speech pathology. NHANES II expanded the target population to an age range of 6 months to 74 years and included persons living in Alaska and Hawaii. It also oversampled several populations, including children between 6 months and 5 years, persons between 60 and 74 years, and persons living in poverty. NHANES III, conducted in 1988–1994, added infants between 2 months and 6 months of age to the target population. This survey oversampled slightly different populations, including children 2 to 35 months of age, persons older than 69 years, African Americans, and Hispanic Americans.[19] Like the NHIS, the NHANES data do not contain a street address and are not useful for analysis at the community level.

Disease Incidence and Prevalence: Cancer

Depending on the location, cancer data are available at national and possibly local levels. On a national level, the Division of Cancer Prevention and Control of the National Cancer Institute conducts the Surveillance, Epidemiology and End Results Program (SEER). Five state cancer registries (Connecticut, Hawaii, Iowa, New Mexico, Utah) and six metropolitan areas (Atlanta, Detroit, Los Angeles, San Francisco/Oakland, San Jose/Monterey, Seattle) provide cancer registry data to the SEER program. This sample covers 14 percent of the U.S. population. Within this sample, SEER monitors persons recently diagnosed with cancer and includes follow-up data on persons previously diagnosed with cancer.[19] The data set has counts and rates of incident (new) cases of cancer by age (18 ranges), race (white/black/other/unknown), gender, year, state and county of residence, and ICD code. To determine incidence, SEER uses denominator data available from the U.S. Bureau of the Census. Using the sample, the program estimates county cancer rates for the entire United States. SEER data are not useful for analyzing cancer data at the subcounty, local level.

During the 1990s, to enhance the existing SEER registries and increase sample size beyond 14 percent of the population, the CDC began developing a National Program of Cancer Registries (NPCR). Congress authorized this work through Public Law 102–515, the Cancer Registries Amendment Act.[19] Eventually, the NPCR will collect cancer incidence data on 93 percent of the U.S. population, including first course of treatment and stage of diagnosis.[19] Many states already have cancer registries. In these states, cancer cases, including detailed information about the cancer and cancer treatment, are reportable by state law. These state registries include demographic and residence address data. In these states, public health practitioners using GIS can study cancer at the community level.[21]

Additional Limitations of Morbidity Data

Most morbidity data include information on race and ethnicity. This information can be quite helpful in identifying risk factors for further investigation and in identifying populations to target for disease prevention and health promotion efforts. For several reasons, however, conclusions drawn from these data can be inaccurate. First, different ethnic populations may have different degrees of access to health care. Some populations may have difficulty obtaining health care, and if they do, they may not have the same access to diagnostic tests as other populations. This can lead to underestimation of disease prevalence in these populations. Second, different programs collect data on race and ethnicity in different ways, making comparisons difficult. For example, the SEER data set contains information on race (white, black, other, and unknown) but not on ethnicity, while the National Center for HIV, STD, and TB Prevention (NCHSTP) data set collects information on race and ethnicity together as a single variable (American Indian/Alaska Native, Asian/Pacific Islander, Black non-Hispanic, White non-Hispanic, or Hispanic). Finally, race and ethnicity are based on self-reports, leading to additional inaccuracies.

HEALTH RESOURCES AND EXPENDITURES

Access to Primary Care and Hospitals

To develop comprehensive community health improvement plans, public health practitioners must address the degree of access to health care for vulnerable populations in their communities. One aspect of access is the physical accessibility of health care resources within a community. Practitioners can use GIS to map the location of hospitals, clinics, dentists, drugstores, and child care facilities, especially in relation to public transportation routes. Several sources of these data are available, including traditional business phone books or CD-ROM telephone books.[19] State hospital associations and state medical associations may have data on hospital and physician street location (by specialty) respectively. Some state agencies, such as the Oregon Office of Health Plan Policy and Research, have estimates of uninsured populations by county.

On a national level, the Health Resources Services Administration (HRSA) provides an updated electronic Area Resource File containing county-level health care resource information. The data include health professions, health facilities, utilization, expenditures, and population.[19] Within HRSA, the Bureau of Health Professions (BHPr) has developed a model to forecast the supply of physicians by specialty and activity. BHPr uses the American Medical Association (AMA) Physician Masterfile in developing this model. On the basis of this model, HRSA publishes a report on physician supply projections by regional areas of the United States. This information is not useful for physician supply projections at the community level.

The BHPr has also developed a model helpful in projecting nursing supply. The model estimates the number of nurses currently licensed to practice and the supply of full- and part-time practicing nurses. Data sources include the National League for Nursing, the National Council of State Boards of Nursing, and the National Sample Survey of Registered Nurses. The model can stratify nurse supply by educational level, including the numbers of nurses with associate degrees, diplomas, baccalaureate degrees, master's degrees, and doctorates.[19] On the basis of this model, HRSA publishes Nurse Supply Estimates by regional areas of the United States. Although these regional data are not helpful at the community level, public health practitioners may find that nursing boards and nursing associations within their state have data on nurse supply based on residence or employment location.

The NCHS publishes the National Health Provider Inventory (National Master Facility Inventory) containing a comprehensive file of inpatient health facilities by large regions of the United States. The inventory categorizes facilities as hospitals; nursing and related care facilities; and other custodial or remedial care facilities. Hospitals included in the database must have at least six inpatient beds; other facilities must have at least three inpatient beds. Reports from state licensing and other agencies on all newly established facilities, a yearly survey of hospitals, and a periodic survey of other facilities keep the inventory current.[19] As a regional inventory, the data file is not useful for community-level resource assessment. However, the same state agencies that report to the NCHS may have local data available for public health practitioner use.

Another NCHS survey, the annual National Home and Hospice Care Survey, begun in 1992, provides data on home health agencies and hospices. Like the National Health Provider Inventory, this survey aggregates data by large regional areas of the United States, making it less useful for community assessments. The survey includes information on the type of care that patients receive, based on a sample of current and discharged patients.[19]

Recently, HRSA has begun working with state and academic partners to develop data on state and national health care and public health workforces.[19] Such workforce data sets, especially if they include residence and work address location, will be useful for state and local health departments in health resource planning.

Health Care Expenditures

In attempting to control the rapidly accelerating cost of health care, it would be helpful to have data on health care expenditures at the local level. Unfortunately, with few exceptions, such local-level data are not yet available. However, public health practitioners can obtain several reports estimating national and state-level health care expenditures. At the national level, the Health Care Financing Administration (HCFA) reports annually estimates of health expenditures by type of expenditure and source of funds. In its report on Estimates of National Health Expenditures, HCFA uses the American Hospital Association (AHA) data on hospital finances as the primary source for estimating expenditures related to hospital care. This information includes expenditures in hospital outpatient clinics and hospital-based home health agencies, the cost of nursing care in hospitals, and the salaries of hospital staff physicians and dentists.[18] HCFA estimates health care expenses outside the hospital, such as home health care and services provided by various health professionals. To do this, HCFA uses data provided by the U.S. Bureau of the Census's Service Annual Survey and the quinquennial census of service industries.[19] Industry data on prescription drug purchases are the source for HCFA estimates of retail drug expenditures. HCFA uses a variety of data sources for other estimates in its report.

In addition to national health expenditures, HCFA uses the same data sources to compile its Estimates of State Health Expenditures. Some health expenditure data are available on a county basis. For example, local health departments providing Women, Infants and Children (WIC) Program nutritional services can report number of clients and expenditures for these services at the county level. In addition to expenditures, state Medicaid agencies have demographic and address data on their recipients. These data can be useful in mapping Medicaid expenditures at the community level.

OTHER HEALTH-RELATED DATA SOURCES USEFUL IN COMMUNITY HEALTH PLANNING

Many other available data sets (see Table 2–4) are helpful in assessing community health. We will list several of them, including occupational health and safety, chemical dependency, mental health, and behavioral risk factors. Public health practitioners should check with the local and state partners, especially state public health agencies, to get a list of other health-related data available for their community.

Injuries, Including Occupational Health and Safety

Local medical examiners have information on preventable work-related fatalities, such as electrocutions, fatal falls at construction sites, deaths in confined spaces, and explosions. In addition to occupational injury data, local medical examiners may have data on motor vehicle crashes, including site and type of roadway.[9] Other sources of data on vehicle crashes and passenger and pedestrian injuries include local and state

Table 2–4 Data for GIS-Based Community Health Planning: Occupational Health and Safety, Substance Abuse, Mental Health/Mental Retardation, Behavioral Risk Factors, and Lifestyle Marketing Data

Category	Source	Data Set Name	Smallest Geographic Unit
Occupational health and safety	National Institute for Occupational Safety and Health Bureau of Labor Statistics	National Traumatic Occupational Fatalities Surveillance System	State
Substance abuse (e.g., drug-related deaths and emergency room visits, alcohol-related deaths and accidents)	Substance Abuse and Mental Health Services Administration	National Household Surveys on Drug Abuse	Four U.S. regions
		Drug Abuse Warning Network	Metropolitan areas
Mental health/mental retardation (e.g., teenage suicides, serious mental retardation in school-age children)	Substance Abuse and Mental Health Services Administration	Monitoring the Future Survey of Mental Health Organizations	National
Behavioral risk factors (e.g., current smokers, sedentary lifestyle, not using seat belt)	Centers for Disease Control and Prevention	Behavioral Risk Factor Survey	State
Lifestyle marketing data	Commercial sources (e.g., CACI International or Claritas)	Neighborhood or lifestyle segmentation	Census tract

police departments, local and state transportation departments, and Emergency Medical Services agencies.[9] The data generally include location of event, allowing local health departments to map these unintentional injuries at the local level. Some states have injury registries, including data on type of injury and location of occurrence and demographic information on the injured person.

The Fatal Accident Reporting System (FARS) gathers data on the most severe traffic crashes that occur each year and result in fatalities. Operational since 1975, FARS contains data on a census of fatal traffic crashes within the 50 states, the District of Columbia, and Puerto Rico. To be included in FARS, a crash must meet two criteria. It must involve a motor vehicle traveling on a traffic-way customarily open to the public, and it must result in the death of a person (occupant of a vehicle or a nonmotorist) within 30 days of the crash. The National Center for Statistics and Analysis (NCSA) conceived, designed, and developed the FARS system to provide an overall measure of highway safety and to help identify traffic safety problems. NCSA also developed FARS to suggest solutions to these problems and to help provide an objective basis on which to evaluate the effectiveness of motor vehicle safety standards and highway safety programs.

As part of the National Traumatic Occupational Fatalities Surveillance Program, the National Institute for Occupational Safety and Health (NIOSH) compiles information on occupational trauma deaths as reported by states on death certificates. NIOSH makes these data available at the state level, so they are not useful in a local analysis. NIOSH selects cases on the basis of several criteria, including age 16 years or older, an external cause of death, and a positive response to the "injury of work" field on the death certificate.[19] The NIOSH mortality data set has counts and rates of death for underlying cause of death based on any of the 92 standard groups of causes. Users can sort these by a single variable such as age (15 ranges); race (white/black/other/ nonwhites); gender; year; state and county of residence; or group of causes. To improve data accuracy, NIOSH has developed guidelines for completion of this item on the death certificate. To calculate rates for the civilian U.S. workforce, the surveillance program uses denominator data from the U.S. Bureau of the Census's County Business Patterns. This data set is supplemented with agriculture employment data supplied from the Census of Agriculture (also from the Bureau of the Census) and public administration data from the Bureau of Labor Statistics' annual average employment data.[19]

Substance Abuse

Tobacco use, the leading actual cause of death, kills over 400,000 persons each year in the United States.[29] Alcoholism, ranking third, kills over 100,000, while illicit drug use ranks ninth and kills over 20,000 each year.[29] Clearly, data on substance abuse are essential for community health assessment and planning.

Since 1971, the Substance Abuse and Mental Health Services Administration (SAMHSA) has conducted the National Household Survey on Drug Abuse. This survey has collected data on trends in the use of marijuana, tobacco, alcohol, and cocaine by persons 12 years of age and older.[19] The survey oversamples younger people (aged 12 to 34), African Americans, Hispanic Americans, and individuals in six selected large metropolitan areas. Because SAMHSA provides the data aggregated by four national regions, the data are not useful for community-level analysis. Some states conduct their own household surveys and may have some data available for local use. Public health practitioners interested in mapping these data should check with their state offices for alcohol and drug abuse programs regarding availability of state and local household drug use data.

The Drug Abuse Warning Network (DAWN), developed in 1978 and revised in 1988, is a large-scale drug abuse data system based on information collected from emergency rooms and medical examiners.[19] DAWN reports these data for metropolitan areas. Information in the system includes drug abuse events resulting in medical emergencies or fatalities. The system has several objectives, including studying drug abuse patterns, identifying trends, identifying substances used, and assessing health outcomes associated with drug abuse.[19]

Another national data source, the Monitoring the Future Study (High School Senior Survey), begun by the National Institutes of Health (NIH) in 1975, is a large-scale annual survey of drug use and attitudes related to drug use. The survey relies on data collected using questionnaires given out in classrooms. In 1991, the survey added eighth- and tenth-grade students.[19] Because data are available at the national level, survey results are not useful for local analysis. As with the household survey, however, some states may perform their own high school drug use surveys and may provide this information at a local level. To see if such data are available, potential data users should check with state agencies on alcohol and drug abuse programs.

Mental Health

Biennially, SAMHSA conducts the Survey of Mental Health Organizations, an inventory of outpatient mental health providers and general hospital mental health services. This survey contains information on patients receiving services provided by these agencies, including demographic, clinical, and treatment characteristics.[19] Because the survey aggregates data into four large regions, the data are not available for local community health assessments. State mental health and Medicaid agencies, however, may have mental health patient diagnostic and utilization data useful for local analysis.

Behavioral Risk Factors

Many important causes of morbidity and mortality, such as cancer and cardiovascular disease, have behavioral risk factors, making these diseases eminently preventable. A 1982 report by the Institute of Medicine estimated that changes in individual behaviors could cause a 50 percent reduction in premature mortality. Local data on risk behavior could help target interventions directed at reducing these risks.

In a partnership between state health departments and the CDC, each state participates in the Behavioral Risk Factor Surveillance System (BRFSS). Each state performs a telephone survey of a state sample of residents, using questions that are uniform across states. Questions include behaviors such as tobacco use, physical activity, and diet. Additional questions about health insurance are helpful in estimating the population without insurance. Although summary data are available at the state level, states and localities can increase the sample size (and add locally relevant questions), allowing for local-level analysis.

States also participate in the Youth Risk Behavior Survey (YRBS). The YRBS, conducted every two years, is a survey of students in grades 9 through 12. In 1997, 39 states, 16 large cities, and 4 territories participated. The average sample size was 2,200. The survey contains questions about many behaviors, including behaviors related to injuries, such as bicycle helmet use; nutrition; sexual behaviors; violence, including weapon carrying; and chemical dependency, such as tobacco, alcohol, and illicit drug use. Survey data are available to each school participating in the survey. State and local departments of education and health can add or delete questions in the core questionnaire to better meet the interests and needs of the state or local school district. Local health departments, through partnerships with their school districts, can use these data to analyze youth risk behavior at the community (high school attendance area) level.

OTHER DATA WITH PUBLIC HEALTH IMPLICATIONS

Some data sets not traditionally considered health related have public health implications and may be useful in GIS applications. For example, at least one state, Oregon, has established juvenile arrest rates as a measure of community well-being.[21] Local law enforcement agencies have arrest data containing information on age, gender, and residence of those arrested and additional information on site and type of alleged crime. With census data as a denominator, GIS can calculate incidence rates for arrests.[21] Other nontraditional data of special interest could include high school dropouts, location of licensed alcohol retail outlets, commuting time, and domestic abuse, including elder, child, and spousal abuse.[21]

ENVIRONMENTAL DATA

The public is more concerned than ever about the risk from exposure to environmental hazards. Although data have been insufficient to quantify fully the relationship between environmental exposure and health outcomes, most epidemiologists believe that exposures to some environmental contaminants are associated with many chronic diseases. Such diseases include cancer, reproductive abnormalities, chronic neurodevelopmental disorders, and dysfunction of the immune and endocrine systems.[3] In the United States, environmental monitoring programs generate large volumes of data (Table 2–5).[3] Unfortunately, the lack of an integrated framework to manage, manipulate, analyze, and present the data has resulted in poor utilization of our environmental data sets. The 1986 Chernobyl accident, resulting in deposition of radioactivity over large areas of northern Europe, highlighted the inadequacies of older tools for handling, manipulating, and analyzing environmental health data.[3] GIS technology, designed to link, analyze, and display multiple data sets, such as morbidity, mortality, and environmental exposure, has the potential to provide the needed integration. We will fully describe the uses of GIS in environmental health in Chapter 4. Here, we will discuss sources of environmental data.

The U.S. Environmental Protection Agency (EPA) maintains many environmental data sets that are useful in geographic analysis and easy to download off the Internet at <www.epa.gov>.[19] We will discuss some of the more widely used and helpful data sets.

The *American Indian Lands Environmental Support Project (AILESP)* has data on air and water contaminant releases for facilities located on or near Native American lands. The data available for the tribal lands include compliance and enforcement histories for the facilities and other environmental data, such as stream reaches with fish consumption advisories, contaminated fish tissues, and contaminated sediments.[19]

The *Toxic Release Inventory (TRI)* is a major EPA database tabulating the releases of toxic chemicals into the environment. The TRI, an outgrowth of the Emergency Planning and Community Right To Know Act of 1986, was the first EPA database planned, designed, and operated for public access. TRI stores information self-reported annually from

Table 2–5 Data for GIS-Based Community Health Planning: Meteorological/Climatological Data and Environmental Hazards

Category	Source	Data Set Name	Smallest Geographic Unit
Meteorological/climatological data	National Climatic Data Center		Local areas
Environmental hazards (e.g., locations of toxic waste sites)	U.S. Environmental Protection Agency	Envirofacts Data Warehouse EPA Spatial Data Library System Better Assessment Science Integrating Point and Non-Point Sources American Indian Lands Environmental Support Project	Local
	Agency for Toxic Substances and Disease Registry	HazDat Environmental exposure registries for selected chemicals (e.g., benzene, trichloroethylene, and dioxin)	Local site specific Registry coverage area

manufacturing industries on the basis of specific industrial classification codes. Facilities are required to report if they manufactured or processed more than 25,000 pounds of a listed chemical during the year, or otherwise used more than 10,000 pounds, and if they have the equivalent of more than 10 full-time employees. Industries must report the on-site releases of toxic chemicals into the air, water, and land and the quantities of these chemicals treated, combusted for energy, and recycled on site. They must also report transfers of wastes that are disposed, treated, combusted for energy recovery, or recycled at a separate facility. The EPA has designated approximately 650 chemicals for reports under TRI. Legislation, including the Clean Air Act, the Clean Water Act, the Safe Drinking Water Act, the Federal Insecticide, Fungicide, and Rodenticide Act, and the Resource Conservation and Recovery Act, has identified many of these chemicals as a public health concern. To get an idea of the size of the database, in 1996, approximately 21,000 manufacturing facilities and 200 federal facilities submitted about 73,000 reports. The TRI database contains information about the location of facilities, including address, EPA region, state, county, ZIP code, and latitude/longitude, allowing for analysis at the local level.

The TRI, the first attempt to quantify toxic chemical pollution, has several limitations. TRI receives reports from only the largest chemical manufacturers, although small polluters, such as dry cleaners and mobile sources, such as cars, contribute substantially to environmental pollution. In addition, reports are most often only estimates of the pollution, since the EPA requires actual monitored data only if they are available. Since the reporting is annual, the report cannot account for changing levels of toxic releases. For example, the total release could have occurred all in one day, or it could have occurred evenly throughout the year. The TRI database, measuring emissions in total pounds, does not account for the relative human toxicity of different toxins. Finally, the EPA has collected TRI data only since 1987, limiting studies for environmentally related illnesses with long latencies. Some of the reporting thresholds, such as release levels, changed during the first two years of the program, from 75,000 pounds in 1987 to 50,000 pounds in 1988 and to 25,000 pounds for 1989 and thereafter. Some of the chemicals of interest currently on the list were not on the list in earlier years. For example, the list of chemicals has grown from 351 in 1987 to 643 in 1996.

The *Aerometric Information Retrieval System (AIRS)* is an EPA database containing information about certain types of air pollutants in the United States. The Air Quality Subsystem (AQS) of AIRS contains measurements of ambient concentrations of pollutants meeting EPA criteria, including carbon monoxide, nitrogen dioxide, ozone, lead, particulate matter, and sulfur dioxide. In addition, AQS contains data on other ambient pollutants, including volatile organic compounds (VOCs) and meteorological data. Thousands of monitoring stations across the United States, operated by the EPA and other federal, state, and local agencies, collect the data. The database contains monitoring site descriptions, including location, raw and summary data, and information on data precision and accuracy (metadata). Data analysis and reporting are possible at the national, regional, state, county, and city levels. Figure 2–10 is an example of a county-level analysis of nitrogen dioxide air pollution.[30]

Limitations of the AIRS-AQS database include its focus only on EPA-criteria pollutants, even though many other chemicals contribute to air quality and health. The number of monitors varies from one area to another, making comparisons difficult. While data are available for years as early as 1957, consistent data have been available only since 1979 because uniform monitoring siting or quality assurance procedures were not available earlier.

The *Safe Drinking Water Information System/Federal Version (SDWIS)* is an EPA national database containing information about the nation's drinking water. For 1996, the most recent year for which annual figures are available, the database included over 172,000 public water systems (PWSs) serving over 90 percent of the U.S. population. PWSs required to report water quality data are those that provide piped water for human consumption to at least 15 service connections or serve an average of at least 25 people for at least 60 days. These facilities must report data on monitored contaminant levels for EPA-regulated contaminants and other contaminants. The 1974 Safe Drinking Water Act, and its 1986 and 1996 amendments, determined the requirements for reporting drinking-water contamination levels. These contaminants include microbiological contaminants, radionuclides, inorganic chemicals, and organic chemicals. Local analysis is possible because spatial information in the database includes PWS address and latitude/longitude. By 2004, reporting rules will require all PWSs to add latitude and longitude information for their water intake source.

Underreporting is a significant limitation of the SDWIS, leading to uneven data. States and regions are responsible for data collection. There are differences among the states in the emphasis they place on data collection efforts and responsiveness to notifications of data errors. Because EPA requires states only to report violations, EPA can know the extent of underreporting only by auditing state records. In addition, the Safe Drinking Water Act allows for modifications in monitoring programs, limiting the comparability of data over time and across public water systems.

Enacted in 1980, the Comprehensive Environmental Response, Compensation and Liability Act (CERCLA) created the EPA Superfund Program. Amended by the 1986 Superfund Amendments and Reauthorization ACT (SARA), the Superfund Program has broad authority to respond to uncontrolled releases of hazardous substances from inactive

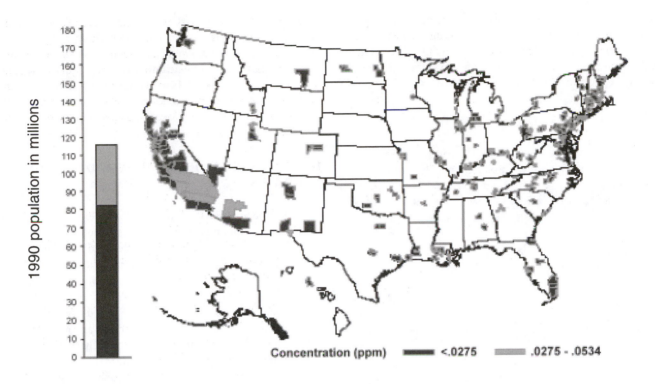

Figure 2–10 Highest NO_2 annual mean concentration by county, 1997

hazardous waste sites that endanger public health. In support of CERCLA, the *Comprehensive Environmental Response, Compensation and Liability Information System (CERCLIS)* is the official repository for all site- and non–site-specific Superfund data. CERCLIS contains information on hazardous waste sites, site inspections, preliminary assessments, and remedial status from 1983 to the present. As of May 1999, the database contained records for 10,625 active sites, with specific information for each site. Descriptions for each site contain name, remedial actions planned, including start and completion dates, costs, principal contaminant(s), and remedies. Additional information includes risk assessment, remedy selection, cleanup actions, community involvement, and removal action at a site. Local analysis is possible because spatial variables in the data set include region, state, city, ZIP code, street name, county, congressional district, metropolitan area, and latitude and longitude. Due to proprietary and enforcement reasons, EPA does not publish some of the Superfund data. Available data are limited to a subset of the comprehensive data that the EPA collects and maintains.

The Agency for Toxic Substance and Disease Registry (ATSDR) developed *HazDat, the Hazardous Substance Release/Health Effects Database.* The purpose of HazDat is to provide access to (1) information on the release of hazardous substances from Superfund sites or from emergency events and (2) information on the effects of hazardous substances on human health. HazDat contains information on the site, including site characteristics, activities, and site events. It also contains information on contaminants found at the site, including contaminant media and maximum concentration levels. HazDat health effect data include impact on population, community health concerns, ATSDR public health threat categorization, ATSDR recommendations, the environmental fate of hazardous substances, exposure routes, and physical hazards at the site/event. In addition, HazDat contains substance-specific information such as the ATSDR Priority List of Hazardous Substances, health effects by route and duration of exposure, metabolites, interactions of substances, susceptible populations, and biomarkers of exposures and effects. HazDat also contains data from the EPA CERCLIS database, including site number, site description, latitude/longitude, and additional site information.

Some states, industrial facilities, the National Institute for Occupational Safety and Health (NIOSH), and the military have developed registries for occupational chemical exposures.[19] This information is useful for studying health outcomes for persons exposed to relatively high level of chemicals. At the community level, local health departments have data on a variety of environmental issues, including restaurant inspection results and drinking-water quality. Local GIS studies of environmental exposures can also gather their own data, such as nitrate levels or VOCs in wells.[31,32]

METEOROLOGICAL DATA

Meteorological data are especially useful for geographic analyses involving releases of toxic chemicals into the air. For example, by incorporating data on local and regional wind conditions, GIS can help estimate potential human exposure downwind from industrial lead emitters[33] or nuclear power plant radioactivity releases, such as the 1986 Chernobyl accident.[3] The National Climatic Data Center (NCDC), the largest and most diverse environmental data center in the world, contains more than 90 percent of the National Oceanic and Atmospheric Administration (NOAA) data. The NCDC inventory includes meteorological and climatological information, environmental satellite data, and NEXRAD weather data and contains the history of U.S. meteorological observations since the 1700s. Data elements include temperature, dew point, relative humidity, precipitation, snowfall, snow depth on ground, wind speed, wind direction, cloudiness, visibility, atmospheric pressure, evaporation, soil temperatures, and various types of weather occurrences such as hail, fog, thunder, and glaze. The weather observations are normally hourly observations but may be more frequent, and there are daily and monthly summaries. Data are available down to the local level in digital and nondigital form. Digital holdings available contain nearly 300 terabytes of information and increase by over 80 terabytes each year.

ADDING LOCATION INFORMATION TO ATTRIBUTE DATA: GLOBAL POSITIONING SYSTEM

Sometimes, especially in studies of environmental risk factors, investigators need to add a geographic reference to their attribute data sets. For example, information on locations of mosquito habitats is essential for malaria control programs. With input from the global positioning system (GPS), GIS technology can map mosquito populations and other important factors.[15] The GPS relies on information relayed by 24 satellites, orbiting at 20,000 km above the Earth. Hand-held ground instruments, receiving signals from these satellites, can precisely calculate their own location with a high degree of accuracy. Investigators in the field can use these devices to identify the location of specific events and risk factors and can incorporate these data into their GIS for mapping.

DATA VERIFICATION: METADATA (DATA ABOUT DATA)

Useful, accurate GIS output is dependent on useful input.[10] Responsible data users must have details about their data. This is true for both spatial and attribute data. Such data about data, commonly termed *metadata*, includes the data's source, quality, timeliness, and reliability.[9,10] Although the Federal Geographic Data Committee (FGDC) has developed metadata guidelines and has required documentation of the quality of data produced by federal agencies, technical documentation is scant for commercially available data. For example, documentation may be lacking on the methodology a vendor uses to derive population estimates.[9]

Exhibit 2–3 is an example of metadata for a spatial database, the TIGER database. Metadata about TIGER includes the data source (U.S. Bureau of the Census), a description of the database, and its purpose. In addition, the TIGER metadata contains information on accuracy and specific features within the database, such as point, vector, line, and polygon information. For GIS users with questions about the TIGER database, the metadata contains contact information at the Bureau of the Census, including a street address, phone number, and e-mail address.

Exhibit 2–4 is a metadata example for an attribute database, the Oregon Birth file. Like the TIGER metadata, the Oregon Birth metadata contain contact information, in this case including the name of the person who maintains the database. Again, the metadata include a description of the database and its purpose and information about the limitations of the data.

Once the spatial and attribute data sets are acquired and stored, and if the attribute data include a geographical reference, such as an address, the mapmaking process can begin.[12] The next chapter will discuss how GIS use spatial and attribute data to make useful maps

Exhibit 2–3 TIGER Metadata

Identification_Information:
  Citation:
    Citation_Information:
      Originator:
        U.S. Department of Commerce
        Bureau of the Census
        Geography Division
      Publication_Date: 1999
      Title: TIGER/Line Files, 1998
      Edition: 1998
      Series_Information:
        Series_Name: TIGER/Line Files
        Issue_Identification: Version (MMYY) represents the
        month and year file created
    Publication_Information:
      Publication_Place: Washington, DC
      Publisher:
        U.S. Department of Commerce
        Bureau of the Census
        Geography Division
Description:
  Abstract:
    TIGER, TIGER/Line, and Census TIGER are registered trademarks of the Bureau of the Census. The 1998 TIGER/Line files are an extract of selected geographic and cartographic information from the Census TIGER database. The geographic coverage for a single TIGER/Line file is a county or statistical equivalent entity, with the coverage area based on January 1, 1998 legal boundaries. A complete set of 1998 TIGER/Line files includes all counties and statistically equivalent entities in the United States, the U.S. Virgin Islands, Puerto Rico, American Samoa, Guam, the Northern Mariana Islands, U.S. Minor Outlying Areas, and the Pacific Island Areas. The Census TIGER database represents a seamless national file with no overlaps or gaps between parts. However, each county-based TIGER/Line file is designed to stand alone as an independent data set or the files can be combined to cover the whole Nation and its territories. The 1998 TIGER/Line files consist of line segments representing physical features and governmental and statistical boundaries. The files contain information distributed over a series of record types for the spatial objects of a county. There are 17 record types, including the basic record, the shape coordinate points, and geographic codes that can be used with appropriate software to prepare maps. Other geographic information contained in the files includes attributes such as feature identifiers/census feature class codes (CFCC) used to differentiate feature types, address ranges and ZIP codes, codes for legal and statistical entities, latitude/longitude coordinates of linear and point features, landmark point features, area landmarks, key geographic features, and area boundaries. The 1998 TIGER/Line data dictionary contains a complete list of all the fields in the 17 record types.
Purpose:
  In order for others to use the information in the Census TIGER data base in a geographic information system (GIS) or for other geographic applications, the Census Bureau releases to the public extracts of the data base in the form of TIGER/Line files. Various versions of the TIGER/Line files have been released; previous versions include the 1990 Census TIGER/Line files, the 1992 TIGER/Line files, the 1994 TIGER/Line files, the 1995 TIGER/Line files, and the 1997 TIGER/Line files. The 1998 TIGER/Line files were originally produced for use by the states participating in the Census 2000 Redistricting Data Program, Phase 2, the Voting District Project (VTDP) to submit their voting districts to the Census Bureau.
Supplemental_Information:
  To find out more about TIGER/Line files and other Census TIGER data base derived data sets visit http://www.census.gov/geo/www/tiger.
Time_Period_of_Content:
  Time_Period_Information:
    Single_Date/Time:
      Calendar_Date: 1998
  Currentness_Reference: 1998
Status:
  Progress: Complete
  Maintenance_and_Update_Frequency:
    TIGER/Line files are extracted from the Census TIGER data base when needed for geographic programs required to support the census and survey programs of the Census Bureau. No changes or updates will be made to the 1998 TIGER/Line files. Future releases of TIGER/Line files will reflect updates made to the Census TIGER data base and will be released under a version numbering system based on the month and year the data is extracted.
Spatial_Domain:
  Bounding_Coordinates:
    West_Bounding_Coordinate: +131.000000
    East_Bounding_Coordinate: –64.000000
    North_Bounding_Coordinate: +72.000000
    South_Bounding_Coordinate: –15.0000000
Keywords:
  Theme:
    Theme_Keyword_Thesaurus: None
    Theme_Keyword: Line Features
    Theme_Keyword: Feature Identifier
    Theme_Keyword: Census Feature Class Code (CFCC)

continues

Exhibit 2–3 continued

Theme_Keyword: Address Range
Theme_Keyword: Geographic Entity
Theme_Keyword: Point/Node
Theme_Keyword: Landmark Feature
Theme_Keyword: Political Boundary
Theme_Keyword: Statistical Boundary
Theme_Keyword: Polygon
Theme_Keyword: County/County Equivalent
Theme_Keyword: TIGER/Line
Theme_Keyword: Topology
Theme_Keyword: Street Centerline
Theme_Keyword: Latitude/Longitude

Theme_Keyword: ZIP code
Theme_Keyword: Vector
Theme_Keyword: TIGER/Line Identification Number (TLID)
Theme_Keyword: Street Segment
Theme_Keyword: Coordinate
Theme_Keyword: Boundary
Place:
　Place_Keyword_Thesaurus:
　　FIPS Publication 6–4
　　FIPS Publication 55
　Place_Keyword_United States
　Place_Keyword: U.S. Virgin Islands
　Place_Keyword: Puerto Rico
　Place_Keyword: Pacific Island Areas
　Place_Keyword: County
　Access_Constraints: None
Use_Constraints:
　None. Acknowledgment of the U.S. Bureau of the Census would be appreciated for products derived from these files. TIGER, TIGER/Line, and Census TIGER are registered trademarks of the Bureau of the Census.
Native_Data_Set_Environment:
　TIGER/Line files are created and processed in a VMS environment. The environment consists of two Alpha Server 8400s clustered together running OpenVMS version 62–1H3 used for production operations. The Census TIGER system is driven by DEC Command language (DCL) procedures which invoke C software routines to extract selected geographic and cartographic information (TIGER/Line files) from the operational Census TIGER data base.
Data_Quality_Information:
　Attribute_Accuracy:
　　Attribute_Accuracy_Report:
　　　Accurate against Federal Information Processing Standards (FIPS), FIPS Publication 6–4, and FIPS55 at the 100% level for the codes and base names. The remaining attribute information has been examined but has not been fully tested for accuracy.
　Logical_Consistency_Report:

The feature network of lines (as represented by Record Types 1 and 2) is complete for census purposes. Spatial objects in TIGER/Line belong to the "Geometry and topology" (GT) class of objects in the "Spatial Data Transfer Standard" (SDTS) FIPS Publication 173 and are topologically valid. Node/geometry and topology (GT)-polygon/chain relationships are collected or generated to satisfy topological edit requirements. These requirements include:
- Complete chains must begin and end at nodes.
- Complete chains must connect to each other at nodes.
- Complete chains do not extend through nodes.
- Left and right GT-polygons are defined for each complete chain element and are consistent throughout the extract process.
- The chains representing the limits of the files are free of gaps.

The Census Bureau performed automated tests to ensure logical consistency and limits of files. All polygons are tested for closure. The Census Bureau uses its internally developed Geographic Update System to enhance and modify spatial and attribute data in the Census TIGER data base. Standard geographic codes, such as FIPS codes for states, counties, municipalities, and places, are used when encoding spatial entities. The Census Bureau performed spatial data tests for logical consistency of the codes during the compilation of the original Census TIGER data base files. Most of the Codes themselves were provided to the Census Bureau by the USGS, the agency responsible for maintaining FIPS 55. Feature attribute information has been examined but has not been fully tested for consistency.
Completeness_Report:
　Data completeness of the TIGER/Line files reflects the contents of the Census TIGER data base at the time the TIGER/Line files (1998 version) were created.
Positional_Accuracy:
　Horizontal_Positional_Accuracy:
　　Horizontal_Positional_Accuracy_Report:
　　　The information present in these files is provided for the purposes of statistical analysis and census operations only. Coordinates in the TIGER/Line files have six implied decimal places, but the positional accuracy of the coordinates is not as great as the six decimal places suggest. The positional accuracy varies with the source materials used, but generally the information is no better than the established national map Accuracy standards for 1:100,000-scale maps from the U.S. Geological Survey (USGS); thus it is NOT suitable for high-precision measurement applications such as engineering problems, property transfers, or other uses that might require highly accurate measurements of the earth's surface. The USGS 1:100,000-scale maps met national map accuracy standards and use coordinates defined by the North Ameri-

continues

Exhibit 2–3 continued

can Datum, 1983. For the contiguous 48 States, the cartographic fidelity of most of the 1998 TIGER/Line files, in areas outside the 1980 census Geographic Base File/Dual Independent Map Encoding (GBF/ DIME) file coverage and selected other large metropolitan areas, compare favorable with the USGS 1:100,000-scale maps. The Census Bureau cannot specify the accuracy of features inside of what was the 1980 GBF/DIME-File coverage or selected metropolitan areas. The Census Bureau added updates to the TIGER/Line files that enumerators annotated on maps sheets prepared from the Census TIGER data base as they attempted to traverse every street feature shown on the 1990 census map sheets; the Bureau also made other corrections from updated map sheets supplied by local participants for Census Bureau programs. The locational accuracy of these updates is of unknown quality. In addition to the Federal, State, and local sources, portions of the files may contain information obtained in part from maps and other materials prepared by private companies. Despite the fact the TIGER/Line data positional accuracy is not as high as the coordinate values imply, the six-decimal place precision is useful when producing maps. The precision allows features that are next to each other on the ground to be placed in the correct position, on the map, relative to each other, without overlap.

Lineage:
  Source_Information:
    Source_Citation:
      Citation_Information:
        Originator:
          U.S. Department of Commerce
          Bureau of the Census
          Geography Division
        Publication_Date: Unpublished material
        Title: Census TIGER data base
        Edition: 1998
      Type_of_Source_Media: On line
      Source_Time_Period_of_Content:
        Time_Period_Information:
          Calendar_Date: 1998
        Source_Currentness_Reference:
          Date the file was made available to create TIGER/ Line
          File extracts:
    Source_Citation_Abbreviation: TIGER
    Source_Contribution:
      Selected geographic and cartographic information (line segments) from the Census TIGER data base.
  Process_Step:
    Process_Description:
      In order for others to use the information in the Census TIGER data base in a GIS or for other geographic

applications, the Census Bureau releases periodic extracts of selected information from the Census TIGER data base, organized as topologically consistent networks. Software (TIGER DB routines) written by the Geography Division allows for efficient access to Census TIGER system data. TIGER/Line files are extracted from the Census TIGER data base by county or statistical equivalent area. Census TIGER data for a given county or statistical equivalent area is then distributed among 17 fixed length record ASCII files, each one containing attributes for either line, polygon, or landmark geographic data types. The Bureau of the Census has released various versions of the TIGER/Line files since 1988, with each version having more updates (features and feature names, address ranges and ZIP codes, coordinate updates, revised field definitions, etc.) than the previous version.
    Source_Used_Citation_Abbreviation: Census TIGER data base
    Process_Date: 1999
Spatial_Data_Organization_Information:
  Indirect_Spatial_Reference:
    Federal Information Processing Standards (FIPS) and feature names and addresses.
  Direct_Spatial_Reference_Method: Vector
  Point_and_Vector_Object_Information:
    SDTS_Terms_Description:
      SDTS_Point_and_Vector_Object_Type: Node, network
      Point_and_Vector_Object_Count: 570 to 56,000
      SDTS_Point_and_Vector_Object_Type: Entity point
      SDTS_Point_and_Vector_Object_Type: Complete chain
      Point_and_Vector_Object_Count: 790 to 83,000
      SDTS_Point_and_Vector_Object_Type: GT-polygon composed of chains
      Point_and_Vector_Object_Count: 290 to 33,000
Spatial_Reference_Information:
  Horizontal_Coordinate_System_Definition:
    Geographic:
      Latitude_Resolution: 0.000458
      Longitude_Resolution: 0.000458
      Geographic_Coordinate_Units: Decimal degrees
Entity_and_Attribute_Information:
  Overview_Description:
  Entity_and_Attribute_Overview: The TIGER/Line files contain data describing three major types of features/entities; Line Features–
    1) Roads
    2) Railroads
    3) Hydrography
    4) Miscellaneous transportation features and selected power lines and pipe lines
    5) Political and statistical boundaries

continues

Exhibit 2–3 continued

Landmark Features–
1) Point landmarks, e.g., schools and churches.
2) Area landmarks, e.g., parks and cemeteries.
3) Key geographic locations (KGLs), e.g., apartment buildings and factories

Polygon features–
1) Geographic entity codes for areas used to tabulate the 1990 census statistical data and current geographic areas
2) Locations of area landmarks
3) Locations of KGLs

The line features and polygon information form the majority of data in the TIGER/Line files. Some of the data/ attributes describing the lines include coordinates, feature identifiers (names), CFCCs (used to identify the most noticeable characteristic of a feature), address ranges, and goegraphic entity codes. The TIGER/Line files contain point and area labels that describe landmark features and provide locational reference. Area landmarks consist of a feature name or label and feature type assigned to a polygon or group of polygons. Landmarks may overlap or refer to the same set of polygons.

The Census TIGER data base uses collections of spatial objects (points, lines, and polygons) to model or describe real-world geography. The Census Bureau uses these spatial objects to represent features such as streets, rivers, and political boundaries and assigns.

Entity_and_Attribute_Detail_Citation: U.S. Bureau of the Census, TIGER/Line files, 1997 Technical Documentation. The TIGER/Line documentation defines the terms and definitions used within the files.

Distribution_Information:
Distributor:
Contact_Information:
Contact_Organization_Primary:
Contact_Organization:
U.S. Department of Commerce
Bureau of the Census
Geography Division
Products and Services Staff
Contact_Address:
Address_Type: Physical address
Address: 8903 Presidential Parkway, WP 1
City: Upper Marlboro
State_or Province: Maryland
Postal_Code: 20772
Contact_Voice_Telephone: (301) 457-1128
Contact_Address:
Address_Type: Mailing address
Address: Bureau of the Census
City: Washington
State_or_Province: District of Columbia

Postal_Code: 20333-7400
Contact_Voice_Telephone: (301) 457-1128
Contact_Facsimile_Telephone: (301) 457-4710
Contact_Electronic_Mail_Address:
tiger@census.gov

Resource_Description: 1998 TIGER/Line Files
Distribution_Liability: No warranty, expressed or implied is made and no liability is assumed by the U.S. Government in general or the Bureau of the Census in specific as to the positional or attribute accuracy of the data. The act of distribution shall not constitute any such warranty and no responsibility is assumed by the U.S. Government in the use of these files.

Standard_Order_Process:
Digital_Form:
Digital_Transfer_Information:
Format_Name: TGRLN (compressed)
Format_Version_Number: 1998
Format_Version_Date: 1998
File_Decompression_Technique: PK-ZIP, version 1.93A or higher
Digital_Transfer_Option:
Offline_Option:
Offline_Media: CD-ROM
Recording_Format: ISO 9660

Fees: The TIGER/Line files are grouped by states or statistical equivalent ($490 for the complete seven-disc set or $70 per CD-ROM/disc). Technical documentation is included on disc or may be downloaded in PDF format over the Internet.

TIGER98: All States (7 CD-ROMs) CD-TGR98-ALL-KIT $490.

TIGER98: CD-TGR98-01 $70; Connecticut, Delaware, District of Columbia, Maine, Massachusetts, Maryland, New Hampshire, New Jersey, New York, Pennsylvania, Rhode Island, Virginia, Vermont, West Virginia, Puerto Rico, and U.S. Virgin Islands.

TIGER98: CD-TGR98-02 $70; Alabama, Florida, Georgia, Mississippi, North Carolina, and South Carolina.

TIGER98: CD-TGR98-03 $70; Illinois, Indiana, Kentucky, Michigan, Ohio, Tennessee, and Wisconsin.

TIGER98: CD-TGR98-04 $70; Iowa, Kansas, Minnesota, Missouri, North Dakota, Nebraska, and South Dakota.

TIGER98: CD-TGR98-05 $70; Arkansas, Louisiana, Oklahoma, and Texas.

TIGER98: CD-TGR98-06 $70; Arizona, Colorado, Idaho, Montana, New Mexico, Utah, and Wyoming.

TIGER98: CD-TGR98-07 $70; Alaska, California, Hawaii, Nevada, Oregon, Washington, and the Outlying Areas of the Pacific.

Ordering_Instructions:
To purchase 1998 TIGER/Line files; order from the U.S. Department of Commerce, Bureau of the Census, by calling

continues

Exhibit 2–3 continued

the Customer Services Center at (301) 457-4100; FAX (301) 457-3842. To obtain more information about ordering TIGER/Line files visit http://www.census.gov/geo/www/tiger.

Turnaround:

Priority Next Day Service; Telephone orders charged to a credit card (Mastercard or Visa) received by 2:00 PM of a business day using priority next day service (excluding Saturday and Sunday) will arrive the next business day. Priority orders are subject to an additional priority fee of $25 per order for priority (overnight) processing of CD-ROM orders. Regular Service; 3 to 5 working days following receipt of payment.

Technical_Prequisites: The 1998 TIGER/Line files contain geographic data only and do not include display or mapping software or statistical data. A list of vendors who have developed software capable of processing TIGER/Line files can be found by visiting http://www.census.gov/geo/www/tiger

Metadata_Reference_Information:

Metadata_Date: 1998
Metadata_Contact:
   Contact_Information:
      Contact_Organization_Primary:
         Contact_Organization:
            U.S. Department of Commerce
            Bureau of the Census
            Geography Division
            Products and Services Staff
      Contact_Address:
         Address_Type: Physical Address
         Address: 8903 Presidential Parkway, WP 1
         City: Upper Marlboro
         State_or_Province: Maryland
         Postal_Code: 20772
      Contact_Voice_Telephone: (301) 457-1128
      Contact_Electronic_Mail_Address: tiger@census.gov
Metadata_Standard_Name: FGDC Content Standards for Digital Geospatial Metadata
Metadata_Standard_Version: 19940608

CHAPTER   REVIEW

1. The five functional components of GIS are
   - Data acquisition and data verification
   - Data storage and database management
   - Data transformation and analysis
   - Data output and presentation
   - User interface
2. GIS require a foundation of spatial (geographic) data. Spatial databases are contained in either a raster or a vector file format. Each has advantages and disadvantages, depending on the study.
3. The raster format stores geographic data as images in a regular grid of cells.
   - Advantages of the raster format include:
     - Raster data are easy to obtain from a digital photograph or satellite image.
     - The database is simple and easy to handle in a computer.
     - The raster format is useful for studies based on environmental features easily scanned (with a computer scanner) from a map, such as vegetation cover.
   - Disadvantages of the raster format include:
     - Each cell has a specific value for each attribute. If the resolution is low, cells can be quite large, leading to inaccuracies.

   - On the other hand, a higher resolution requires a greater number of cells, increasing the size of the database (with concomitant computer storage requirements) and computer computational time.
   - Linear and demographic data, such as street names and addresses, are not easy to store in raster format, making raster data less useful in community health applications that require analyses based on political boundaries and demographics.

4. In a vector database, points, lines, and polygons represent geographic features.
   - A major advantage of the vector format is that the vector format can define the exact boundaries of areas of any shape. This is particularly useful for community health applications where political and social geographic boundaries, such as states, cities, counties, legislative districts, and neighborhoods, are essential.
   - Disadvantages of the vector format include
     - Its complexity and size
     - The inability to easily store details of an image
     - Its assumption that features are uniform within the polygon

Exhibit 2–4 Oregon Birth File Metadata

Health Data Resources
KEY: 1=Yes; 0/Blank=No/Na
Resource Name: Birth Certificate Statistical File
Primary Category: Health
Contact Person:
Cathy Riddell, Research Analyst, Oregon Health Div., Center for Health Statistics
800 NE Oregon Street, Room 225, Portland, 97232
503-731-4491
Catherine.A.Riddell@state.or.us
Purpose: Coded from birth certificates representing all births occurring in Oregon and all births occurring out-of-state to Oregon residents. Used to measure progress toward health-related Oregon Benchmarks and *Healthy People 2000* Objectives and other uses.
Audience: General public, local health departments, and state and federal agencies.

Type of data: (1=Yes, 0=No) Complete Count:	1
Registry Data:	0
Sample Survey Data:	0
Other:	0

How often is the data resource updated? Other
For which years are the data collected? 1903 through YTD

Demographic detail collected (1=Yes, 0=No) Address:	1
Age:	1
Age group:	1
Date of birth:	1
Education:	1
Ethnicity:	1
Gender:	1
Income:	0
Race:	1

Other demographics:
Restrictions on the data resource because of confidentiality: Personal identifiers are not released.
Smallest geographic detail collected: ZIP code
Largest geographical detail collected: Other
Unique features: LBW; PNC; congenital anomalies & other conditions of the newborn; medical factors of pregnancy; method of delivery; complications of labor and delivery; smoking, drinking, other drug use during pregnancy.
Format: Database: mainframe and clientserver (1989-present)
Spreadsheet:
Word Processing Document:
World Wide Web: http://www.ohd.hr.state.or.us/chs/welcome.htm
Hard Copy: 1
Other Format:
Limitations on the data resource: Small numbers at county/ZIP code level. Hispanic ethnicity was not recorded prior to 1981; during 1981–1988, Hispanic ethnicity was recorded as a race category; since 1989, Hispanic ethnicity has been included in all race categories.
Regular reports/publications produced from this data resource: Oregon Vital Statistics Annual Report Vol. 1; Oregon Vital Statistics County Data; electronic publication.
Procedure for making a request, if possible: FAX detailed request to (503) 731-3076—include phone number where you can be reached.
Other comments about the data resource: Census tract data available for Portland and Multnomah County.

5. Modern GIS technology has the ability to store and manipulate data in both raster and vector formats.
6. Public health GIS users can obtain spatial data from several sources, including local, state, and federal governmental agencies and commercial vendors. The most commonly used spatial database is the U.S. Bureau of Census's Topologically Integrated Geographic Encoding and Referencing (TIGER) files.
7. Two fundamental geographic characteristics that developers of GIS applications must consider are scale and projection.
   - *Scale* refers to the ratio between the size of an object (or the length of a distance) on a map and the size of the object (or the actual distance) in the real world.
   - *Projection* is the mathematical model that transforms three-dimensional features on the earth's curved surface to a two-dimensional map.

   Different spatial databases must have the same scale and projection to be viewed and mapped together.
8. After obtaining the spatial data, the next step in a GIS analysis is to obtain the attribute data and link them to the spatial database. Attribute data relate to any public health issue of interest and can include disease information, such as reported cholera cases and social and environmental data. To map an attribute like cholera, the attribute data must link with the spatial data. To do this, the attribute data set must include a geographic reference, such as a state, county, ZIP code, or street address. Data containing street addresses allow for the most detailed analysis.

9. Depending on the state and locality, many data sets are easily obtainable, such as vital statistics data (perinatal and mortality), health care expenditures, access to primary care, hospital discharge data, and behavioral risk factor data. Demographic data, available from the U.S. Bureau of the Census, are essential for calculating incidence and prevalence of health-related conditions for diverse populations.

10. Some data sets not traditionally considered health related have public health implications and may be useful in GIS applications. Examples include law enforcement data (arrests), high school dropouts, location of licensed alcohol retail outlets, commuting time, and domestic abuse reports, including elder, child, and spousal abuse.

11. GIS analyses of environmental data, such as the Toxic Release Inventory, can help epidemiologists understand complex relationships between environmental exposures and chronic disease, such as cancer.

12. Responsible data users must have details about their data. Data about data, commonly termed *metadata*, include the data's source, quality, timeliness, and reliability.

REFERENCES

1. K.C. Clarke et al. "On Epidemiology and Geographic Information Systems: A Review and Discussion of Future Directions." *Emerging Infectious Diseases* 2, no. 2 (1996): 85–92.

2. M. Blakemore. "Geographic Information Systems," in *Dictionary of Human Geography*, ed. R.J. Johnston et al. Oxford, England: Blackwell, 1986.

3. U.S. Tim. "The Application of GIS in Environmental Health Sciences: Opportunities and Limitations." *Environmental Research* 71 (1995): 75–88.

4. P.A. Burrough. *Principles of Geographical Information Systems for Land Resources Assessment*. Oxford, England: Clarendon Press, 1986.

5. T.R. Smith et al. "Requirements and Principles for the Implementation and Construction of Large-Scale Geographic Information Systems." *International Journal of Geographic Information Systems* 1 (1987): 13–31.

6. J.C. Antenucci et al. *Geographic Information Systems: A Guide to the Technology*. New York: Chapman & Hall, 1991.

7. K.C. Clarke. *Analytical and Computer Cartography*, 2d ed. Englewood Cliffs, NJ: Prentice Hall, 1995: 137.

8. U.S. Department of Health and Human Services. *Healthy People 2010* (conference ed., 2 vols.). Washington, DC: USDHHS, 2000.

9. M.Y. Rogers. "Getting Started with Geographic Information Systems (GIS): A Local Health Department Perspective." *Journal of Public Health Management and Practice* 5, no. 4 (1999): 22–33.

10. A.L. Melnick and D.W. Fleming. "Modern Geographic Information Systems: Promise and Pitfalls." *Journal of Public Health Management and Practice* 5, no. 2 (1999): viii–x.

11. S. Wilkinson et al. "Lead Hot Zones and Childhood Lead Poisoning Cases, Santa Clara County, California, 1995." *Journal of Public Health Management and Practice* 5, no. 2 (1999): 11–12.

12. S. McLafferty and E. Cromley. "Your First Mapping Project on Your Own: From A to Z." *Journal of Public Health Management and Practice* 5, no. 2 (1999): 76–82.

13. M.F. Vine et al. "Geographic Information Systems: Their Use in Environmental Epidemiologic Research." *Environmental Health Perspectives* 105, no. 6 (1997): 598–605.

14. S.E. Thrall. "Geographic Information System (GIS) Hardware and Software." *Journal of Public Health Management and Practice* 5, no. 2 (1999): 82–90.

15. U. Kitron. "Landscape Ecology and Epidemiology of Vector-Borne Diseases: Tools for Spatial Analysis." *Journal of Medical Entomology* 35, no. 4 (1998): 435–445.

16. G.E. Glass et al. "Environmental Risk Factors for Lyme Disease Identified with Geographic Information Systems." *American Journal of Public Health* 85, no. 7 (1995): 944–948.

17. H.J. Scholten and M.J.C. de Lepper. "The Benefits of the Application of Geographical Information Systems in Public and Environmental Health." *World Health Statistics Quarterly* 44 (1991): 160–170.

18. C.M. Croner et al. "Geographic Information Systems (GIS): New Perspectives in Understanding Human Health and Environmental Relationships." *Statistics in Medicine* 15 (1996): 1961–1977.

19. C.V. Lee and J.L. Irving. "Sources of Spatial Data for Community Health Planning." *Journal of Public Health Management and Practice* 5, no. 4 (1999): 7–22.

20. W.J. Clinton. "Coordinating Geographic Data Acquisition and Access: The National Spatial Data Infrastructure. Presidential Executive Order 12906." *Federal Register* 59 (April 13, 1994): 17671–17674.

21. A. Melnick et al. "Community Health Mapping Engine (CHiME) Geographic Information Systems Project." *Journal of Public Health Management and Practice* 5, no. 2 (1999): 64–69.

22. M.F. MacDorman and G.A. Gay. "State Initiatives in Geocoding Vital Statistics Data." *Journal of Public Health Management and Practice* 5, no. 2 (1999): 91–93.

23. J. Slosek et al. "Hospitalizations for All Injuries, Average Annual Rates per 1,000 Adults, Ages 25–44 by ZIP Code, Boston, Massachusetts, 1994–96." *Journal of Public Health Management and Practice* 5, no. 2 (1999): 29–30.

24. D.C. Goodman and J.E. Wennberg. "Maps and Health: The Challenges of Interpretation." *Journal of Public Health Management and Practice* 5, no. 4 (1999): xiii–xvii.

25. J. Wennberg, series ed., and M. Cooper, ed. "The Quality of Medical Care in the United States: A Report on the Medicare Program," in *The Dartmouth Atlas of Health Care in the United States 1999*, 3d ed. Chicago: American Hospital Association, 1999.

26. U.S. Preventive Services Task Force. *Guide to Clinical Preventive Services*, 2d ed. Alexandria, VA: International Medical Publishing, 1996.

27. T.L. Schlenker et al. "Incidence Rates of Hepatitis A by ZIP Code Area, Salt Lake County, Utah, 1992–1996." *Journal of Public Health Management and Practice* 5, no. 2 (1999): 17–18.

28. Centers for Disease Control, Epidemiology Program Office. "Nationally Notifiable Infectious Diseases: United States 2000." <www.cdc.gov/epo/dphsi/infdis.htm>. Last update October 22, 2000; last access March 17, 2001.

29. J.M. McGinnis and W.H. Foege. "Actual Causes of Death in the United States." *Journal of the American Medical Association* 270, no. 18 (1993): 2207–2212.

30. U.S. Environmental Protection Agency, Center for Environmental Information and Statistics. *Major Findings from the CEIS Review of EPA's Aerometric Information Retrieval System–Air Quality Subsystem (AIRS-AQS) Database.* April 2, 1999. <www.epa.gov/ceisweb1/ceishome/ceisdocs/airs-aqs/airs-aqs.pdf>.

31. M. Ralston. "Elevated Nitrate Levels in Relation to Bedrock Depth, Linn County, Iowa, 1991–1996." *Journal of Public Health Management and Practice* 5, no. 2 (1999): 39–40.

32. J. Pruitt. "Monitoring Volatile Organic Compounds in Private Wells Near a Community Landfill by Tax Parcel, Harford County, Maryland, 1986–1998." *Journal of Public Health Management and Practice* 5, no. 2 (1999): 41–42.

33. D. Wartenberg. "Screening for Lead Exposure Using a Geographic Information System." *Environmental Research* 59 (1992): 310–317.

CHAPTER 3

GIS Data Transformation: Making Maps

Chapter 2 described the spatial and attribute databases needed to perform a GIS analysis. Once these data sets are in place, the mapmaking process can begin. Making maps, or cartography, is the primary purpose of GIS technology. Using a childhood lead-poisoning project as a case study, and a few other examples, this chapter will describe how to use the stored spatial and attribute data sets to create maps for public health applications.

For our case study, we will consider a diverse city or county with a history of having significant numbers of children exposed to lead. The local public health department is interested in reducing the number of children with lead poisoning. Because it has a limited budget, the health department would like to target its lead-screening and abatement programs to geographic areas where children with high blood lead levels live. Additionally, the health department would like information on the location of potential sources of environmental lead exposure, including streets, highways, old housing, and potentially contaminated industrial sites. We will explore how GIS-produced maps can elegantly display this information.

GEOCODING

The first steps in the mapmaking process are to determine what spatial and attribute data sets would be helpful and then to link them. In this case study, the appropriate spatial database would be TIGER because TIGER is inexpensive, includes detailed street and address range information and political boundaries, and is often used by sister county and city agencies. The appropriate attribute database would be reports of childhood lead toxicity. To map reported lead cases, the data must include a geographical reference, a field in the database that identifies a location. In this case study, the lead report data include the residential address of each child reported with elevated lead levels.

The next step in making a map is geocoding, the process by which the GIS software matches each record in an attribute database with the geographic file. The GIS software converts each address in the attribute file to a point, such as latitude and longitude, on a map. Figure 3–1 illustrates how the matching process works.[1] First, the attribute data, such as an electronic file of lead poisoning case reports, must contain an address field. The GIS application must also contain a spatial database, such as TIGER, which includes a digital representation of street segments. The digital street segments include coordinates (latitude and longitude) for addresses at each end of each street segment. The GIS software matches the address number in each record of the attribute database to an address range in the digital map. Then, by interpolation, the software estimates where the address might be located between the two coordinates at the two ends of the address range. In our example, the GIS software compares each residential address in the lead report file with the corresponding information in the TIGER spatial database. A match occurs when the two agree.[2,3] Through matching, the software assigns each reported lead-poisoning case with a latitude and longitude point on the map. All GIS software has the capacity to match addresses.[2]

Matching is a time-consuming process, especially in areas with rapid growth and in rural locations.[4] Typically, only one-half to two-thirds of addresses match in the first attempt. Obviously, without any corrections, any resulting output would have gross inaccuracies. The next step, then, is to examine all the unmatched records for errors, correct the errors, and increase the match rate. Frequently, in the attribute database, simple errors in spelling or abbreviation of street

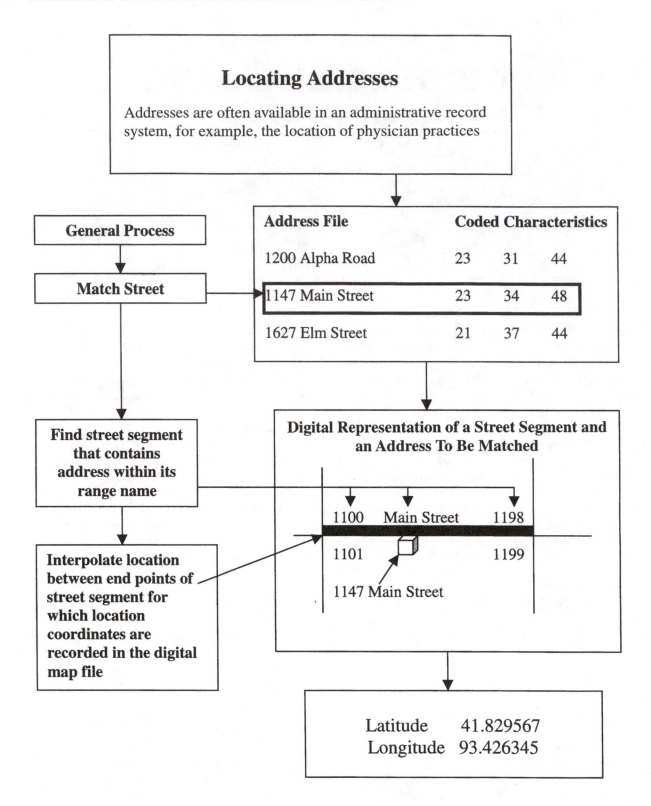

Figure 3–1 The process for finding a location for an address

names are responsible and are easy to correct. For example, the lead report file may list an address as "North Elm Street," while the spatial database lists the same address as "N. Elm Street."[1] Wholly incorrect street names pose a more significant challenge. Inaccuracies may also exist in the spatial database, especially if it is outdated. For example, new housing developments often result in new roads that will not be present in an old spatial file.[5] When cases need to be geocoded individually or reviewed through nonelectronic (hard-copy) sources, the geocoding process can be extremely time consuming. For example, geocoding 6,545 motor vehicle crashes in DeKalb County, Georgia, required one month of staff time.[4] Other errors in the attribute data include addresses that are difficult or impossible to match, such as post office boxes (especially in rural areas).[5] For example, a trailer park address may be acceptable for mail delivery but may not be included in the spatial database.[4] After correcting obvious errors, a typical match rate should exceed more than 90 percent. Match rates lower than 90 percent are an indication of errors requiring further study.[2]

EVENT MAPPING

Once stored and geocoded, the data are ready for analysis and display. The power of GIS technology stems from its ability to allow users to analyze and display health-related data in new and effective ways.[6] We will discuss several of them. The simplest form of display is analogous to a pushpin depiction—events, such as reported cholera cases, displayed as dots on a map, a "dot-density map."[7] In our lead example, the local health department might want to create a map showing the home locations of children with high blood lead levels. In Figure 3–2, areas with larger numbers of children with reported high blood lead levels show up as clusters of triangular-shaped black dots.[2] Neighborhoods with large numbers of children with elevated blood lead levels are easy to see.[2] In some cases, the clustering can be so dense that it obscures specific locations. Fortunately, GIS software can solve this problem by allowing the user to zoom in within a geographic area of the map, to move from a larger general view to a more detailed view, revealing the detailed, local geography of reported lead cases.[2,4]

Like other epidemiologic studies, this map raises additional questions. For example, was clustering a reflection of high prevalence of elevated blood lead levels or a reflection of greater screening efforts? A second map, in which circular clear dots display all children screened, answers this question, revealing the varying patterns of children with high and low blood lead levels (see Figure 3–3).[2] This analysis illustrates the power of GIS, the notion that a picture is worth ten thousand words. Compared to numerical tables, this simple visual presentation elegantly conveys a great deal of infor-

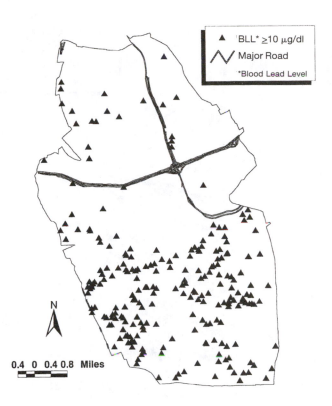

Figure 3–2 Children with elevated blood lead levels

mation showing that prevalence of lead poisoning varies by neighborhood.

The choice of triangular black dots for lead cases and circular clear dots for all children screened illustrates the importance of carefully choosing symbols.[2] GIS software allows for countless varieties of symbol sizes, shapes, and colors. By varying symbol size, the user can create contrast. In a proportional (or graduated) symbol map, the size of the symbol is proportional to the number of events at a given location.[2] For example, in Figure 3–4, the size of the circles is proportionate to the number of vehicle crashes at given locations.[4] Shapes can be geometric, such as triangles, circles, or squares, or they can be actual pictures, such as hospitals or clinic buildings.[2] Picture symbols may be more understandable, but geometric symbols are easier to read and distinguish.[2] Color choice is important for both symbols and backgrounds, such as polygons. Because color can differ in both hue and intensity, it allows for endless possibilities in map presentations.[2] We will discuss many of these in subsequent chapters. Another type of map, a chart/graph map, can display bar charts, line charts, or pie charts instead of symbols.[7] For example, a map of counties can include bar charts superimposed on each county, where the height of the bar

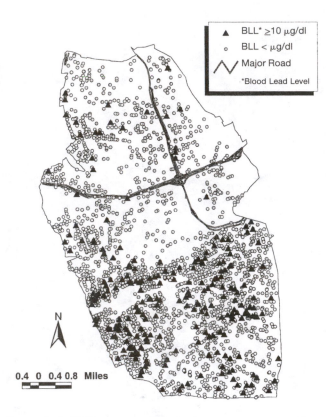

▲	BLL* ≥10 µg/dl
○	BLL < µg/dl
∧∨	Major Road
	*Blood Lead Level

0.4 0 0.4 0.8 Miles

Figure 3–3 Children screened for lead

represents the number of children within each county with reported high lead levels.

The map of lead cases and children screened in Figure 3–3 uses symbol shape and size to create contrast. The residences of children with low lead levels appear as small circular dots, while those of children with elevated levels are slightly larger triangles. The larger, darker triangles direct the viewer's gaze to the neighborhoods where a greater proportion of children with high lead levels live.[2] GIS software allows the user to try many combinations of symbol shape, size, and color to produce the most easily understandable map. The user can view these combinations on the screen, make adjustments on the fly, and decide on the optimal layout before printing.[2]

OVERLAYS

GIS can perform much more complex tasks than simple mapping of events.[6] The overlay capability of GIS allows the user to display more than one attribute or theme on a map at a time.[7] In our lead example, the health department might be interested in looking at potential risk factors for lead exposure, such as socioeconomic status. Available socioeconomic variables include poverty, education level, and age of housing.[8] Housing age is especially relevant in measuring the risk of childhood lead exposure because houses built before 1950 are more likely to contain lead paint.[4] The Centers for Disease Control and Prevention (CDC) has identified older housing as the most significant risk factor for lead exposure in young children. Clearly, the local health department might be interested in identifying the location of older housing in targeting lead exposure prevention efforts. If housing data were available, a GIS map could overlay the triangular black dots of reported childhood lead cases with the location of houses built before 1950. In this case, dots of different colors and shapes could represent older housing.

Besides the visual presentations, GIS can facilitate a multilayer geographic analysis.[4] In our lead example, suppose that the local health department wants to identify individual newborns with the greatest risk of lead paint exposure. Birth certificates include residential address of the mother. Using the birth certificate street address data, the GIS software can assign each birth record to a census block group. Then the software can link the data layer with the geocoded residential street address location of new births with another data layer containing the block group information about the percentage of pre-1950 housing. The system can then issue a report listing names and street addresses of newborns living in census block groups with elevated risk of lead paint exposure.

CHOROPLETH MAPS

As noted in Chapter 2, some attribute databases may not contain actual address information but may instead have information at larger, or aggregate, geographical areas, such as block groups, census tracts, districts, or counties. The smallest level of aggregation for which data are available is the baseline aggregation.[9] For example, housing data may not contain street addresses but may include block group. In this case, the GIS software can match the housing data to the TIGER spatial database, but by block group rather than street address. This is possible because the housing and TIGER databases include a common field, the block ID number.[2] The GIS user could overlay the reported lead cases with a map showing the percentage of homes built before 1950 by census block group or aggregates of census block groups such as census tracts.[2] Each census block group polygon (or larger polygons made up of combinations of block groups) could be colored, shaded, or patterned (e.g., striped) on the basis of its range of percentage of housing built before 1950. This type of thematic map, in which the appearance of a given area, or polygon, is varied to depict variations of fea-

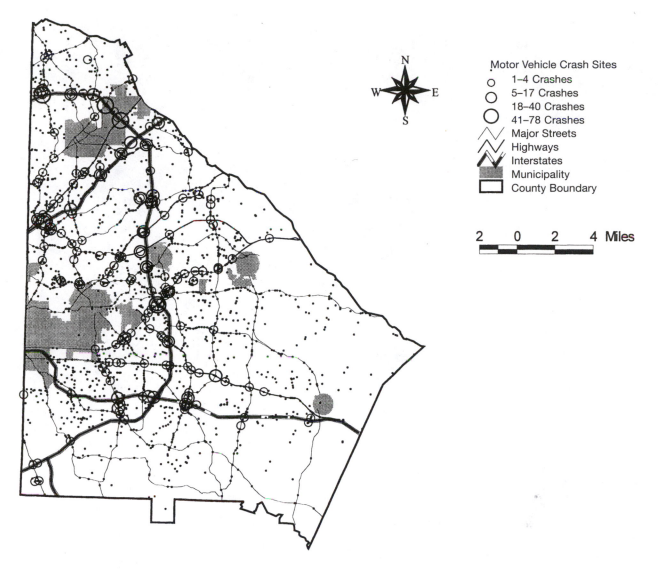

Figure 3–4 Location of motor vehicle crashes (based on a 20 percent sample of 32,808 crashes included in county public safety records) in DeKalb County, Georgia, 1995

tures or themes such as the percentage of older housing stock, is called a choropleth map. Public health planners in Duval County, Florida, used overlays to create such a map. Census block groups were shaded on the basis of the percentage of older housing, with reported childhood lead-poisoning cases displayed as black dots (see Figure 3–5).[10] This map was quite useful in focusing blood lead–screening efforts.

Public health applications use choropleth maps frequently for several reasons. First, many attribute databases do not contain a specific address field, preventing point location on a map. For example, the housing database in our lead screening study contains information only by area (block group). In many cases, data are only available at much larger aggregate levels, such as census tract, county, or state, allowing display only at these levels or higher. In addition,

data collected and presented without point location are less likely to violate anyone's privacy and confidentiality. As we will discuss in Chapter 8, however, when small numbers are involved, the possibility exists that the aggregated data can identify individuals.[5]

Choropleth Map Presentations: Intervals

The map with percentage of older housing by census block groups in Figure 3–5 illustrates another, and perhaps the most important, use of choropleth maps. Choropleth displays are essential for visually comparing proportions, such as incidence rates and prevalence. GIS software can display such proportions in different ways, including equal intervals and

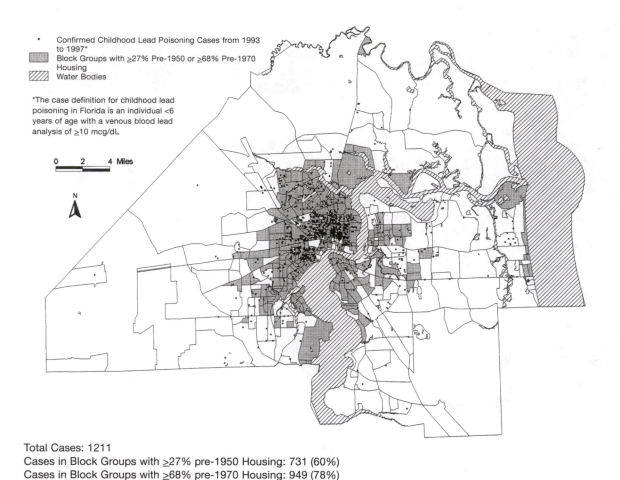

- •   Confirmed Childhood Lead Poisoning Cases from 1993 to 1997*
-   Block Groups with ≥27% Pre-1950 or ≥68% Pre-1970 Housing
-   Water Bodies

*The case definition for childhood lead poisoning in Florida is an individual <6 years of age with a venous blood lead analysis of ≥10 mcg/dL

0   2   4   Miles

N

Total Cases: 1211
Cases in Block Groups with ≥27% pre-1950 Housing: 731 (60%)
Cases in Block Groups with ≥68% pre-1970 Housing: 949 (78%)
Cases in Block Groups with ≥27% pre-1950 housing or ≥68% pre-1970 Housing: 994 (82%)

Figure 3–5 Development of childhood blood lead screening guidelines, Duval County, Florida, 1998

---

quantiles. The simplest method, equal intervals, displays equal ranges of values as specific colors, shades, or patterns. Figure 3–6 is an example of a choropleth map based on equal intervals.[11] In this map, the age-adjusted homicide rate in Kansas City ranges from 2 per 100,000 to 106 per 100,000. The Kansas City Health Department divided this range into four classes of equal intervals of 25 and patterned ZIP code polygons based on these equal intervals. GIS software allows users to select any number of classes. In this example, the Kansas City Health Department could have used eight different patterns to illustrate classes of equal intervals of 13. In creating classes, users should avoid overlapping classes, such as "54 to 79 per 100,000" and "79 to 104 per 100,000," because the overlap creates confusion as to which class "79 per 100,000" belongs. One way to resolve this is to extend the number of decimal places, such as 54.0 to 79.0 and 79.1 to 104.0.[12]

A significant limitation of the equal-interval method is that it does not work well with extreme data values or with highly skewed data.[2] When working with skewed data, the quantile method is a better choice. With quantiles, the map divides the range into classes so that an equal number of polygons fall in each class. The size of each class is based on the number of total classes. Figure 3–7 is an example of a quantile map.[13] In this study, the rate for childhood asthma hospitalization in King County, Washington, ranges from 0 per 100,000 to 1,210 per 100,000. If the cartographers had used the equal-interval method, with four equal intervals of approximately 300, most of the ZIP code polygons would have been one color, at the lower end of the range. With the quantile method, this map splits the data into four quartiles so that an equal number of polygons fall into each class. The resulting map has an equal distribution of color. GIS software allows for an almost unlimited number of quantiles. On the basis of the divisibility of total number of polygons, the cartographer must decide on the number of classes to use. If the number of classes does not divide evenly into the number of polygons, the cartographer should try to spread

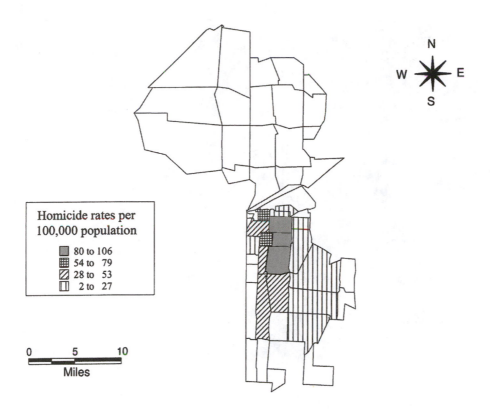

Figure 3–6 Rates are not shown for ZIP codes with 5 or fewer cases. The average age-adjusted homicide rate for all ZIP codes in the Kansas City area is 30 homicides per 100,000 population.

any unevenness among the classes.[12] Figure 3–7 illustrates a limitation of quantile maps in that areas with very similar proportions can end up in different classes,[2] while areas with very different proportions can end up in the same class. In this example, the range of asthma hospitalization rates in the highest quartile exceeds the range of all the other quartiles.

GIS software allows for many other options besides equal intervals and quantiles for defining and describing polygons.[2] For quantitative data, cartographers can customize their own class-interval breaks or even define polygons based on statistical significance.[3] For example, polygon shades can represent whether rates within polygons such as counties are statistically greater than, equal to, or less than a standard rate, such as a state rate. Cartographers must be careful how they choose class intervals because their choice can fundamentally change the appearance and the "message" of the map.[2] Before making their final choice, cartographers should experiment with different class intervals, seeing how each map represents actual data values.[2]

Choropleth maps are also useful for displaying nonquantitative information. For example, in Figure 3–8, a GIS marketing application uses patterns and shades to define "lifestyle clusters" such as "Aging Couples in Inner Suburbs" and "Upscale Suburban Fringe Couples."[14]

Other Choropleth Map Characteristics: Color, Shading, and Polygon Size

Besides class intervals, the choice of shading, color, pattern, size, and shape of polygons can greatly influence the appearance and message of the map. Maps can be either black and white or colored. In either case, most maps are easier to interpret if they contain a single color that varies in intensity.[2] In most cases, polygon values are proportional to their hue. Lighter hues represent polygons with lower values, whereas progressively darker hues represent progressively

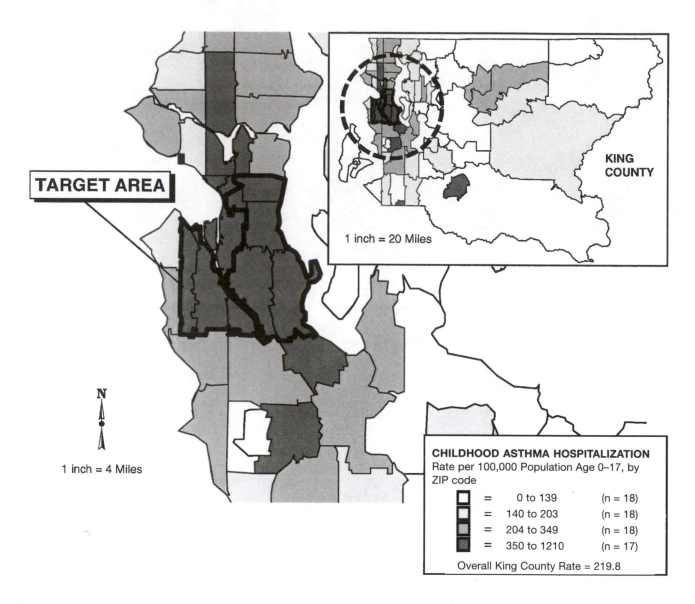

TARGET AREA

KING
COUNTY

1 inch = 20 Miles

N

1 inch = 4 Miles

CHILDHOOD ASTHMA HOSPITALIZATION
Rate per 100,000 Population Age 0–17, by
ZIP code

☐ =	0 to 139	(n = 18)
☐ =	140 to 203	(n = 18)
☐ =	204 to 349	(n = 18)
☐ =	350 to 1210	(n = 17)

Overall King County Rate = 219.8

Figure 3–7 Childhood asthma hospitalization rates by ZIP code of residence, King County, Washington, 7-year average, 1990–1996

higher values. One caveat is to avoid using 100 percent black as a shade because it can visually dominate the map.[12] An exception to the single-color rule is found in maps designed to show comparisons, especially statistical comparisons, to a population value.[2] For example, a map comparing census tract teen birthrates with a state or national rate could use different colors to illustrate tracts with rates statistically higher than, equal to, or lower than the state or national rate. For most maps, the size and shape of the polygons should be roughly equal.[12] Polygons much larger than others can domi-

nate the map, while dissimilar shapes can lead to misinterpretations of patterns. Figures 3–9 and 3–10 illustrate why the number of polygons is also critical.[12] Because Delaware has only three counties, a map of county per capita income gives little information about how income varies within the state. In comparison, a map of per capita income by county for Georgia, with many more counties than Delaware, provides much more information on income distribution. The influence of metropolitan Atlanta on income distribution is clearly visible on this map.

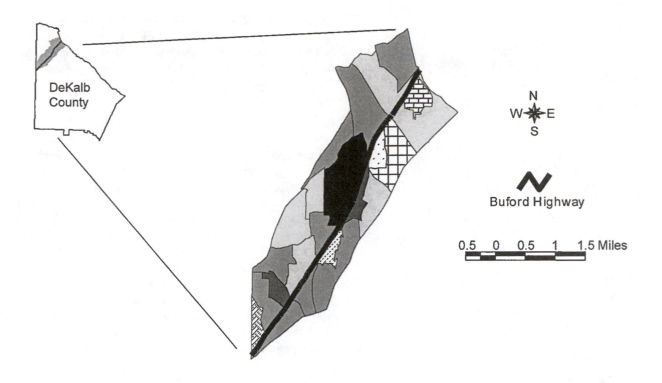

Cluster Group	Smoke 40+ Cigarettes per Day	Smoked Last Year	Med. Ins. through Medicaid	Domestic Beer Last Week	Any Lottery Purchase in Last Month	Top Media	Bottom Media
Low-Income Hispanic Families	195	141	213	112	97	Nostalgia TV	Classical radio
Aging Couples in Inner Suburbs	156	108	128	115	125	Pay-per-view TV	Nostalgia TV
Young Blue-Collar/ Service Families	153	109	69	95	100	Spanish radio	Black radio
Young Mobile City Singles	68	127	61	138	98	TV M–F 12:30–1 am	News radio
Middle-Income Empty Nesters	100	103	133	100	114	Nostalgia TV	Spanish radio
Young Midscale Suburban Couples	68	110	47	110	113	Classical radio	TV M–F 1–2 am
Upscale Suburban Fringe Couples	21	98	55	94	116	Nostalgia radio	Spanish radio
Upwardly Mobile Singles and Couples	81	87	76	121	93	Jazz radio	Country Music TV
Upscale White-Collar Couples	34	78	30	94	101	Classical radio	Nostalgia TV

Figure 3–8 Using marketing information to focus smoking cessation programs in specific census block groups along the Buford Highway corridor, DeKalb County, Georgia, 1996

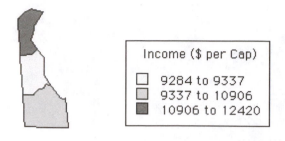

Figure 3–9 Map of county per capita income for the state of Delaware

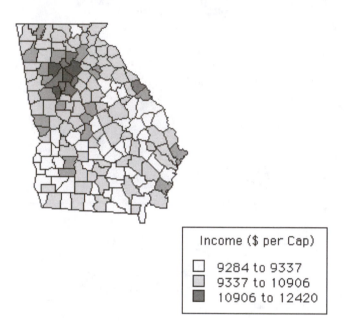

Figure 3–10 Map of county per capita income for the state of Georgia

QUERYING: DISTANCE AND BUFFERING

Distance

GIS analyses can respond to questions, or queries, about distance and travel time measurements, such as the distance from a household to the nearest toxic waste site or the travel time for emergency vehicles to reach a specific neighborhood.[3] As we will explore in subsequent chapters, distance measurements are useful for environmental exposure measurements and for evaluating and improving health care ac-

cess. For example, a local health department outreach worker could use GIS to determine the distance, travel time, and directions from a low-income, non–English-speaking household to the nearest specific-language–capable primary care facilities.[15]

Buffering

Buffering is another powerful feature of GIS analysis. Using this feature, GIS can create polygons based on the distance from a target object,[6] such as a power transmission line or a toxic industrial emitter. If climatological data were available (and incorporated into the GIS), the buffer area can include the geographic region for toxic dispersal, based on wind speed, wind direction, precipitation, and other climatologic variables. Users can query the number of events (and underlying population, for proportions) within the buffer area. Buffers are particularly useful in identifying people at risk of exposure to environmental hazards. For example, John Snow could have drawn circles around the Broad Street pump and calculated the number of ill and well people within each circle. A GIS study of childhood lead risk could define a 25 m zone around main roads to identify areas with potentially high levels of lead-contaminated soil from past use of leaded gasoline[16] (see Figure 3–11). The same study could then identify and locate children living within these areas who would benefit from lead screening. Another study used buffering to evaluate potential health risks and health risk perceptions of minority populations living within 0.2 miles of businesses that stored hazardous chemicals (see Figure 3–12).[17]

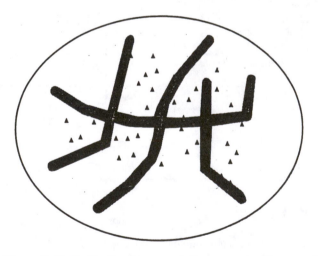

Figure 3–11 Buffer functions can define a geographic area of a desired width around a point, line, or area (e.g., a 25 m zone around main roads to identify areas with potentially high levels of lead-contaminated soil from past use of leaded gasoline)

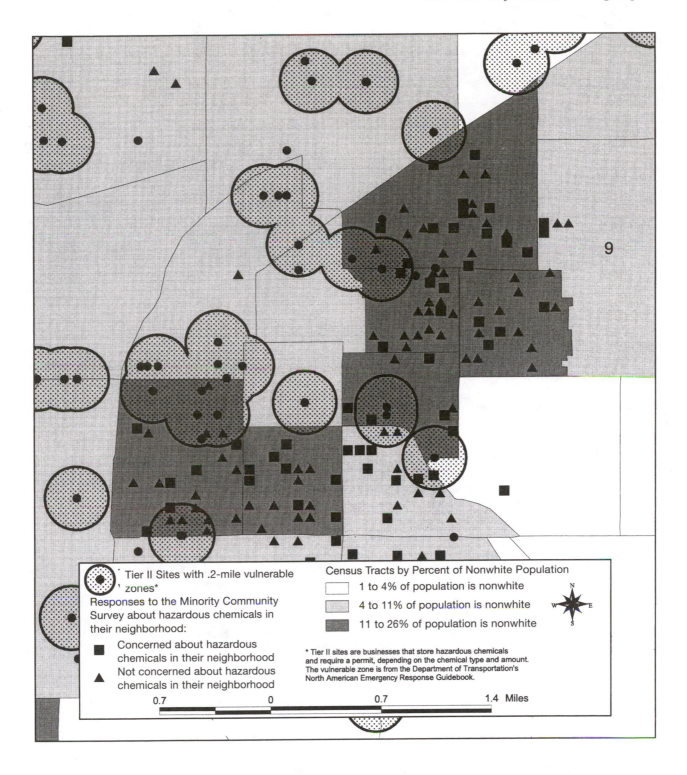

Figure 3–12 Responses to the Survey of Environmental Health Hazard Risks in the Minority Community, in relation to the primary minority census tracts and the evacuation zones for Tier II Sites in Lincoln, Nebraska, February 1999

STATISTICAL ISSUES

Rates

Usually, health outcomes cluster geographically because of underlying population characteristics, not because of the geography itself.[5] This can be a problem in choropleth mapping because the proportion, and the ultimate map shading, may be due more to these underlying characteristics than to the geography. In such cases, the use of crude rates can lead to misinterpretation. For example, crude rates of breast cancer are likely to be higher in areas with a higher proportion of women, especially older women, because older women are more likely diagnosed with breast cancer.[9] A map of breast cancer rates would really demonstrate the age and gender distribution of the population, rather than showing areas with higher breast cancer risks. Similarly, maps of rates of other diseases that vary by underlying population characteristics, such as sickle cell anemia, can lead to misinterpretation. As in other epidemiologic applications, a solution to this problem is adjustment for the underlying population characteristics. In our breast cancer example, age-adjusted rates are necessary.

For adjustment in single large areas, directly standardized rates are appropriate because the results are comparable with rates calculated in other studies using the same standard population.[9] However, studies simultaneously mapping and comparing adjusted rates in many small areas should use indirectly standardized rates because directly standardized rates are statistically unstable in small areas.[9] Most GIS software can calculate crude rates. Those interested in formulas for the methodology of indirect standardization can consult several statistical references.[9,18] Using these formulas, simple spreadsheet software or statistical software is sufficient for calculation of adjusted rates. The adjusted rates are easily importable into the GIS software for mapping.[9] Figure 3–13 is an example of a map showing indirectly age- and gender-associated relative risks for lung cancer in New Mexico.[9]

Spatial Aggregation

In addition to underlying population characteristics, rates can vary due to random geographic variation. This is especially true with polygons containing small numbers of events. Statistically, rates for small areas, such as census blocks, are unstable even when one is using indirect standardization. A solution to this problem is to aggregate the data into larger geographic areas, also known as higher-level aggregation.[9] For instance, reported sexually transmitted disease data are usually collected at the street address level and are available by block group. However, actual numbers at this level may be so small that it would make more sense to map rates of

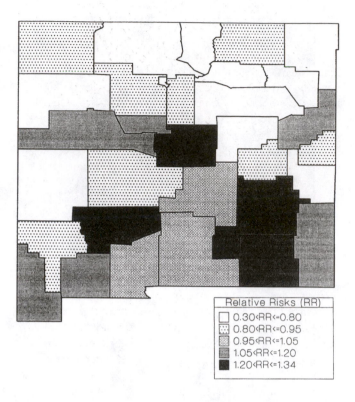

Figure 3–13 Indirectly age- and gender-adjusted relative risks of lung cancer incidence in New Mexico, 1973–1991. The data, containing a total of 9,254 cases, were collected by the New Mexico Tumor Registry for the National Cancer Institute's Surveillance, Epidemiology and End Results (SEER) program.

sexually transmitted disease at the census tract or even county level. Higher-level aggregation comes with a trade-off, the loss of local-level information. Whatever the level of aggregation, random geographic variation is always a possible cause of rate differences across polygons. Fortunately, statistical tests for spatial randomness are available to evaluate this possibility.[9]

Smoothing

One limitation of choropleth maps is that they assume uniformity of features within each polygon, even though there may be extreme variation. For example, within the shaded areas of Figure 3–5, although these entire block groups have high percentages of older housing, the age of individual houses within each block group may vary considerably. Another problem with choropleth maps is that they assume sharp changes across their borders when in fact the underlying distribution changes gradually and continuously. For our lead example, suppose that the local health department created a choropleth map showing rates of childhood lead poisoning for census tracts within the county. Like other health problems, such as communicable disease, lead poisoning does not generally follow administrative or political boundaries.[9] For our example, also suppose that a cluster of lead-poisoning cases is present very locally in four adjacent census block groups, each belonging to a different census tract. An analysis at the larger census tract level will dilute the block group–level data and miss the cluster entirely. If the census tract is the baseline level of aggregation, the only way to solve this problem will be to go back and collect the data at a lower level of aggregation, such as block group or event street address. Once the lead-poisoning data are available at the lower level of aggregation, calculating rates for overlapping rather than nonoverlapping areas can solve this problem. The result is a map with smoothed rates.[9]

Figure 3–14 illustrates the simplest technique for creating smoothed rates.[9] The first step is to create a spatial filter, a set of overlapping circles of fixed size that are centered on a regular grid of points.[9] The next step is to calculate the rate within each circle, assigning the rate to the center of the circle. Because the circles overlap, neighboring circles have similar rates, resulting in a smoothed map. Using GIS software, the cartographer can create a continuous surface map, or isopleth map, based on contours,[9] similar to altitude contour maps used by mountain climbers. In this case, the contours reflect the proportion of the attribute of interest, such as the prevalence of childhood lead poisoning. In contrast to choropleth maps that display attributes uniformly within polygons, isopleth maps display attributes based on contours.

Figure 3–15, a map illustrating the estimated percentage of uninsured adults in Ingham County, Michigan, is an ex-

ample of an isopleth map developed by smoothing.[19] The height of this map's surface at each point where grid lines intersect represents the estimated percentage of adults without health insurance within a one-mile diameter circle around the point. In this case, the "mountain" represents the concentration of uninsured adults in Lansing, Michigan. Using our lead example, mountains in a continuous surface map would represent concentrations of children with lead poisoning.

The cartographer must specify two parameters to create smoothed maps. These parameters are the distance between grid points and the circle radius. There are advantages and trade-offs in choosing these parameters. Shortening the distance between grid points retains information that is more detailed but increases the computer workload. As long as the distance between grid points is much smaller than the typical distance between the baseline aggregated areas, the specified distance does not matter much. For example, suppose that in a smoothed map of prevalence of childhood lead poisoning, census tracts were the baseline level of aggregation. Considering that typical census tracts are several square miles in area, it would not matter much if grid point distances varied from ¼ to ½ mile.

The radius of the circle determines the degree of smoothing. As the circle radius increases, the degree of smoothing increases. When there is baseline aggregation, increasing the circle size increases the chance that a circle border may cut through an aggregated area. One way to solve this problem is to assign the aggregated area to fall within or outside the circle on the basis of the location of the center of the aggregated area.[9] In calculating smoothed rates, most studies count all observations within each circle equally, whether or not they are close to the center. Another alternative is to weight observations that are closer to the circle higher than those that are further away. For further information, several references provide detailed methods for performing these calculations.[9,20] As with grid point distances, there are advantages and trade-offs in choosing smoothing scale. As smoothing increases, the map may miss some interesting features. As smoothing decreases, and the number of observations within the smaller circle decreases, the resulting smoothed rates will retain a lot of "noise."[9]

Before deciding on the final map, cartographers choosing to create a smoothed map should investigate map appearance at different levels of smoothing.[9] Different smoothers applied to the same data set can create maps revealing different features, resulting in potentially different interpretations. To avoid misinterpretation, tests for spatial randomness are necessary.[9]

A geographic study of breast cancer treatment provides another example of smoothing. Several years ago, the Iowa State Cancer Registry reported that Iowa women had a higher

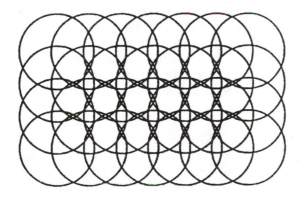

Figure 3–14 A set of overlapping circles used to construct a smoothed map of rates. The rate calculated for each circle is assigned to the center of that circle.

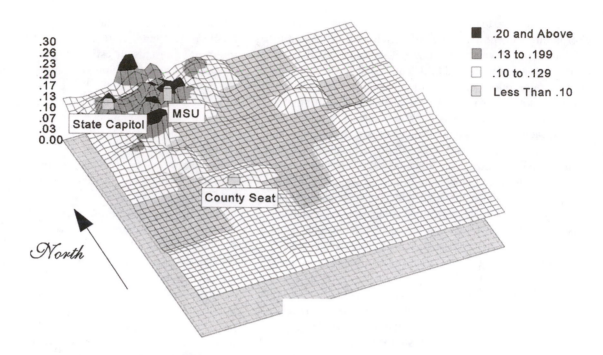

Note: These estimates were made using "synthetic" methods. About 14 percent of the population lack insurance. Concentrations of uninsured are found in north and southeast Lansing. About 15 percent of students lack insurance.

Figure 3–15 Percentage of adults without health insurance in Ingham County, Michigan, 1994

rate of total mastectomy for localized, early breast cancer compared to women in other states. This was occurring in spite of an earlier National Institute of Health (NIH) recommendation that less aggressive breast-conserving treatment rather than mastectomy was the treatment of choice for most women with early-stage breast cancer.[21] The NIH defines breast conservation treatment (also known as lumpectomy, segmental mastectomy, or partial mastectomy) as excision of the primary tumor and adjacent breast tissue followed by radiation therapy. The concern over the high mastectomy rate led Iowa health officials to question whether total mastectomy rates were unusually high throughout the state or whether there were areas within Iowa that were responsible. Using GIS technology, investigators at the University of Iowa tried to answer this question. First, they drew maps of Iowa ZIP codes with an overlay of localized breast cancer cases.[22] Figure 3–16 is a map of southeastern Iowa ZIP codes, with the size of gray circles proportionate to the number of localized breast cancer cases. Within many of the ZIP codes, the numerator (number of breast cancer cases) was too small for calculating stable mastectomy rates. To calculate rates, investigators had to aggregate the data spatially by county. Figure 3–17 is the resulting choropleth map, with the mastectomy rates (the number of women having mastectomy per 1,000 women with localized breast cancer) by county. This map has an overlay of the location of radiation treatment facilities that could be used by women undergoing breast conservation treatment. Like other choropleth maps, this map assumes that mastectomy rates change sharply across county borders when in fact the underlying distribution changes gradually and continuously. Compare this with Figure 3–18, a smoothed map of the same data. To create the smoothed map, University of Iowa investigators used spatial filters, illustrated by the large, clear circles in Figure 3–16. Although the smoothed map does not answer the question of why mastectomy rates are high in Iowa, it does raise an interesting hypothesis: proximity to radiation treatment facilities may be associated with lower total mastectomy rates.[22]

Probability Maps

Returning to our lead example, let us suppose that the county health department is interested in whether specific areas within the county have significantly increased incidence rates of elevated childhood lead levels. One way to do this would be to test whether the observed number of cases of childhood lead poisoning in each area was statistically sig-

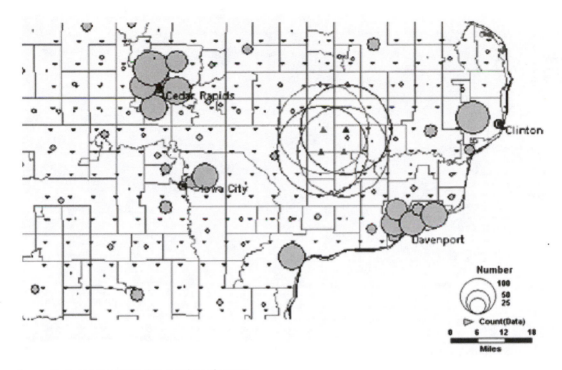

Note: Size of gray circle is proportional to number of cases.

Figure 3–16 Number of cases of localized breast cancer, by ZIP code area, southeastern Iowa, 1991–1996

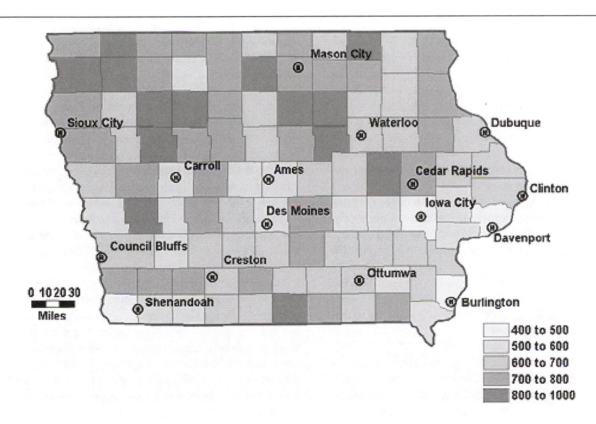

Figure 3–17 Number of women selecting mastectomy per 1,000 cases of localized breast cancer, by county, Iowa, 1991–1996

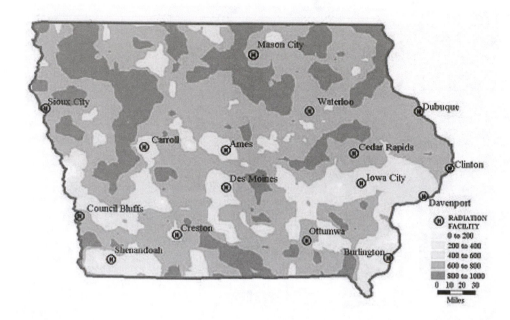

Figure 3–18 Smoothed (spatially filtered) map of number of women selecting mastectomy per 1,000 cases of localized breast cancer, Iowa, 1991–1996

nificantly greater than the expected number of cases. Instead of mapping the incidence rates of lead poisoning, the health department could map the *p* value for each area. The resulting map, a probability map, generally applies to traditional choropleth maps, with each polygon representing a *p* value. Using the smoothing process, the health department could also create continuous contour maps with *p* values rather than rates.[9] Probability maps can provide a useful complement to maps of rates, but they come with an important caveat. Whenever multiple simultaneous statistical tests are performed, there is a possibility that one or more of the tests will show significance even when the results are due solely to chance. This problem is solvable with additional statistical procedures, such as Bonferroni adjustments[23] or a spatial scan statistic.[9]

Statistical Tests

A Spatial Scan Statistic

Clearly, multiple testing can lead to misinterpretation, especially when those interpreting the tests are falsely led into believing that statistical significance proves "something is there when it's not."[9] To prevent such misinterpretation, cartographers creating maps based on multiple testing have a responsibility to determine whether such significant results are indeed due to chance. Two types of tests for spatial randomness can solve this problem. The first test, the spatial scan statistic,[9] is a cluster detection test. It is useful for determining the existence of statistically significant clusters while pinpointing their locations. The test methodology is similar to that described for creating smoothed rates (see Figure 3–14). Instead of using overlapping circles of fixed size, this test uses a larger set of overlapping circles of many different sizes[9] (see Figure 3–19). The first step is to calculate the likelihood associated with the observed number of events (such as reported elevated lead levels) in each circle. The next step is to pick the circle with the highest likelihood. This cluster is the most likely cluster, the one least likely to have occurred by chance.

The purpose of determining the most likely cluster is to solve the problem of multiple testing. Instead of testing multiple polygons for significance (as in the probability map) and running into the possibility that one or more significant findings are really due to chance, this one cluster provides a single test statistic for the entire map. Unlike a probability map, however, no mathematical formula exists for the probability distribution of the test statistic, so it is impossible to calculate the *p* value analytically. Fortunately, free software, SaTScan, is available for download through the National

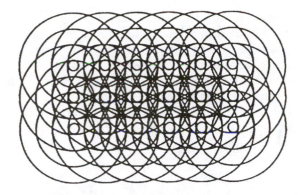

Figure 3–19 A small sample of the many overlapping circles used by the spatial scan statistic

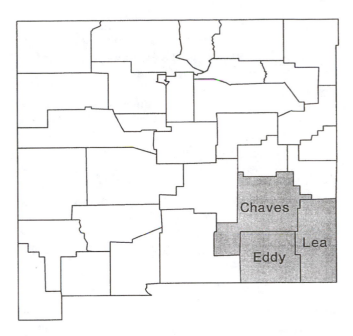

Figure 3–20 Application of the spatial scan statistic on lung cancer incidence in New Mexico, 1973–1991. The most likely cluster is shown in the southeast corner, consisting of Chaves, Eddy, and Lea Counties (RR = 1.26). The *p* value is 0.0001. Due to this Chaves-Eddy-Lea cluster, we can reject the null hypothesis of a geographically random distribution of lung cancer in New Mexico.

Cancer Institute for performing the necessary Monte Carlo simulation calculations.[9] The address of the Web site is <http://dcp.nci.nih.gov/bb/satscan.html>.

Figure 3–20 is an example of the spatial scan statistic applied to the New Mexico lung cancer incidence data in Figure 3–13. In this example, the most likely cluster is located in an area containing Chaves, Eddy, and Lea Counties in the southeastern part of the state. The rate of lung cancer in this cluster is 26 percent higher than the state rate, with a *p* value of 0.0001. Because the comparison is between this single area and the state, one can reject the null hypothesis of no geographic clustering of lung cancer incidence in New Mexico. This conclusion is independent of the case distribution in any other part of the state and applies only to the comparison between this single area and the state of New Mexico. Because of the baseline aggregation into counties, the cluster is not a perfect circle. The central locations (centroids) of the three counties are within the same circle.[9] In addition, the method uses many windows that overlap with the most likely cluster and thus have only slightly lower likelihood values. As a result, for studies done at lower levels of aggregation, the exact borders of the most likely cluster are uncertain.

Global Clustering

Unlike the spatial scan statistic, the second type of test for spatial randomness is based on global rather than local clusters. This type of test, global clustering, analyzes whether clustering occurs throughout an area without pinpointing the location of any specific clusters. Two events occurring close together, such as two cases of childhood lead poisoning, count as a cluster no matter where they occur on the map. Such clustering is common with many communicable diseases

where person-to-person transmission occurs. One specific test for global clustering is the *k*–nearest neighbor test.[9,24,25] The first step in performing the test is to specify a value *k*. For each event *j*, such as a reported childhood lead case, the next step is to calculate how many other events occur among the *k* nearest neighbors. The number of such neighbors summed over all events becomes the test statistic. One can reject the null hypothesis of no clustering if each event has more other events as close neighbors than there would be without clustering.[9] Stat! software capable of calculating the *k*–nearest neighbor test is available through BioMedware.[26] Tango's excess events test is another useful test for global clustering.[9,27] Further information is available from Tango at the Institute of Public Health in Tokyo, Japan.

MODELING

One strong point of GIS technology is its ability to predict disease risk on the basis of simultaneous evaluation of multiple risk factors. In many cases, especially those involving diseases (such as communicable diseases) with short latencies, investigators clearly understand the epidemiology of the disease with its associated risk factors.[28] In these situations, a geographic analysis based on simple overlays is enough to identify the predicted distribution of disease. For example, one investigator used information on the breeding, feeding, and flight habits of a mosquito, a malaria vector, and the locations of villages, combined with satellite image–determined environmental features, to predict the risk of malaria in coastal regions of Mexico.[28,29] In such cases, the investigators, knowing the risk factors, just use the query function of GIS to identify where the risk factors exist.

For many other health conditions, however, investigators do not have as complete an understanding of associated risk factors. In these situations, investigators can use GIS technology as an "exploratory tool to develop and test hypotheses"[28(p.16)] about potential risk factors. For example, a case-control study of Lyme disease (see Chapter 4) used GIS to model Lyme disease risk on the basis of where cases and controls lived in relation to environmental variables associated with the tick vector and deer reservoir. Using logistic regression, investigators developed a map of predicted Lyme disease risk, based on the regression coefficients of these environmental variables. The following year, the investigators tested this model, finding that new cases were 16 times more likely to occur in high-risk compared to low-risk areas.[28] Although such models can be useful, investigators must use caution because the models can be unstable when the number of potential variables is equal to or greater than the number of cases of disease.[28] In addition, the traditional statistical methods used in developing these models assume that each observation is independent when (especially with communicable disease) this is unlikely to be true. On the contrary, many factors associated with specific health outcomes have some underlying spatial correlation. Students interested in further information on how this can affect their data can consult an appropriate reference on spatial autocorrelation.[28,30]

The statistical methods that we have described in this chapter should serve as an introduction to basic concepts and methods of spatial statistics. Many other spatial statistical methods not described here are useful in epidemiologic and community health GIS applications. Practitioners and students interested in more advanced methods for spatial smoothing using empirical Bayes estimators should consult Devine et al.[9,31] For determining whether diseases cluster around health hazards such as toxic emitters, focused tests are useful.[9,32,33] Spatial regression is useful in analyzing disease rates in relation to geographically specified exposures such as air pollution or neighborhood socioeconomic status.[9,34] For those interested in studying the spatial distribution of health over time, statistical techniques are available for analyzing spatio-temporal data.[9,35]

CHAPTER   REVIEW

1. Making maps, or cartography, is the primary purpose of GIS technology. The first steps in the mapmaking process are to determine what spatial and attribute data sets would be helpful and then to link them.

2. The next step in making a map is geocoding, the process by which the GIS software matches each record in an attribute database with the geographic file. The GIS software converts each address in the attribute file to a point, such as latitude and longitude, on a map.

3. Matching is a time-consuming process, especially in areas with rapid growth and in rural locations. Typically, only one-half to two-thirds of addresses match in the first attempt. To improve accuracy, cartographers must examine all the unmatched records for errors, correct the errors, and increase the match rate.

4. Once stored and geocoded, the data are ready for analysis and display. The simplest form of display is to display events, such as reported cholera cases, as dots on a map, a "dot-density map."

5. GIS software can display events as symbols of different sizes, shapes, and colors. Varying symbol size creates contrast. In a proportional (or graduated) symbol map, the size of the symbol is proportional to the number of events at a given location. A chart/graph map uses bar charts, line charts, or pie charts in place of symbols.

6. With overlays, cartographers can display more than one attribute or theme on a map at a time.

7. Choropleth maps, a specific type of thematic map, alter the appearance of geographic areas, or polygons, to depict variations of features or themes such as the percentage of older housing stock. Choropleth maps are essential for visually comparing proportions, such as incidence rates and prevalence. GIS software can display such proportions in different ways, including equal intervals and quantiles. Besides intervals, the choice of shading, color, pattern, size, and shape of polygons can greatly influence the appearance and message of the map.

8. GIS analyses can respond to questions, or queries, about distance and travel time measurements, such as the distance from a household to the nearest toxic waste site, or the travel time for emergency vehicles to reach a specific neighborhood. Using buffering, cartographers can create polygons based on the distance from a target object, such as a power transmission line or a toxic industrial emitter.

9. Usually, health outcomes cluster geographically because of underlying population characteristics, not because of the geography itself. This can be a problem in choropleth mapping because the proportion, and the ultimate map shading, may be due more to these underlying characteristics than to the geography. In such cases, the use of crude rates can lead to misinterpretation. As in other epidemiologic applications, a solution to this problem is adjustment for the underlying population characteristics. For adjustment in single large areas, directly standardized rates are appropriate because the results are comparable with rates calculated in other studies using the same standard population. However, studies simultaneously mapping and comparing adjusted rates in many small areas should use indirectly standardized rates because directly standardized rates are statistically unstable in small areas.

10. Rates can also vary due to random geographic variation, especially in areas with small numbers of events. Statistically, rates for small areas, such as census blocks, are unstable even when using indirect standardization. A solution to this problem is to aggregate the data into larger geographic areas, a practice known as higher-level aggregation. Higher-level aggregation comes with a trade-off, the loss of local-level information.

11. One limitation of choropleth maps is that they assume uniformity of features within each polygon, even though there may be extreme variation. Another problem with choropleth maps is that they assume sharp changes across area borders when in fact the underlying distribution changes gradually and continuously. A solution to these problems is to calculate rates for overlapping rather than nonoverlapping areas. The result is a map with smoothed rates. Using GIS software, the cartographer can create a continuous-surface map, or isopleth map, based on contours, similar to altitude contour maps used by mountain climbers. The contours reflect the proportion of the attribute of interest, such as the prevalence of childhood lead poisoning.

12. Probability maps are special kinds of choropleth maps in which polygons are shaded on the basis of whether the number of events (or cases) within each polygon is statistically significantly greater than the expected number of cases. Each polygon shade or color represents a p value. Probability maps can provide a useful complement to maps of rates, but they come with an important caveat. Whenever multiple simultaneous statistical tests are performed, there is a possibility that one or more of the tests will show significance even when the results are due solely to chance. This problem is solvable with additional statistical procedures, such as Bonferroni adjustments or tests for spatial randomness.

13. In numerous cases, especially those involving diseases (such as communicable diseases) with short latencies, health officials clearly understand the epidemiology of the disease with its associated risk factors. In these situations, a geographic analysis based on simple overlays is enough to identify the predicted distribution of disease. For countless other health conditions, however, we do not have as complete an understanding of associated risk factors. Using GIS technology, epidemiologists can develop models to test hypotheses about potential risk factors for many of these health conditions, leading to better prevention and control strategies.

REFERENCES

1. G. Rushton. "Methods To Evaluate Geographic Access to Health Services." *Journal of Public Health Management and Practice* 5, no. 2 (1999): 93–100.

2. S. McLafferty and E. Cromley. "Your First Mapping Project on Your Own: From A to Z." *Journal of Public Health Management and Practice* 5, no. 2 (1999): 76–82.

3. C.M. Croner et al. "Geographic Information Systems (GIS): New Perspectives in Understanding Human Health and Environmental Relationships." *Statistics in Medicine* 15 (1996): 1961–1977.

4. M.Y. Rogers. "Getting Started with Geographic Information Systems (GIS): A Local Health Department Perspective." *Journal of Public Health Management and Practice* 5, no. 4 (1999): 22–33.

5. A.L. Melnick and D.W. Fleming. "Modern Geographic Information Systems: Promise and Pitfalls." *Journal of Public Health Management and Practice* 5, no. 2 (1999): viii–x.

6. K.C. Clarke et al. "On Epidemiology and Geographic Information Systems: A Review and Discussion of Future Directions." *Emerging Infectious Diseases* 2, no. 2 (1996): 85–92.

7. S.E. Thrall. "Geographic Information System (GIS) Hardware and Software." *Journal of Public Health Management and Practice* 5, no. 2 (1999): 82–90.

8. C.V. Lee and J.L. Irving. "Sources of Spatial Data for Community Health Planning." *Journal of Public Health Management and Practice* 5, no. 4 (1999): 7–22.

9. M. Kulldorff. "Geographic Information Systems (GIS) and Community Health: Some Statistical Issues." *Journal of Public Health Management and Practice* 5, no. 2 (1999): 100–106.

10. C. Duclos et al. "Development of Childhood Blood Lead Screening Guidelines, Duval County, Florida, 1998." *Journal of Public Health Management and Practice* 5, no. 2 (1999): 9–10.

11. J. Cai and Q.B. Welch. "Age-Adjusted Homicide Rates by ZIP Codes, Kansas City, Missouri, 1991–1995." *Journal of Public Health Management and Practice* 5, no. 2 (1999): 27–28.

12. G. Rushton and M. Armstrong. "GIS in Public Health: GIS Procedures-Mapping." 1997. <www.uiowa.edu/~geog/health/mapping/num.html>.

13. D. Solet et al. "VISTA/PH Software for Community Health Assessment." *Journal of Public Health Management and Practice* 5, no. 2 (1999): 60–63.

14. M.Y. Rogers. "Using Marketing Information To Focus Smoking Cessation Programs in Specific Census Block Groups along the Buford Highway Corridor, DeKalb County, Georgia, 1996." *Journal of Public Health Management and Practice* 5, no. 2 (1999): 55–57.

15. G.I. Thrall. "The Future of GIS in Public Health Management and Practice." *Journal of Public Health Management and Practice* 5, no. 4 (1999): 75–82.

16. M.F. Vine et al. "Geographic Information Systems: Their Use in Environmental Epidemiologic Research." *Environmental Health Perspectives* 105, no. 6 (1997): 598–605.

17. P.H. Bouton and M. Fraser. "Local Health Departments and GIS: The Perspective of the National Association of County and City Health Officials." *Journal of Public Health Management and Practice* 5, no. 4 (1999): 33–41.

18. R.C. Elandt-Johnson. "Rates, Standardized," in *Encyclopedia of Statistical Sciences*, eds. S. Kotz and N.L. Johnson. New York: John Wiley, 1986: 632–635.

19. M. Cheatham. "Percent of Adults without Health Insurance in Ingham County, Michigan, 1994." *Journal of Public Health Management and Practice* 5, no. 2 (1999): 53–54.

20. K. Kafadar, "Smoothing Geographical Data, Particularly Rates of Disease." *Statistics in Medicine* 15 (1996): 2539–2560.

21. National Institutes of Health. "Treatment of Early-Stage Breast Cancer." *NIH Consensus Statement Online* 8, no. 6 (June 18–21, 1990): 1–19. <http://text.nlm.nih.gov/nih/cdc/www/81txt.html>.

22. G. Rushton and M. Michele. "Women with Localized Breast Cancer Selecting Mastectomy Treatment, Iowa. 1991–1996." *Public Health Reports* 114 (1999): 370–371.

23. A. Melnick et al. "Clackamas County Department of Human Services Community Health Mapping Engine (CHiME) Geographic Information Systems Project." *Journal of Public Health Management and Practice* 5, no. 2 (1999): 64–69.

24. A.D. Cliff and J.K. Ord. *Spatial Processes: Models and Applications.* London: Pion, 1981.

25. J. Cuzick and R. Edwards. "Spatial Clustering for Inhomogeneous Populations." *Journal of the Royal Statistical Society* B52 (1990): 73–104.

26. G.M. Jacquez. *Stat! Statistical Software for the Clustering of Health Events.* Ann Arbor, MI: BioMedware, 1994.

27. T. Tango. "A Class of Tests for Detecting 'General' and 'Focused' Clustering of Rare Diseases." *Statistics in Medicine* 14 (1995): 2323–2334.

28. G.E. Glass. "Geographic Information Systems," in *Infectious Disease Epidemiology Theory and Practice,* eds. K.E. Nelson et al. Gaithersburg, MD: Aspen Publishers, Inc., 2000; 231–254.

29. L.R. Beck et al. "Assessment of a Remote Sensing-Based Model for Predicting Malaria Transmission Risk in Villages of Chiapas, Mexico." *American Journal of Tropical Medicine and Hygiene* 56 (1997): 99–106.

30. D.A. Griffith. *Spatial Autocorrelation: A Primer.* Washington, DC: Association of American Geographers, 1987.

31. O.J. Devine et al. "Empirical Bayes Methods for Stabilizing Incidence Rates before Mapping." *Epidemiology* 5 (1994): 622–630.

32. J.F. Bithell. "The Choice of Test for Detecting Raised Disease Risk Near a Point Source." *Statistics in Medicine* 14 (1995): 2309–2322.

33. A. Lawson and L. Waller. "A Review of Point Pattern Methods for Spatial Modeling of Events around Sources of Pollution." *Environmetrics* 7 (1996): 471–488.

34. R. Haining. "Spatial Statistics and the Analysis of Health Data," in *GIS and Health,* eds. A. Gatrell and M. Loytonen. London: Taylor & Francis, 1998; 29–47.

35. M. Kulldorff et al. "Evaluating Cluster Alarms: A Space-Time Scan Statistic and Brain Cancer in Los Alamos." *American Journal of Public Health* 88 (1998): 1377–1380.

Public Health GIS Applications: Environmental Health

ENVIRONMENTAL EXPOSURE AND DISEASE RISK

Perhaps the most direct uses of GIS technology are as tools for understanding diseases or disease risks directly related to environmental exposures[1] and as tools for targeting public health interventions based on these risks. The development of GIS technology is timely, for the level of public concern about risks from environmental exposure has increased significantly over the past few decades.[2] Most environmental epidemiologists believe that exposures to environmental contaminants contribute to many chronic diseases, including cancer, reproductive and other endocrine dysfunctions, neurodevelopmental disorders, and abnormalities of the immune system.[2] Increasingly, the public is asking environmental epidemiologists to determine whether exposure to specific contaminants has caused specific adverse health outcomes at local, regional, and national levels.[2] The 1986 Chernobyl nuclear accident and other recent environmental catastrophes have increased public questioning regarding the degree of environmental exposure and its relation to chronic disease.[2]

To answer these questions, epidemiologists need accurate exposure information. Usually this is the most difficult, expensive, and time-intensive piece of any study.[3] Before the development of modern GIS technology, studies relied on indirect or surrogate measures of exposure.[4] For example, interviews on occupation in the shipbuilding industry provided surrogate measures of asbestos exposure data for case-control studies.[4] Now, with available GIS technology, epidemiologists can combine existing databases, including environmental data, to make better estimates of exposure levels.[3] This information is essential for protecting the public's health.

The sample inventory of attribute data sources in Chapter 2 illustrates that historically, environmental and public health surveillance programs have generated large amounts of data. Many different agencies at the local, state, and federal levels have collected and maintained environmental exposure and health data in different formats in different locations. Without an integrated framework to manage, manipulate, analyze, and present the data, many of these data sets have languished in obscurity. By combining available morbidity, mortality, and demographic data with available environmental data, GIS technology has the potential to solve this problem and begin addressing the public's concerns. In this chapter, we will use several examples involving different types of environmental exposures to illustrate this potential of GIS technology.

NONIONIZING RADIATION EXPOSURES: IDENTIFYING EXPOSED COHORTS FOR FURTHER STUDIES

One recent public concern has been the question of an association between nonionizing radiation, such as electric and magnetic fields, and the incidence of cancer.[5] This concern increased significantly following publication of a study investigating the association between residential exposure to electric and magnetic fields and childhood cancers in Denver, Colorado.[5,6] Since that study, several other studies have led to conflicting results. Although occupational case-control studies have demonstrated increased rates of leukemia and brain cancer deaths in workers exposed to electric and magnetic fields, the exposure estimates, based on job titles and not actual work, were inaccurate. Additionally, the failure of these studies to account for other exposures and confounders has prohibited drawing any definitive conclusions.[5]

In contrast to occupational exposures, residential exposures to magnetic fields may be easier to estimate on the basis of the measured distance between residence and high-voltage transmission lines. The geographic querying capabilities of GIS technology, including the capability to measure distance and create buffer zones, are uniquely suited for this type of analysis. In addition, because GIS software can integrate many different data sets, it can evaluate potential confounders of any exposure-disease relationship, such as demographic and other socioeconomic variables. A pilot study in New Jersey illustrated this potential use of GIS software.[5]

The first step in the pilot study was to digitize the location of a high-voltage transmission line. Using electrical utility company maps, the investigators specified the geographic coordinates of the towers and stored the data in a vector format. The vector format permitted drawing the transmission line between the specific points of the towers. The next step was to superimpose this digitized information on a spatial file, the U.S. Bureau of the Census TIGER files. This displayed the transmission line in relation to other physical and political features, such as rivers, roads, and census blocks, block groups, and tracts. The third step was to incorporate

U.S. Bureau of the Census demographic data. Next, on the basis of the transmission line power, the investigators specified a 100 m buffer zone on either side of the transmission line. This buffer contained the population with a specific level of exposure. Obviously, the investigators could change the size of the buffer on the basis of the level of exposure they wished to evaluate. Using GIS software, the investigators were able to determine the area and proportion of each census block within the buffer. Finally, by using the incorporated demographic data, the investigators evaluated the demographic characteristics of the cohort population contained within or intersecting the buffer area and could compare this with unexposed populations living outside the buffer area.[5]

Figures 4–1 and 4–2 are maps illustrating the transmission line superimposed on township and U.S. Bureau of the Census block group boundaries, respectively.[5] Some of the census block groups were completely contained within the buffer, while the proportion of others contained within the buffer zone varied. If they desired, the investigators could refine their analysis further by using aerial photographs to determine whether individual housing units in blocks intersecting the buffer lay within or outside the buffer zone.[5]

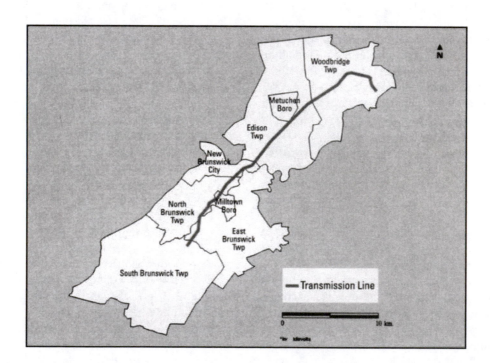

Figure 4–1 A map of a high-voltage transmission line digitized and superimposed on township boundaries generated using U.S. Bureau of Census TIGER files

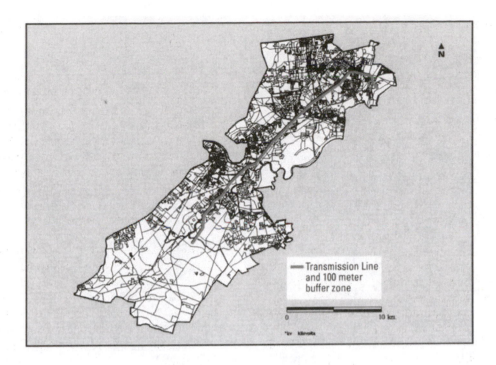

Figure 4–2 The map and line shown in Figure 4–1 digitized and superimposed on U.S. Bureau of the Census block boundaries generated from the U.S. Bureau of Census TIGER files, with a 100 m buffer on either side of the line

Table 4–1 illustrates the demographic and perceived housing value characteristics of cohort populations living in towns and living in blocks intersecting and completely outside the buffer zone.[5] The results show that demographic values, including age and race, were similar among towns and inside and outside the buffer zone. Interestingly, perceived housing values differed more within towns than they did for blocks within the buffer zone.

In the past, most environmental epidemiological studies relied on case-control designs to evaluate the association between rare cancers and nonionizing radiation exposures. Because these case-control studies selected subjects on the basis of disease and not exposure to nonionizing radiation, they were limited in accurately characterizing exposures and in evaluating unusually high levels of exposure. Using GIS technology, this pilot study found hundreds of potential subjects living within 100 m of a high-voltage transmission line in New Jersey. In addition, the study found that this population did not differ sociodemographically from the rest of the population, making the individuals within this population attractive for a future cohort study. Similar population cohorts, exposed to high levels of magnetic radiation, exist elsewhere due to the wide distribution of high-voltage transmission lines. GIS technology now provides the means for iden-

tifying individuals exposed to high residential levels of nonionizing radiation for cohort studies because it can easily locate and characterize these cohorts on the basis of potentially confounding socioeconomic variables.[5]

AIR EMISSIONS

Ionizing Radiation: Using GIS To Target Communities for Health Screening

One study illustrates the use of GIS technology in modeling disease risk and identifying an at-risk cohort for further evaluation on the basis of exposure to radioactive iodine, Iodine-131 (I-131). Between 1945 and 1951, the Hanford Nuclear Reservation, located in eastern Washington State, released large quantities of I-131 into the air.[7] At the time, Hanford produced plutonium used in nuclear weapons. After the release, the resulting plume deposited the radioactive iodine across a large area. Consumption of milk contaminated with I-131 was the route of exposure for people living in the region. Those living in an area where they were likely to drink contaminated milk as young children are at lifetime risk for developing thyroid and parathyroid disease, including thyroid cancer.

Table 4–1 Population Characteristics by Town: Overall and with 100 m Buffer

Township	No. of Blocks	Population	Housing Units	% under 18	% over 65	% White	% Black	% Owner Occupied	Mean Cost ($)	Mean Rent ($)
East Brunswick	–	43,548	15,395	24.0	8.7	88.1	2.2	81.7	203,700	725
Blocks intersecting buffer	10	731	248	24.6	10.7	94.1	0.4	90.3	274,979	535
Edison	–	88,680	32,832	21.7	10.7	79.5	5.6	64.7	204,500	659
Blocks intersecting buffer	50	6,436	2,678	19.5	9.4	86.1	4.1	62.7	177,405	588
North Brunswick	–	31,287	12,186	20.4	9.2	80.1	11.1	61.2	199,300	681
Blocks intersecting buffer	15	2,003	369	13.3	6.6	86.9	3.9	97.3	268,968	1,175
South Brunswick	–	25,792	9,962	25.2	6.5	84.1	6.2	70.5	201,600	724
Blocks intersecting buffer	1	152	55	20.4	15.1	94.7	0.7	81.8	233,400	520
Woodbridge	–	93,086	34,498	19.3	13.0	86.6	6.5	70.7	163,400	644
Blocks intersecting buffer	53	5,853	2,643	18.0	13.4	85.8	4.5	60.4	127,062	602
Mean difference among towns				3.1	3.0	4.7	3.7	9.4	17,320	45
Mean difference between town and buffer				3.2	3.0	6.2	3.6	13.7	47,236	200

In this study, investigators used GIS technology, with the appropriate data sets, to predict which populations were at increased risk and would consequently benefit from a screening program. The study used spatial data in raster format based on a 10 km by 10 km grid overlaying a 75,000-square-mile area in Washington, Oregon, and Idaho. Using available data by year, age group, and milk source, Batelle Corporation investigators (working for the National Center for Environmental Health of the Centers for Disease Control and Prevention [CDC]) developed a model map displaying isopleths of median thyroid dose estimates[7] (see Figure 4–3). Investigators established eligibility criteria for medical screening and evaluation of a target population of 14,000, based on a median thyroid dose estimate of at least 10 rads. Figure 4–3 shows two regions, based on the model, where children living in 1945 could have received such a dose. Dose estimates are highly dependent on age because younger children were more likely to drink milk. The larger polygon represents an area where younger children (ages 0–4 years) would have received median thyroid doses of 10 rads or higher. Older children (ages 5–19 years) were at risk in a smaller area, closer to the facility, because they would have received comparable doses by drinking a smaller amount of more highly contaminated milk. Adults in both regions, drinking even less milk, would have received only one-tenth the dose estimates for children and would not need medical screening. The Agency for Toxic Substance and Disease Registry (ATSDR) is using this map to educate the public on their eligibility for the screening program.[7]

Asthma

Asthma, the most common chronic illness in childhood, affects an estimated 4.8 million children in the United States aged less than 18 years (6.9 percent of all U.S. children).[8] In 1993, asthma accounted for an estimated 198,000 hospitalizations and 342 deaths among persons aged less than 25 years.[8] Asthma is a multifactorial disease that has been associated with familial, infectious, allergenic, socioeconomic, psychosocial, and environmental factors.[8,9] Decreases in lung function and exacerbations of asthma have been associated with exposure to automobile-produced pollutants, including nitrous oxide and particulates.[8,9]

A San Diego study illustrates the potential of GIS technology in integrating several data sets and in using locally available data not ordinarily considered health related to gain a new understanding of asthma and raise questions for further study. Using a case-control design, the study evaluated the association between childhood asthma and traffic flow.[10] The spatial data source was a 1:24,000–scale street network layer obtained from the San Diego Association of Governments (SANDAG) in San Diego, California. Several sources contributed to the multiple layers of attribute data. For asthma cases and controls, investigators obtained data from the Medi-Cal (California's Medicaid program) paid-claims database. This database, maintained by the California Department of Health Services, contains information on all Medicaid beneficiaries in California. The data set contains information on each patient's name, address, date of birth, gender, race/ethnicity, and medical diagnosis (at the time of the study, based on ICD-9 codes); the date of the patient's visit; and the type of medical visit.[10] Cases were based on physician, inpatient, and hospital visits with a diagnosis of asthma in a child aged 14 years or younger between January 1993 and June 1994 for San Diego County. Controls included an equivalent random sample of children with any other diagnosis in the same geographic area over the equivalent time. Because medical providers saw some of the cases and con-

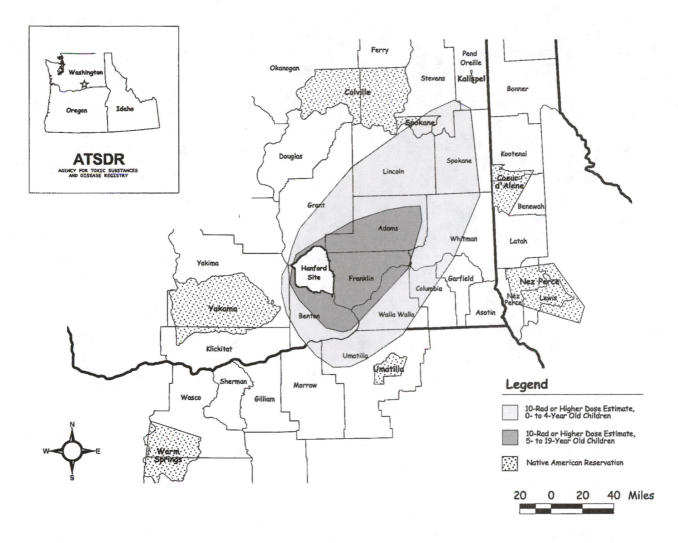

Figure 4–3 Locations around the Hanford Nuclear Facility where average milk consumption by children in 1945 would have resulted in an estimated median Iodine-131 dose to the thyroid of 10 rad or higher, Washington

trols more than once, the study counted only the first visit. Geocoding of cases and controls resulted in a match rate of 85.2 percent.

The next level of attribute data was the traffic data. SANDAG maintains a database containing information on average daily traffic (ADT) flow linked to the 1:24,000–scale street network layer.[10] To create the database, city and county governments use traffic counters, who collect the data for almost all the highways and major roads in San Diego County. In addition, some traffic counters collect data on a smaller proportion of local roads. To ensure comprehensiveness of the traffic flow data, investigators added another attribute data set, the ADT values for state highways and collector roads, obtained from the California Department of Transportation (CALTRANS). ADT values, calculated from a

minimum of 48 hours of weekday traffic flow, are defined as the average number of cars per weekday.

Census data served as the next level of attribute data. To identify a block group for each case and each control residence, investigators linked each residence address to SANDAG block group boundary layers. Then, investigators used 1990 census data to add several other variables of interest for each block group. The variables included percentages of unemployment, childhood poverty, educational status, urban/rural status, median household income, and type of home heating fuel used (electricity, gas, coal, or wood).[10]

Once they had incorporated all layers of attribute data, investigators began their analysis by creating buffers around each case and control geocoded residence (see Figure 4–4). They chose a 550-foot buffer based on models of air emis-

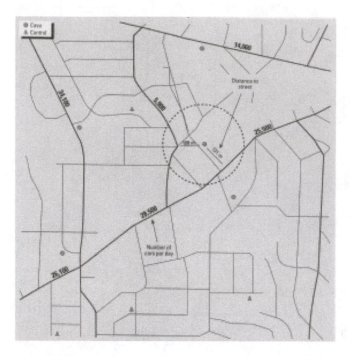

Figure 4–4 Buffer (550 ft; 168.8 m) encircling cases and controls to capture traffic flow

sion decay with distance from traffic. Within each buffered region, they captured all street segments for which they had ADT data. Using these data, they determined the distance from each case and control residence to each street segment and the average daily traffic count for each of these segments within each buffered region.[10]

The next step in the analysis was to compare cases and controls on the census block group socioeconomic variables and on individual variables, such as age, gender, race/ethnicity, and visit type (based on the Medi-Cal claims data). Investigators compared cases and controls on traffic variables, including differences in ADT for the street with the highest ADT within each buffer region, the closest street to each residence, and the sum of all streets within each buffer region. Because air pollution dispersion is a function of distance and climatic conditions, such as wind speed, investigators were able to apply weights to their traffic flow data and look at different models of potential exposure. Investigators also tested for spatial clustering of cases irrespective of proximity to traffic by using a form of a nearest neighbor statistical test (see Chapter 3). Next, the investigators tried to determine whether the ADT was associated with medical visits for asthma rather than the asthma diagnosis itself. To

do this, investigators compared ADT at closest streets to each residence, and all streets within the buffer, for cases with two or more medical visits and cases with only one visit during the study period.[10]

Data analysis failed to show any association between children's asthma risk and traffic counts near their homes, even after using different pollution dispersion models and controlling for confounders in a multivariate model.[10] However, for children already diagnosed with asthma, proximity to streets with higher traffic counts was associated with increased numbers of medical care visits. Investigators concluded that air pollutants associated with traffic might exacerbate rather than cause asthma. The investigators pointed out several limitations with their study. They had no information on duration of exposure, individual exposure from other sources or sites, or the presence of other potential confounders, such as secondhand smoke exposure.[10]

In spite of these limitations, this investigation illustrates the potential of GIS technology in case-control studies involving environmental exposure. The integrative capabilities of GIS technology allowed linkage of traffic data, home addresses, socioeconomic data, and medical diagnostic data. Because it tied traffic data to each individual case, the study provided a reasonable estimate of individual exposure, avoiding some of the bias inherent in ecologic studies.[10] In addition, because the study based exposure estimates on actual traffic counts, rather than questionnaires on proximity to traffic, it avoided the information bias inherent in self-reports.[10]

LEAD

Exposure to lead, an environmental toxin, can cause serious damage to the development of children. Even low levels of exposure can cause decreased growth, hearing, and intelligence. Higher levels of exposure can result in encephalopathy (brain disease), including seizures, and death.[11,12] Blood lead levels as low as 10 μg/dl can cause problems, and the higher the level, the greater the risk.[12] Unfortunately, lead is widely distributed throughout the environment, including air, dust, and water,[13] especially in urban areas. Its widespread use in paint, batteries, solder, and gasoline provides many potential sources for exposure for children and adults.[14]

Like other illnesses due to environmental exposure, lead poisoning is preventable. In 1991, the CDC recommended screening for all children at age one year (universal screening) and high-risk children (targeted screening) as early as age six months.[12] Consequently, traditional lead-screening programs relied on targeting an at-risk population when possible, sampling blood lead, and identifying individual cases of toxicity. But for communities interested in reducing the communitywide risk of childhood lead poisoning, these programs, designed to test and treat affected individuals, had significant limitations. First, programs based on individual sampling missed potentially affected neighbor children and clusters, making community evaluation difficult or impossible. While these screening programs detected many cases, their rate of detection was low because those children at the highest risk of exposure often had the least access to primary health care.[13] Second, programs relying only on sampled children were likely to miss information on factors associated with lead exposure, such as housing age or water supply, that could be useful in identifying high-risk neighborhoods[13] for communitywide interventions. Finally, although communities found universal screening highly desirable, many communities lacked the resources to target everyone.

Not surprisingly, a 1994 national survey found that lead programs screened only one-fourth of all young children. Even worse, these programs screened only one-third of poor children, who were at higher risk of exposure than other children.[15] Clearly, alternative public health strategies, directed at populations with the highest risk and incidence, would be beneficial for communities interested in maximizing benefits while conserving resources.[13] In 1997, the CDC issued new guidelines for targeting lead-screening programs based on such strategies. The guidelines recommended that state health officials develop a statewide plan for childhood lead screening. Based on the desirability of targeting high-risk populations, the recommendations stated that the plan should divide the state, if necessary, into areas with different recommendations for screening and should address screening recommendations for each area. The guidelines defined the type of screening, universal or targeted, on the basis of specific geographic criteria, including childhood blood lead levels and housing age (see Table 4–2).

The CDC recommended screening all children (universal screening) in higher-risk areas. Higher-risk areas were defined as having at least 27 percent of the housing built before 1950 and/or having at least 12 percent of 1- and 2-year-old children with blood lead levels of at least 10 μg/dl. For intermediate-risk areas, where less than 27 percent of the housing had been built before 1950 and the prevalence of elevated blood levels was between 3 and 12 percent or was unknown, they recommended targeted screening. The CDC defined targeted screening as screening of children who were receiving services from public assistance programs and children whose parents answered "yes" or "don't know" to questions about personal risk.[15] In addition, the guidelines recommended targeted screening in areas where at least 27 percent of housing had been built before 1950 and where reliable and representative prevalence data revealed a prevalence of less than 12 percent.[15]

Table 4–2 Guidelines for Choosing an Appropriate Recommendation for Screening Children with Elevated Blood Lead Levels (BLLs)

% Children, Ages 12–36 Months, with BLLs ≥ 10 μg/dl	% Housing Built before 1950	Recommended Screening
≥ 12	—	Universal
<12	≥ 27	Universal (or targeted—see discussion)
3–12	<27	Targeted
<3	<27	See discussion
Unknown	≥ 27	Universal
Unknown	<27	Targeted

On the basis of these criteria, the CDC recommended geographically "pinpointing" small areas where lead exposure was likely because analysis of small areas might reveal "pockets of risk" invisible within a larger area of analysis. They also recommended avoiding analysis of areas, such as census tracts, whose boundaries would not be recognizable by health care providers or parents. As an example, the CDC included a GIS analysis of South Carolina in the guidance, showing high-risk areas for universal screening based on housing age (see Figure 4–5). The maps illustrate that analysis at the county level misses pockets of higher risk as revealed by GIS analysis at the ZIP code and census tract levels.

As one alternative approach to individual sampling–based lead-screening programs, GIS technology, with its capacity to organize and integrate many data sources, can help evaluate local, community risks for lead exposure. Many data sets, maintained by many different agencies, contain information on known lead exposure risk factors, including ethnicity, socioeconomic status, lead-contaminated soil, housing age, water pipes with corrosive water, and location of industrial lead sources.[13] For example, GIS can incorporate census data, housing data, Environmental Protection Agency (EPA) Toxic Release Inventory (TRI) data, and climatic data (wind speed and direction) and, using buffering, can develop a predictive model for community exposure risk.[13,15]

Wartenberg provides an example of how such an approach using GIS technology might work.[13] Consider a 16–square-block region for a lead-screening program. With limited resources, the health department is interested in prioritizing its screening program to high-risk blocks. For this simple example, the health department has incorporated a couple of attribute data sets into its GIS, socioeconomic status (see Figure 4–6) and lead soil contamination. In a real-life situa-

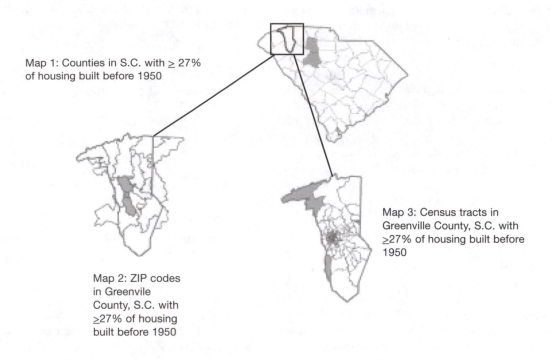

Map 1: Counties in S.C. with ≥ 27% of housing built before 1950

Map 2: ZIP codes in Greenvile County, S.C. with ≥27% of housing built before 1950

Map 3: Census tracts in Greenville County, S.C. with ≥27% of housing built before 1950

Figure 4–5 Housing built before 1950 in South Carolina: geographic analysis at three different levels—county, ZIP code, and census tract. (Shading indicates ≥27% of housing built before 1950.)

tion, a typical health department could incorporate additional data sets containing other relevant variables, including housing age, water-supply lead concentration, and ethnicity. For our simple example, the region also contains an industrial lead emitter, and the health department used GIS to model the plume of air emissions from the facility (see Figure 4–7). Table 4–3 lists the scores for each variable—socioeconomic status, soil, and air—for each block on the basis of the GIS model. The total score, equal to the risk estimate, is simply the sum of the individual scores for each variable for each block. Figure 4–8 is a map of these scores by block.

On the basis of this map, the local health department could prioritize its lead-screening program to blocks with the highest total risks, while minimizing its travel time and expense. In this example, the health department should target blocks 4 and 10 first, followed by blocks 9 and 14, and then blocks 5 through 8 and 13.[13] The health department could also use its GIS to identify clusters of cases of lead poisoning. As a simple example, Figure 4–9 is a map plotting individual cases as black dots.[13] The map indicates that there is a cluster of cases in the neighborhood around block 10. However, this is difficult to confirm without denominator information be-

cause the blocks within this neighborhood may contain a higher overall population than other blocks in the 16-block region. Of course, the health department could add denominator data to determine actual rates.

Next, assume that the health department has added population data and that the population in the region is even, with 100 residents on each block. On the basis of blocks 1 through 8, we could assume a background rate of 2 per 800. In this scenario, the probability of a block having more than 1 case is approximately 0.02, and the probability of a group of eight blocks with more than six cases is approximately 0.01. On the basis of this information, the health department may want to investigate further the apparent excess number of cases in the neighborhood in the lower half of the region involving blocks 9 through 16.[13]

Additionally, the health department could use GIS technology to compare the number and location of actual cases with its predicted risk model. Table 4–4 compares the distribution of cases in Figure 4–9 with the distribution of risk scores in Figure 4–8. The model's higher risk blocks tend to have more cases, but the relationship is not exact. Small numbers of cases and overall population may be responsible for

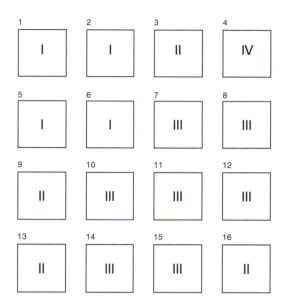

Figure 4–6 A hypothetical map of socioeconomic status in a neighborhood. Each box represents a subarea within the neighborhood. The small number to the upper left of each box is an index number for identification. The Roman numeral inside each box is the socioeconomic status, which is scaled from 1 to 4, with 1 being the highest. There is a hypothetical factory to the upper right of the neighborhood.

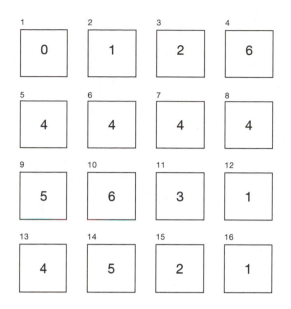

Figure 4–8 A hypothetical map of lead exposure risk score in the neighborhood shown in Figure 4–6. This score combines the socioeconomic status data and the soil and air contamination data. The risk scores range from 0 to 6, with 6 being the highest risk. See text for details.

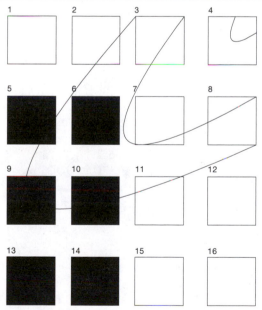

Figure 4–7 A hypothetical map of soil and air contamination in the neighborhood shown in Figure 4–6. The shaded boxes have contaminated soil. The plume of air contaminants is shown by the elliptical curves emanating from the factory. The curves represent contours of decreasing concentrations, the one closest to the factory representing a value of 3, the next a value of 2, and the one reaching farthest into the neighborhood a value of 1. The units are arbitrary.

Table 4–3 A Hypothetical Region for Lead Screening

Region	SES	Soil	Air	Score
1	0	0	0	0
2	0	0	1	1
3	1	0	2	3
4	3	0	3	6
5	0	3	1	4
6	0	3	1	4
7	2	0	2	4
8	3	0	2	5
9	1	3	1	5
10	2	3	1	6
11	2	0	1	3
12	1	0	0	1
13	1	3	0	4
14	2	3	0	5
15	2	0	0	2
16	1	0	0	1

Note: SES (socioeconomic status) is derived from U.S. Bureau of the Census files (0 = high; 3 = low). Soil is derived from local soil quality files (0 = clean; 3 = contaminated). Air is derived by specifying a buffer from a point source (0 = no effect; 3 = maximum effect). Score is the sum of SES, Soil, and Air.

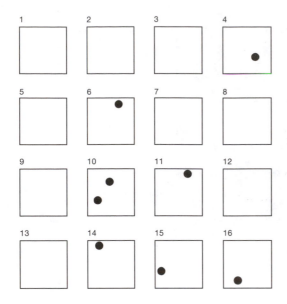

Figure 4–9 A hypothetical map of lead exposure cases in the neighborhood shown in Figure 4–6. Each solid circle represents a case.

Table 4–4 A Frequency Distribution of Lead Exposure Cases by Risk Score

Risk Score	Number of Blocks	Number of Cases	Overexposure Rate (Cases per Block)
0	1	0	0.00
1	3	1	0.33
2	2	1	0.50
3	1	1	0.33
4	5	1	0.20
5	2	1	0.50
6	2	3	1.50
Total	16	8	0.50

some of this variation. Alternatively, the model itself may need refining by addition of more variables associated with exposure risk. Once the health department adds the additional data sets, it could use its GIS to create new predictive models and then test these with case observations in other areas of the region. In this iterative manner, the health department could continually create increasingly accurate predictive models useful for targeting screening programs in other areas.[13]

The New Jersey Department of Environmental Protection and Energy (NJDEPE) has developed a pilot project using such methods to identify communities for lead prevention efforts.[14] The pilot took advantage of the capacity of GIS technology to integrate many different data sets from several different agencies. Pilot project developers chose the Newark/East Orange/Irvington area because it contained large numbers of children with elevated blood levels and a large number of industrial, residential, and vehicular sources of lead (see Figure 4–10). TIGER line files, supplemented with ETAK, a commercial database, supplied the spatial data, providing census tract boundaries, roads, waterways, and other geographic features. The project incorporated several attribute databases. First, the pilot added a data set containing blood lead–screening records, supplied by the New Jersey Department of Health (NJDOH). These records contained address information, allowing case assignment to specific locations. The records also contained information on date of birth, gender, and the date of the blood sample. Investigators defined cases of elevated lead as individuals with blood levels of at least 15 μg/dl. Using GIS software, investigators then assigned each case to its specific census tract. Figure 4–11 is a choropleth map using patterns to differentiate census tracts by numbers of cases.

The pilot project then added two more layers of attribute data supplied by NJDEPE. First, investigators added data on the location of industrial lead emitters, supplied by the 1987 TRI (see Chapter 2). Next, the NJDEPE's 1989 Site Status Report provided data on location of hazardous waste site locations. These data sets contained information on the name of each facility, the amount of lead released, and the medium (air, water, etc.) into which the facility released the lead. Figure 4–12 is a map showing the location of lead-containing waste sites and industrial lead emitters.

Another agency, the New Jersey Department of Transportation (NJDOT), provided an additional layer of attribute data containing traffic volume estimates. The NJDOT reports vehicle miles traveled by type of road for each New Jersey municipality. Investigators combined this information with ETAK spatial files to display this information on a map (see Figure 4–13).

Figure 4–14 shows how the overlay feature of GIS technology can compare the number and location of actual lead-poisoning cases with a predicted risk model on one choropleth map.[14] Census tracts with a greater predicted risk, based on large numbers of preschool children and pre-1940 housing, have a speckled pattern. Census tracts with above-average frequencies of cases of elevated lead levels, based on their containing 13 or more individuals with high blood lead levels, have a striped pattern. The map also contains location of potential environmental lead sources, including roads, hazardous waste sites, and industrial lead emitters. In

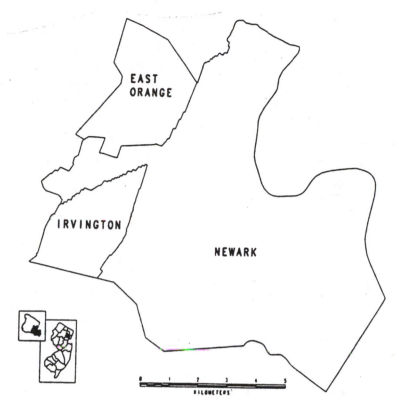

Figure 4–10 Municipalities selected for lead exposure and screening pilot project: Newark/East Orange/Irvington study area, New Jersey

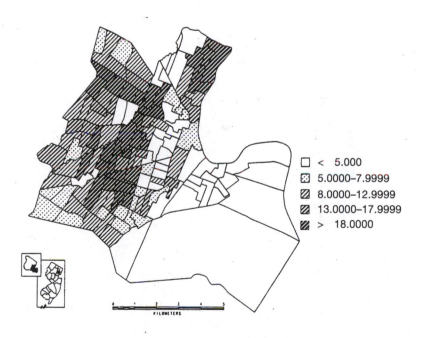

Figure 4–11 Number of individuals with high initial blood lead levels in Essex County, New Jersey, 1983–1990. A reading of 15 µg/dl or more is considered high.

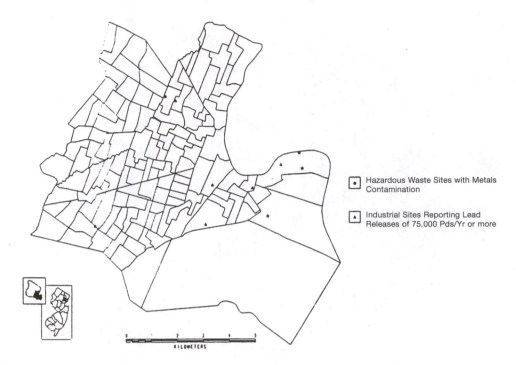

Figure 4–12 Metals waste sites and industries that are major users of lead in Newark/East Orange/Irvington study area, New Jersey. Sources are NJDEPE Site Remediation Program and Toxic Release Inventory.

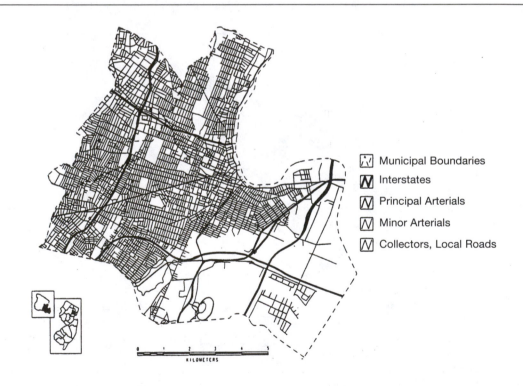

Figure 4–13 Roads and relative traffic volume in Newark/East Orange/Irvington study area, New Jersey. Sources are NJDOT data and ETAK files.

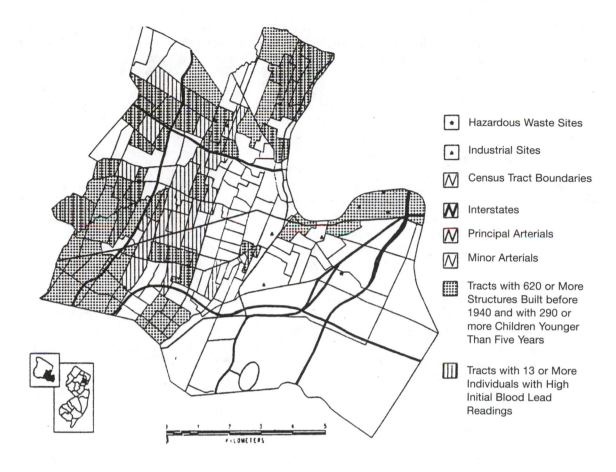

Figure 4–14 Occurrences of high blood lead, expected versus actual, for Newark/East Orange/Irvington study area, New Jersey

some areas, such as northeastern Newark and tracts extending into East Orange, the patterns overlap, pointing out census tracts that have both predicted high risk and large numbers of actual cases. In other areas, such as the border of Newark with Irvington, several counties with low predicted risk contain large numbers of cases. However, the opposite is true for southwestern Irvington, where many model-predicted high-risk census tracts do not have large numbers of cases. One possibility for this inconsistency is variability associated with small numbers. Alternatively, like other ecologic analyses, the results suggest questions about other possibilities. For example, other variables, such as access to lead screening, lead in drinking water, socioeconomic status, education, and ethnicity may be associated with reported elevated lead levels. The TRI and hazardous waste site data may have omitted several categories of environmental lead sources, such as abandoned industrial sites, vacant houses, and illegal smelting activities. Using GIS technology, investigators can find and add databases containing such information and generate new and improved models of lead risk that they can later compare with actual cases. As the models get better,

they become more useful for targeting lead prevention efforts.

As a follow-up to the pilot project, the NJDEPE began looking at other potential variables. For example, the NJDEPE Bureau of Safe Drinking Water evaluated the presence of lead in the drinking water of 22 New Jersey public schools.[14] Some of the systems had elevated lead levels, most from first-flush samples. At least one school had drinking water levels exceeding EPA standards even after the water had been running. The project can incorporate these data into its GIS so that the predicted risk model includes data on drinking-water exposure at school by children living in each census tract. Another variable that investigators can add to their model is air exposure to lead. The NJDEPE maintains a database containing permitted levels of air emissions and an air-monitoring system for lead. Still another variable that might help predict lead exposure is soil exposure associated with residual lead contamination from urban industrial sources. Investigators can measure lead concentrations in soil samples taken from areas near industrial sites. As with the drinking-water data, the project can incorporate air and soil information into its GIS, along with climatic data and assumptions on lead deposition, to create better risk models.[14] These improved models can then be useful for other communities interested in targeting their educational and lead-screening efforts.

In 1997, the North Carolina Ad Hoc Study Group on Lead Screening Guidelines showed how a GIS analysis, incorporating the CDC guidelines, could be helpful in developing a statewide lead-screening plan.[16] The Study Group used two attribute databases for its analysis. They obtained housing age data from the U.S. Bureau of the Census and lead-screening data from the North Carolina Childhood Lead Poisoning Prevention Program. The lead program had been collecting and maintaining data on childhood blood lead levels for the previous five years. Because the lead-screening data were aggregated to the city, county, and ZIP code levels, the study was unable to do a geographic analysis below the ZIP code level. Even if lead reports by street address had been available, matching lead records at the street address level would have been difficult because many rural counties in North Carolina lacked numbered street addresses. In addition, the study group felt that patients and physicians would be able to recognize ZIP code boundaries more easily than census tract or census block group boundaries.[16] For example, when North Carolina health care providers perform lead blood tests, they request patients to report their residence ZIP code on the lead-screening form. Also, determining whether a child required a test, on the basis of living in a high-risk area, would be performed more easily by asking about ZIP code of residence than by determining census tract or block group information.[16]

To perform the analysis, the Study Group used a spatial database containing five-digit ZIP code boundaries obtained from a commercial source, Geographic Data Technology, Inc. (GDT). In the first step of the analysis, the Study Group created a map of North Carolina ZIP codes with at least 27 percent of houses built before 1950. Of the 729 mappable ZIP codes, 123 (16.9 percent) met this criterion. These were not concentrated in any particular area of the state. Many counties had no ZIP codes with older housing.

Next, using the census data, the Study Group produced a map of North Carolina Census block groups with at least 27 percent of houses built before 1950. Of the 5,695 block groups, 1,534 (26.9 percent) met this criterion. Unlike the ZIP code map, the new map showed that only one county contained no block groups with older housing. After completing this map, the Study Group became concerned that the ZIP code analysis had missed many areas with older housing. To correct this, they used GIS software to overlay the ZIP code map on the block group map, allowing them to determine which ZIP codes contained whole or partial block groups with older housing. The overlay analysis revealed that

466 (63.9 percent) of the 729 ZIP codes contained block groups (whole or partial) with older housing. The Study Group used the map resulting from this analysis as a "base map" to designate ZIP code areas for universal screening.[16]

In the next two steps of the analysis, the Study Group used the lead report database to set criteria for adding or deleting some of these 466 ZIP code areas from designation as areas for universal screening. Using GIS software, they mapped the prevalence of elevated blood lead levels for 91,780 one- and two-year-olds, based on 1995–1996 data from the universal screening program. They overlaid this map, showing ZIP codes with at least a 12 percent prevalence of lead levels of at least 10 μg/dl, on the base map. Next, for each ZIP code, the Study Group computed confidence intervals for the elevated lead level prevalence. They deleted ZIP codes with at least 100 children screened where upper limits of the confidence interval revealed less than 12 percent elevated blood lead levels.

Figure 4–15 is the resulting map with the final screening recommendations.[16] On this map, the shaded polygons are 415 (56.9 percent) of the 729 ZIP code areas designated for universal screening. The other 314 nonshaded ZIP code polygons are areas in which children should receive targeted screening. On the basis of this analysis, the Study Group developed a Lead Risk Assessment Questionnaire for clinical staff to determine which children required lead screening. The questionnaire contained six questions—one on residence ZIP code and the other five on lead poisoning risk. Two of the risk questions specifically asked about age of housing. All children in the universal screening ZIP codes required testing. Children living in targeted ZIP codes did not require testing if the answers to the risk questions were negative.[16]

As we noted in Chapter 3, spatial aggregation to areas as large as ZIP codes or even smaller census tracts comes with a trade-off. Within these large areas, there can be a great deal of variation in housing age and sociodemographic factors.[16] Analysis at this level can potentially miss many children with high risks for lead exposure. Street address matching, with analysis at a lower level of aggregation, such as census block groups, is preferable for designating high-risk areas for universal lead screening but requires good spatial data with street address information in the attribute database.[16]

A Florida analysis, at a smaller area level, shows how GIS technology can be useful for developing childhood blood lead–screening guidelines tailored to specific local needs. For many communities, the 1997 CDC guidelines recommending screening on the basis of a 1950 housing age cutoff make sense because houses this age and older are more likely to contain paint with high levels of lead.[16,17] However, paint continued to contain dangerous amounts of lead until the

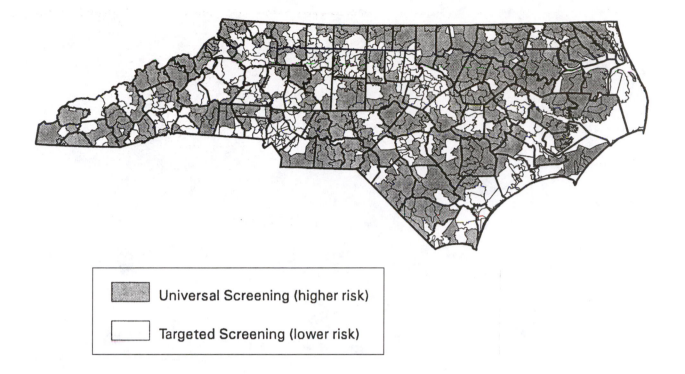

Figure 4–15 Final lead screening recommendations for North Carolina ZIP codes, 1997

mid-1970s. In other communities, especially in places like Florida, where the growing population purchased many new houses between 1950 and 1970, many other children exposed to paint are at risk of lead poisoning.[16] The Bureau of Environmental Epidemiology of the Florida Department of Health was able to use GIS technology as a tool to help develop screening guidelines appropriate for Florida, based on this additional population of children at risk for lead toxicity from exposure to pre-1970 housing. Figure 4–16, a choropleth map of Duval County, Florida, depicts census block groups as polygons and reports childhood lead-poisoning cases as black dots. (Cases are individuals under six years of age with venous blood lead levels of at least 10 µg/dl.) To create the map, investigators linked U.S. Bureau of the Census housing data with lead-poisoning data. Then they used GIS software to develop the combination of percentages of housing age per block group that best fit with the distribution of residences of reported lead cases. Shaded block groups have either 27 percent or more pre-1950 housing or 68 percent or more pre-1970 housing. This map was then useful in focusing screening programs that maximized the number of at-risk children tested while minimizing the use of scarce health department resources.[17]

A similar project in Santa Clara County, California, used three variables—pre-1950s housing, children under six years

of age, and poverty—to define lead "hot zones."[18] For the map in Figure 4–17, investigators defined lead hot zones as census tracts above the 50th percentile for all three variables. They obtained attribute data for the map from the U.S. Bureau of the Census. The black dots represent reported lead cases, with their size related to the number of cases in each census tract. Although the risk of lead poisoning is probably associated with more than the three variables used, the local public health department found that the map proved useful in directing its prevention efforts and in making screening recommendations to local health care providers.[18]

A time series of maps of the geographic distribution of mean childhood blood lead levels shows how GIS technology can help monitor health risks for communities exposed to lead in their environment.[19] The Bunker Hill Mining and Metallurgical Complex site encompasses 21 square miles along Interstate 90 in the Silver Valley area of Shoshone County in northern Idaho. The site includes the now active Bunker Hill Mine and the inactive metallurgical and smelting facility (together called the Bunker Hill Complex) and the cities of Kellogg, Pinehurst, Smelterville, and Wardner. These cities have a combined population of over 5,000.[20]

In 1917, the Bunker Hill lead smelter began producing lead, cadmium, silver, and alloys of these heavy metals. Smelter operations resulted in fugitive and stack emissions

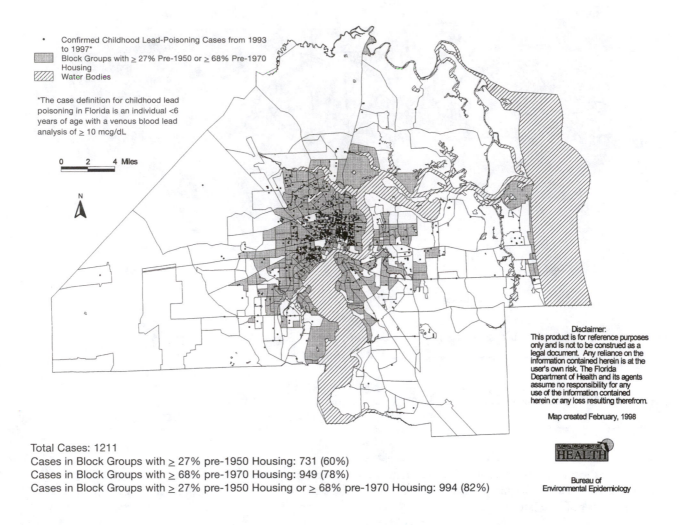

Figure 4–16 Development of childhood blood lead-screening guidelines, Duval County, Florida, 1998

of metals and sulfur dioxide. To reduce the amount of heavy metals released into the air, the smelter used pollution control devices, known as bag houses, to recover metals from furnace stack emissions. In September 1973, a fire destroyed most of the bag house at the lead smelter operated by Gulf Resources and Chemical Corporation (Gulf). The company decided to bypass the bag house and continued to produce lead. This decision resulted in a dramatic increase in emissions. During the first three months of 1974, the facility emitted approximately 73 tons of lead per month into the environment, heavily contaminating air and soil in the Silver Valley region. In 1974, the average blood lead level for children under 12 years of age within the site boundaries was 65 micrograms of lead per deciliter of blood, over six times the CDC's current level of concern. Residential area soil analyses revealed higher lead levels in communities close to the smelter. The Bunker Hill facility closed in 1981. In 1983, the EPA placed the 21–square-mile site, including the Pinehurst, Page, Smelterville, Kellogg, and Warner communities, on the National Priorities List.

The site has widespread lead contamination from mine tailings, emissions from the Bunker Hill smelter complex, and blowing dust from tailings piles and other barren areas. Barren hillsides and open areas within the site contribute to erosion and blowing-dust problems. As a result, extensive soil contamination remains in the residential areas in the affected communities, as well as in the surrounding nonpopulated areas. In addition, there are high lead levels in house dust. Historical mining activities and continued leaching of metals from mine and mill wastes contribute to extensive heavy-metals contamination of groundwater and surface water. Cleanup is occurring. The bulk of the Smelter

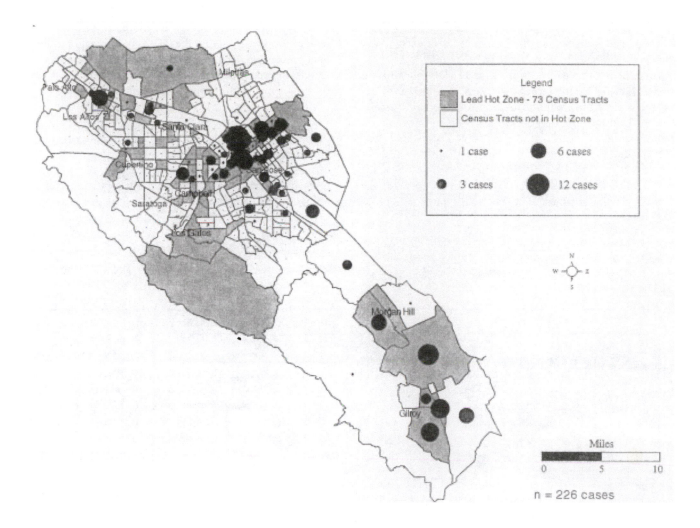

*Census tracts in the lead hot zones ranked above the 50th percentile on all three indicators: poverty, population under age six, and pre-1950 housing.

Figure 4–17 Lead hot zones and childhood lead-poisoning cases, Santa Clara County, California, 1995

Complex has been demolished, and a Closure Cap area is being constructed. In addition, the EPA is beginning the removal of contaminated soils from the surrounding gulches for consolidation under the Closure Cap.[19]

The ATSDR performed two cohort studies on potential health effects from lead exposure, one involving smelter workers and the other involving children living in the area at the time of high lead releases. The first study looked at females who had worked in the smelter in the 1970s and compared them with an unexposed population.[19,21] The workers had significantly higher amounts of lead in their bones and decreased bone formation and density. In addition, the former workers had more neurological symptoms and reported being diagnosed more often with hypertension, anemia, arthritis, and osteoporosis.[19,21] The second study looked at previous and current site residents who were children at the time of the peak lead releases, comparing them with an unexposed population of Spokane, Washington, residents. The exposed cohort had significantly increased neurological symptoms, poorer performance on neurobehavioral tests, more difficulty conceiving children, increased anxiety, and more reported illnesses, such as anemia, hypertension, and arthritis.[22]

Considering these findings, the ATSDR questioned whether GIS technology might assist in monitoring the affected communities, helping to determine populations eligible for health evaluation and referral. Using mean blood levels as an indicator of risk, the choropleth maps in Figure 4–18 display mean blood lead levels for children aged 9 months to 9 years in these communities over several years.[19] Cross-sectional surveys of the five communities over six years supply the attribute data. The maps categorize poly-

gons by shades and patterns on the basis of public health intervention levels set by the CDC guidelines for childhood lead prevention. As these maps clearly display, mean blood lead levels declined markedly for all five communities over the six-year period, although data were not available for two of the intervening years for Pinehurst. The proportion of surveyed children with levels in the most serious categories (those above 40 μg/dl) ranged from 60 to 100 percent for all communities in 1974. This range decreased to 0 to 1.8 percent in 1983.[19] Such geographic analyses, using GIS technology, are very helpful in determining populations for evaluation even 15 years later.

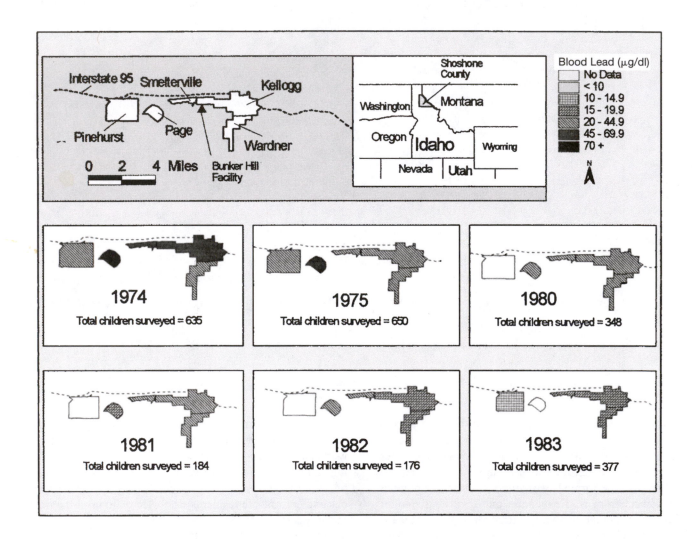

Figure 4–18 Geographic distribution of mean blood lead levels by year in children residing in communities near the Bunker Hill Lead Smelter Site, 1974–1983

DRINKING-WATER POLLUTION: USING GIS TO TARGET INTERVENTIONS TO PROTECT COMMUNITIES FROM HEALTH RISKS DUE TO SEPTIC CONTAMINATION, NITRATES, AND VOLATILE ORGANIC COMPOUNDS

The Pollution Prevention Act of 1990 (U.S. Code Title 42, Chapter 133) defines pollution prevention as any practice that reduces the amount of any hazardous substance, pollutant, or contaminant entering any waste stream or otherwise released into the environment (including fugitive emissions) before recycling, treatment, or disposal. According to the definition, pollution prevention reduces the hazards to public health and the environment associated with the release of such substances, pollutants, or contaminants.[23] Pollution prevention is a logical use for GIS for several reasons. First, GIS overlays of environmental, health, and demographic data can identify persons and communities at risk of environmental exposure from industry. Public health officials can share this information with businesses to encourage them to use less toxic chemicals. Second, GIS technology can help officials identify and characterize many non–manufacturing-related potential sources of drinking water pollution, such as sewers, landfills, underground storage tanks, and chemical storage facilities. Using GIS mapping technology, public health officials can evaluate groundwater quality and define populations at risk for exposure—for example, when an industrial plant releases a plume of hazardous materials into the groundwater supply.[23] Third, environmental health GIS applications can provide health departments with a revenue source because the resulting geographic analysis is useful for private environmental consulting firms.[23]

In 1998, the EPA gave the National Association of County and City Health Officials (NACCHO) a grant to study the use of GIS in pollution prevention, including how to integrate the technology with existing local health department programs. Later that year, NACCHO conducted three local health department case studies using GIS for pollution prevention. Study sites included Needham, Massachusetts; Lincoln-Lancaster, Nebraska; and Hutchinson, Kansas. These three case studies showed how GIS technology could help health officials identify communities at disproportionate risk, protect public wellheads and surface water from failing septic systems, and provide assistance to businesses and the public to reduce pollution risk.[23] The Needham study, described below, and the Hutchinson study, described later in this chapter, addressed septic and volatile organic compound (VOC) pollution respectively. Later in this chapter, we will describe how the Lincoln study tackled the issue of communities at disproportionate risk, or environmental equity. These studies also illustrate that even small health departments have the capacity to use GIS technology to protect their communities from environmental pollutants.

Septic Pollution

Needham, Massachusetts, with a population of 28,000, is a small suburban community located 10 miles west of Boston. It has a small local health department, with five staff and an annual budget of $300,000. Before 1997, failing household septic (waste) systems posed a threat to municipal drinking water wells and surface water. In 1997, the Massachusetts Department of Environmental Protection (DEP) gave the Needham Health Department (NHD) a $20,000 grant to implement a management and loan program that provided incentives for inspections and upgrades of these failing systems. To accomplish this, the NHD used GIS technology to identify household septic systems for priority targeting. The GIS software mapped households with septic systems and overlaid environmentally sensitive areas containing surface water and wellheads (see Figure 4–19). The map helped the NHD prioritize areas for pollution prevention and allocate loan funds to household septic systems that posed the greatest risk. The State Water Pollution and Abatement Trust and the DEP then offered residents with failing septic systems in sensitive areas long-term, low-interest loans to upgrade their systems.

To create the map in Figure 4–19, the NHD used TIGER files (for Norfolk County, Massachusetts) as the spatial foundation database. Attribute data came from several sources, including the Board of Health, the Conservation Commission, and the Department of Public Works. Data included household septic system locations, type, pumping history, date of upgrades, and date of last inspection. The NHD employed two college interns to sort through hard-copy records and enter the necessary information into a Microsoft Excel spreadsheet. The NHD also worked with these agencies to identify environmentally sensitive areas. Once the data were entered, the NHD used its GIS to map wellhead protection zones II and III, draw a 500-foot buffer around the Charles River, and plot household septic systems. The NHD then used this map to prioritize failing septic systems for its program.

Of the 10,000 homes in Needham, 800 used septic systems. The NHD mailed packets to all septic system owners containing the map, education on proper septic system maintenance, and information on the availability of the low-interest loan program to fix failing systems within the protection zones. Additionally, the NHD convened public meetings to discuss the map and the program. Because of these efforts, 30 residents informed NHD that they were interested in applying for the loans. As funds were limited, the NHD used its GIS application to prioritize septic systems for the program. For septic system owners located within the most sensitive environmental areas, the NHD provided additional information, including how to have their system inspected. The NHD also encouraged these owners to apply for the low-interest loans to upgrade their septic system if it was failing.

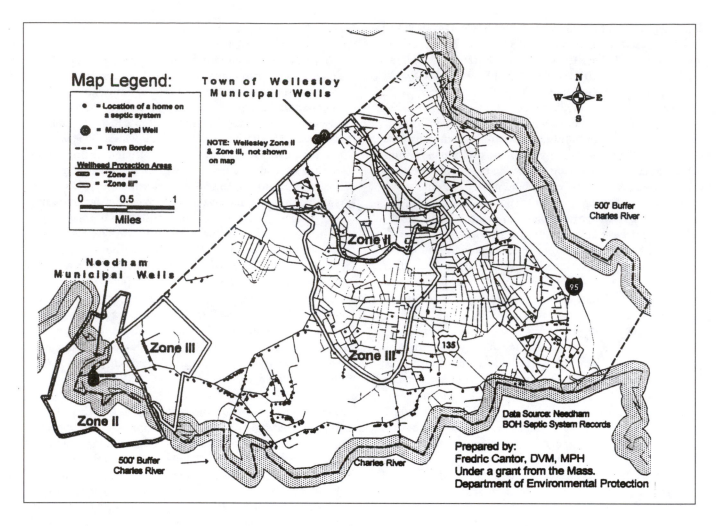

Figure 4–19 Wellhead and source water protection zones in Needham, Massachusetts, January 1999

As funds allow, the NHD is giving additional residents a chance to participate in the loan program.

The cost of developing the Needham GIS application was within the reach of a typical small health department. Hardware included a $3,500 desktop, 200-megahertz (MHz) personal computer (PC) with a CD-ROM drive, color printer, and scanner. GIS software (MapInfo Professional 4.1), including the TIGER files, cost the NHD $1,200, and the health department director spent $700 on a basic GIS training course. Community notification and education cost the NHD an additional $1,060 for printing and mailing.

This low-cost GIS application has had additional benefits for Needham residents and officials. They now know the number of residential septic systems within their community, and they understand the impact that failing systems can have on their health and environment. The GIS application will help health officials to track and educate owners of fail-

ing septic systems and, if necessary, take enforcement actions. Additionally, by mapping environmentally sensitive areas containing private septic systems, the GIS application will be useful in identifying priority areas for expansion of the Needham sewer system. Future versions of the GIS application could incorporate additional environmental health risks, such as underground storage tanks and hazardous waste sites.[23]

Nitrates

Babies consuming formula prepared from drinking water with high concentrates of nitrates are at risk for methemoglobinemia, a condition characterized by low levels of oxygen in the blood. Relatively moderate exposures to nitrates can subject these infants to significant morbidity and even mortality. In agricultural areas with porous soils, fertilizer use can result in groundwater contamination with nitrates, leading to contamination of well water. As illustrated in a GIS analysis conducted in Iowa, shallower depths to bedrock level are associated with higher nitrate levels[24] (see Figure 4–20).To create this map, the Linn County, Iowa, Health Department first measured nitrate levels in well water samples taken between 1991 and 1996. They combined these data with depth information on the bedrock layer that they obtained from the Iowa Geological Survey. Such maps are useful for zoning and planning the location of additional wells to reduce the risk of drinking-water contamination for new residents.

A Chautauqua County, New York, Health Department study illustrates how health departments can use GIS technology to identify and target infants at risk of exposure to prevent them from developing this condition (see Figure 4–21).First, the health department identified and mapped the location of nitrate-contaminated groundwater in Clymer, a town in rural, southwestern New York. Much of the town obtained drinking water from a public well. Private homes in outlying areas, including homes within the Clymer Water District, obtained their drinking water from private wells. Because public and private wells tapped into the same aquifer, they were both subject to the same contamination. Next, after incorporating the New York State Electronic Birth Certificate Database into its GIS application, and by overlaying the groundwater map with the location of families with newborns, the health department instantly identified newborns

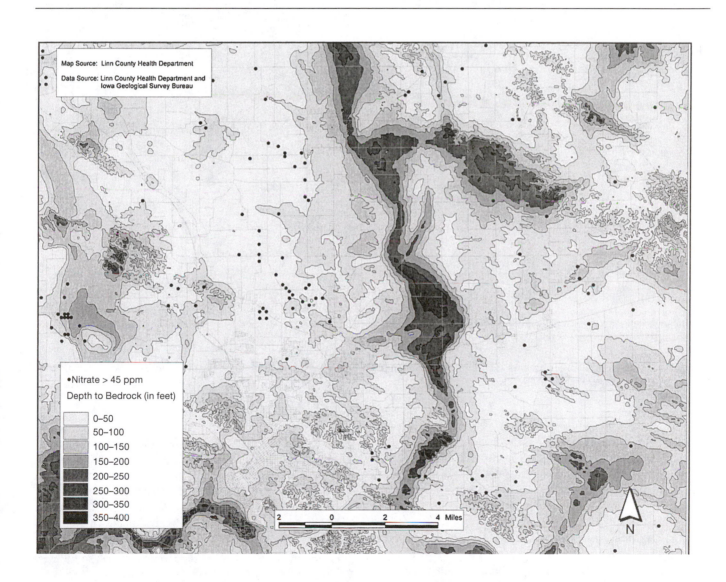

Figure 4–20 Water Pollution: Elevated nitrate levels in relation to bedrock depth, Linn County, Iowa, 1991–1996

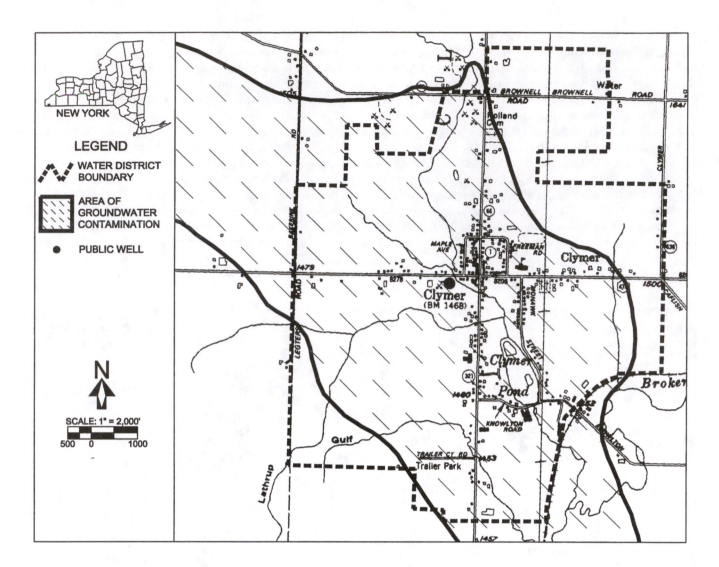

Planimetric base map is from NYSDEC 7.5 Minute Quadrangle Images. Residences, symbolized by small filled squares, are served either by the public well or individual private wells.

Figure 4–21 Public notification to families with newborns at risk for methemoglobinemia from drinking-water exposure, Clymer, New York, 1996–1998

at risk of exposure. This allowed the health department to notify these families of the risk, protecting the infants. Additionally, the health department used the map to notify and educate health care providers and water customers in the area.[25]

Volatile Organic Compounds

Drinking-water wells, frequently subject to contamination by improperly disposed hazardous chemicals,[26] can pose a threat to human health. The ATSDR and other environmental and public health agencies have recommended against the use of wells contaminated by hazardous substances in concentrations that approach or exceed levels potentially associated with adverse health outcomes. In addition, the CDC has recommended that public health and environmental officials require the proper closure of contaminated drinking-water wells after providing alternative uncontaminated water supplies. Specifically, the closure orders should include requirements for properly sealing contaminated drinking-water wells, such as filling the well completely with concrete, cement grout, neat cement, or clays. To prevent further human exposure, the alternative sources of water could require the construction of new water supplies.[26,27]

Unfortunately, because our public health system does not routinely monitor private residential wells, human exposures to high concentrations of contaminants can occur before public health officials detect the contamination. Exposure to some of these hazardous materials such as VOCs, by inhalation, ingestion, or skin contact, can increase the risk of cancer or other adverse health effects to people who rely on the wells for drinking water.[26] A study in Maryland demonstrates that GIS technology may be helpful in identifying potentially contaminated private wells even when routine private well monitoring is unavailable.[28]

The Harford County, Maryland, Health Department has routinely sampled groundwater for VOCs to identify areas of groundwater pollution in need of remediation. Through this sampling program, the health department detected 13 organic compounds, including tetrachloroethene, trichlorofluoromethane, dichloroethene, and trichloroethane, in groundwater located near a community landfill.[28] Because of concerns about the potential spread of contamination, the health department sampled groundwater in tax parcels either adjacent to, down gradient from the landfill or at the request of property owners. Using GIS software, the health department then mapped the results for parcels containing private wells within one mile of the landfill, summarizing samples collected from 1986 to 1998. Figure 4–22 is a choropleth map with parcel polygons shaded on the basis of groundwater VOC contamination. Further studies identified VOC levels above the EPA's maximum contamination limit in three private water supplies located within the sampled parcels. VOC contamination may have reached one of these wells, in the southwest quadrant, due to contours of the land, with groundwater flowing into it from the landfill. Contamination of the other two wells, in the northeast quadrant, was probably associated with a nearby leaking underground storage tank. This monitoring program using GIS technology has been effective in targeting potentially contaminated wells for evaluation, and the health department's groundwater protection program continues to monitor contaminated tax parcels and adjacent parcels.[28]

Some communities, such as Hutchinson, Kansas, with a population of 40,000, are completely dependent on groundwater for their drinking-water supply. In such communities, GIS technology is an effective tool for planning for water system development because it is useful in developing models predicting future sites of groundwater VOC contamination. Figure 4–23 is a map of Hutchinson and surrounding areas, showing current and predicted future groundwater sources for municipal wells.[29] The health department produced this map for planning and educational purposes. Although Hutchinson has 20 municipal wells, it is unable to use three of them due to VOC contamination. Produced in 1998, the map predicts the source of Hutchinson's water over the ensuing five years. To make this map, health department officials used several data sets, including transportation, hydrology, tax parcels, and public wells and zones of capture. To create five-year zones (in 300-day intervals) of capture, the health department developed a computer model using particle tracking to simulate groundwater movement as a consequence of natural flow and groundwater withdrawal by the public water system and industrial and irrigation wells. The concentric lines around each well represent the area of the underground aquifer needed to provide 300 days of pumping, while the shaded areas represent the aquifer portion needed for the next five years, approximately 1,800 days of pumping. The lines flowing out from each well represent the path of a water molecule traveling toward the well. These models are useful for planning on how to protect the only source of drinking water for this community, an aquifer vulnerable to VOC contamination due to sandy soils and a shallow water table.[29]

ENVIRONMENTAL EQUITY: COMMUNITIES AT DISPROPORTIONATE RISK

During the past two decades, the publication of studies identifying an unequal distribution of environmental hazards across racial, ethnic, and socioeconomic groups have led to nationwide concerns about environmental inequity.[30] Contributing to these concerns have been the disparities between health status indicators, such as morbidity and mortality, and social class and ethnicity. For example, people from households with an annual income of at least $25,000 live an average of three to seven years longer, depending on gender and race, than people from households with annual incomes of less than $10,000.[31] In addition, the African American infant mortality rate is more than twice that for the white population. Compared to whites in the United States, African Americans have a 40 percent greater death rate from heart disease and a 30 percent greater death rate for all cancers.[31] These disparities have not been due just to differences in access to health care. For example, even though African American women have a higher mammography-screening rate compared to whites, their death rate from breast cancer is higher.[31]

Although such health status disparities, which have continued to increase, are undoubtedly due to the interaction of many factors, such as health care access, genetic variations, health behaviors, and occupation, they are probably also due to differential environmental exposures. The *Healthy People*

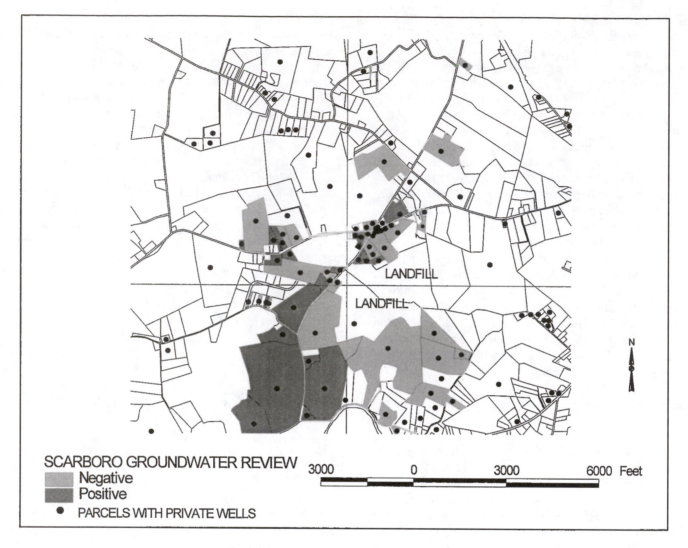

Figure 4–22 Monitoring volatile organic compounds in private wells near a community landfill by tax parcel, Harford County, Maryland, 1986–1998

2010 report holds individual behaviors and environmental factors responsible for about 70 percent of all premature deaths in the United States.[31] Specifically, *Healthy People 2010* states:

> The physical environment can harm individual and community health, especially when individuals and communities are exposed to toxic substances; irritants; infectious agents; and physical hazards in homes, schools, and worksites. Developing and implementing policies and preventive interventions that effectively address these determinants of health can reduce the burden of illness, enhance quality of life, and increase longevity.[31(pp.18–19)]

In 1987, in a report frequently cited in environmental equity literature, the Commission for Racial Justice of the United Church of Christ (UCC) documented an association between the presence of hazardous waste sites (specifically waste treatment, storage, and disposal facilities, or TSDFs) and racial and socioeconomic characteristics of surrounding communities.[30,32,33] The UCC study used two sources of data containing the location of the waste sites, the Environmental Information Limited's Directory of Industrial and Hazardous Waste Firms, and the EPA's computerized database, the 1986 Hazardous Waste Data Management System (HWDMS). On the basis of these data sets, the study evaluated the location of hazardous waste facilities in relation to five-digit ZIP code population data. Variables of interest in-

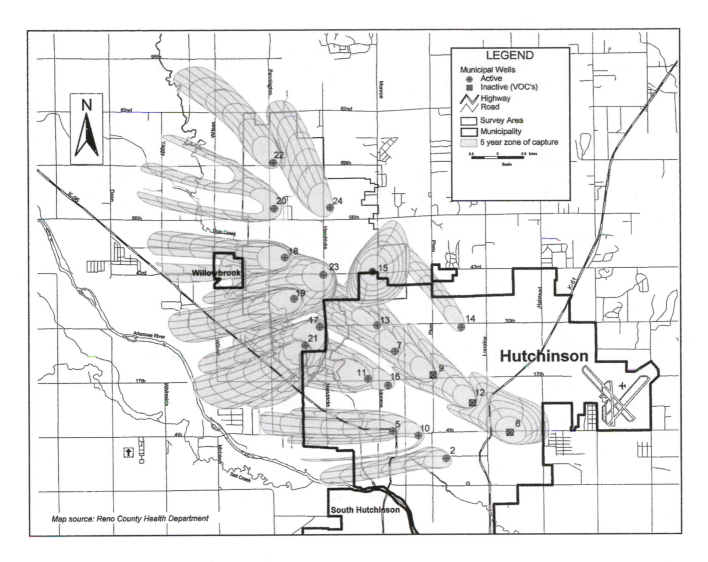

Figure 4–23 A computer simulation of groundwater withdrawal patterns for public water supply wells, Hutchinson, Kansas, 1998–2003

cluded percentage of minority population and two surrogate measures of socioeconomic status: mean household income and mean value of owner-occupied housing. The final report stated that ZIP codes with one commercial TSDF operating in 1986 had percentages of minority populations twice those of ZIP codes without operating TSDFs. In addition, the report stated that the percentage of the minority population was more significant than socioeconomic factors. Their conclusion: "Race proved to be the most significant among variables tested in association with the location of commercial hazardous waste facilities."[32,33(p.xiii)]

This study and others, in addition to the activities of the burgeoning environmental justice movement, have contributed to a national debate about the extent to which low-income and minority populations suffer disproportionately from exposure to environmental hazards.[30] In 1994, President Clinton responded with Executive Order 12898, requiring all federal agencies to adopt the principle of environmental justice as part of their mission. Each federal agency would accomplish this "by identifying and addressing, as appropriate, disproportionately high and adverse human health or environmental effects of its programs, policies, and activities on minority populations and low-income populations in programmatic decisions."[34] The executive order created an interagency working group to assist in coordinating research by, and stimulating cooperation among, the EPA, the Department of Health and Human Services, and the Department of Housing and Urban Development. To comply with the order, the EPA created the office on Environmental Justice.

To evaluate whether environmental risks to health vary by race, ethnicity, and socioeconomic status, we need to know whether these populations suffer from an increased exposure to environmental hazards. Answers to these questions could lead to policies that prevent such disparate exposures, leading to reduced health disparities.[35] Over the past few years, the development of GIS technology has helped federal, state, and local agencies and academic institutions investigate potential environmental inequities because questions about whether minorities suffer disproportionately from exposure to environmental hazards are inherently spatial. GIS technology is particularly suited to help answer spatial questions such as "Who lives how far from the hazards, and why are communities and hazards located where they are?"[30(p.18)] Specifically, GIS technology has the capacity to

- Integrate multiple sources of data, such as population data and environmental data
- Employ spatial analysis techniques, such as overlays and buffering
- Develop and evaluate models of exposure, such as plume dispersion models
- Portray the results of any evaluation in an easy-to-understand, visual format[30]

Given these capacities, the EPA has begun to promote the use of GIS technology to evaluate the extent to which environmental hazards disproportionately affect communities.[36]

While some GIS studies have found that racial/ethnic minorities and low-income populations suffer disproportionately from exposure to environmental toxins, others have found no associations, and some have even found that white and higher-income communities suffer more. These inconsistencies have several probable causes, including

- The spatial resolution and scale of the geographic area studied
- The type/quality of data used (e.g., accurate address information)
- The measures of exposure

Several investigations have shown that the spatial resolution and the geographic scale of GIS environmental equity studies can affect the results. At the smaller, census tract resolution, a South Carolina study found no significant association between racial minorities or low-income populations and the location of toxic facilities. However, using the larger, county resolution, the same study found a significantly positive association between urban, white, middle-income counties and toxic facilities.[30,37] Another study, in Pittsburgh, found that as the spatial resolution changed from census block

groups to census tracts to ZIP codes, the association strengthened between the presence of minorities and the number of nearby toxic sites. Conversely, these changes in spatial resolution weakened the associations between the number of nearby toxic sites and per capita income and population density.[30,38] One reason for these differences is that the larger the spatial resolution, the greater the heterogeneity of the population in the area. Fortunately, GIS technology can solve this problem, but only if the incorporated population and environmental toxin data contain accurate address information. If they do, GIS applications can analyze geocoded data at much finer levels of resolution, including block groups and blocks.

Studies in Minnesota and Ohio illustrate how the scale of analysis can influence the results of environmental equity studies. In the Minneapolis area, analysis at a county-level scale found a stronger relationship between minority populations and toxic sites, while the same analysis at a city-level scale found a stronger association between income and toxic site locations.[30,39] The Ohio study found a positive association between minority populations and toxic sites (and toxic release volumes) at the state level, with the opposite (inverse) association at the metropolitan (Cleveland) scale. Interestingly, at the metropolitan scale, as in Minneapolis, the Ohio study found a positive association between low-income populations and the location of toxic sites in the Cleveland area.[40]

The most common approaches to evaluating environmental equity using GIS technology are similar to the 1987 UCC approach and are based on the proximity of specific populations to environmental hazards. The "spatial coincidence" method compares the racial/ethnic makeup of populations in geographic areas (such as census tracts or block groups) containing potential environmental hazards, such as TRI facilities, with the racial/ethnic makeup of populations living in hazard-free areas.[30] (See Chapter 2 for a discussion of TRI facilities.) An alternative method uses buffering, by comparing the racial/ethnic makeup of populations living at varying distances around hazardous sites.[30] Buffers can be linear—for example, varying distances surrounding a high-power transmission line—or they can be circular—for example, circles of varying sizes around a toxic emitter (see Figures 3–11 and 3–12).

Figure 4–24 illustrates the two methods. Polygons represent block groups within the city of Minneapolis, with superimposed numbers representing the percentage below poverty for each specific block group. In the simplest, spatial coincidence method, the percentage of the population that is low income within the block group containing the TRI facility is the measure of environmental equity: in this case, 26 percent. The alternative method, using a buffer, incorporates all block groups overlapping the buffer into the analyses by studying the portion of the block groups within the buffer.

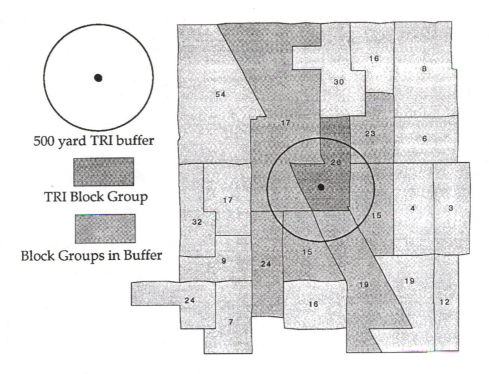

Figure 4–24 Two measures of proximity: spatial coincidence and buffering

In this example, the environmental equity measure would be lower than 26 percent because the additional overlapping block groups have lower percentages of low-income residents.

Besides economic measures, polygon shades can also represent the racial/ethnic makeup of specific geographic areas. Figure 4–25, another map of Minneapolis, shades block group polygons depending on the percentage of the block group population that is African American. This map is possible because the incorporated block group data contain information on race/ethnicity, including African American, American Indian, Hispanic American, and Asian American populations, in addition to age and income. The EPA's TRI database supplied the location of TRI facilities for the map. Figure 4–25 indicates that the African American population is concentrated in two areas, south and northwest of the center of the city. Cities characterized by such segregated patterns serve as good cases for studies of environmental equity because of the large spatial variation in population characteristics. The circles on the map represent TRI facilities, which appear to cluster in the northeast part of the city and in a secondary site west of the Mississippi River and just north of the central city.

Table 4–5 compares populations inside (nearby, or "proximate") with populations outside block groups containing TRI

facilities. The numbers represent the percentage of populations below the poverty level by race/ethnicity, age (children below age five), and total population for the block groups. Dividing the percentage of the population of interest within block groups containing TRI facilities by the percentage outside those block groups gives the proximity ratio: a simple measure of environmental equity.

The results suggest that within Minneapolis, populations living in block groups with TRI facilities have a higher likelihood of being poor (as defined by living below the poverty level) than those living in block groups without TRI facilities. While this is true for the total population, the likelihood is strongest for the white population, which is twice as likely to be poor if living in block groups with TRIs. Compared to Asian Americans, American Indians, and African Americans, this likelihood is also stronger for Hispanic Americans and young children, although not as strong as for the white population. Although, like other GIS studies, this simple spatial coincidence study does not provide reasons for these differences, it does imply a complex relationship between race/ethnicity, income, and location of TRI facilities. Investigators suggested that understanding the industrial history of the city may explain some of these relationships.[30,39]

How would the study results differ if investigators used the alternative, buffering methodology? Figure 4–26 illus-

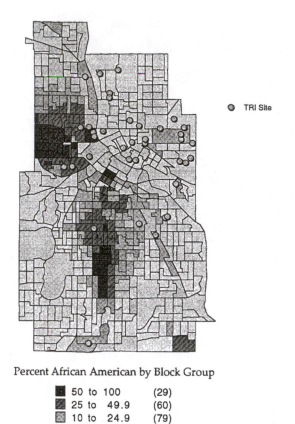

Percent African American by Block Group

■	50 to 100	(29)
▨	25 to 49.9	(60)
▨	10 to 24.9	(79)
▢	5 to 9.99	(63)
▢	0 to 4.99	(245)

● TRI Site

Figure 4–25 City of Minneapolis, percent African American and TRI sites. Numbers in parentheses represent counts of block groups in each category.

in Figure 4–26 shows only 1,000-yard buffers, they performed the analyses for several size buffers, including 100 yards, 500 yards, and 1,000 yards. Next, they identified the block groups either entirely or partially within each buffer and used the population information on these block groups to estimate the characteristics of the populations within each buffered area. To develop these estimates, investigators summed the population estimates for block groups weighted by their fraction inside the buffer.

Table 4–6, using a format similar to that of Table 4–5 in the spatial coincidence analysis, compares populations inside (proximate) with populations outside buffers around TRI facilities. The numbers in the table represent the percentage of populations below the poverty level by race/ethnicity, age (children below age 5), and total population within and outside each buffer. Dividing the percentage of the population of interest within the buffers containing TRI facilities by the percentage outside those buffers gives the proximity ratio: the measure of environmental equity.

Table 4–6 and Table 4–7, a summary table, show that the results vary by buffer size and methodology. At the 100-yard distance, the proximity ratios are similar to those in the coincidence method, with whites having the highest ratio, followed by Hispanics. Extending the buffer to 500 yards causes virtually no change, probably because block groups themselves are not much larger than the area within the 500-yard buffer (see Figure 4–24). At the 1,000-yard distance, however, the results differ from the other buffers and the coincidence analysis. At this distance, the proximity ratio markedly increases for all population subgroups, with especially large increases for American Indians, Asian Americans, and Hispanic Americans. Buffers this large are significantly larger than block groups and in fact contain several block groups. Of course, extending the buffer much further, to the city limits of Minneapolis, would reduce the proximity ratio to unity because the poverty rates within a buffer this large would represent the average poverty rate for the entire city.

Obviously, results from studies using this methodology could vary greatly in any direction depending on the prede-

trates the buffering approach to the same Minneapolis data. This time the polygon shades depict the percentage of the population in each block group living below the poverty line. Investigators first assigned predetermined, circular buffers of various distances around each TRI site. Although the map

Table 4–5 Poverty Rates, Proximate and Nonproximate Block Groups, for Different Races and Young Children

Proximity Measure	Whites	African Americans	American Indians	Asians	Hispanics	Population Aged 0–5	Total
Within TRIBG	22	43	64	52	47	47	30
Outside TRIBG	11	40	52	45	26	32	18
Proximity ratio*	1.98	1.07	1.23	1.15	1.80	1.47	1.67

*The proximity ratio is the ratio of the within-TRIBG (Toxic Release Inventory block groups) poverty rate and the outside-TRIBG poverty rate.

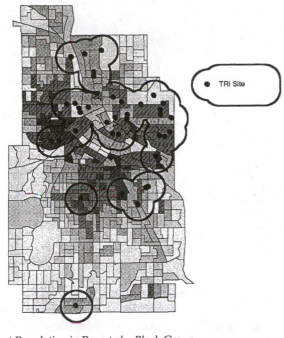

Percent Population in Poverty by Block Group

■ 50 to 100   (36)
▨ 25 to 49.99 (102)
▨ 10 to 24.99 (121)
▨ 5 to   9.99 (78)
▨ 0 to   4.99 (138)

Figure 4–26 City of Minneapolis, percent population in poverty and 1,000-yard TRI buffers

termined buffer. In this study, increasing the buffer sizes resulted in an increasing measure of inequity. Once the buffer size reached a certain distance, we would expect the proximity ratio to decrease until the buffer contained the entire city, and this distance probably differs from locality to locality. In spite of this, because the same pattern persisted at all three smaller distances, the study suggests an association between income and residential proximity to TRI facilities. For all populations, people living closer to such facilities were more likely to be living below the poverty line. However, the proximity ratios for racial groups with the highest overall poverty rates (African Americans, American Indians, and Hispanic Americans) were lower than those for the white population, suggesting that the pattern may not be as significant for these groups.

When studies find associations between poverty and residential proximity to TRI facilities, how do we know they are significant? One way to evaluate the significance of positive results is to perform randomization tests for environmental equity.[30] Such methods test the hypothesis that the proximity ratios are larger than what we would observe if TRI facilities had been randomly distributed within the city. In other words, are these associations between poverty and residence near TRI facilities higher than one would expect by chance?[30]

Minneapolis investigators used a simple approach to evaluate the significance of their results. They began by randomly assigning the 38 TRI sites in Minneapolis to new locations. To do this, they selected Cartesian coordinates for each site's location from a random number distribution. The only constraint was that the location had to be within the municipal boundaries of the city. Each choice of 38 sites served as one random configuration, and they repeated this process 1,500

Table 4–6 Poverty Rates Inside and Outside Buffers, for Different Subpopulations

Proximity Measure	Whites	African Americans	American Indians	Asians	Hispanics	Population Aged 0–5	Total
Within 100-yard buffer	22	52	61	58	48	49	32
Outside 100-yard buffer	12	41	54	46	29	33	18
Proximity ratio	1.83	1.27	1.13	1.26	1.66	1.48	1.78
Within 500-yard buffer	22	51	64	57	40	51	33
Outside 500-yard buffer	11	40	52	43	27	31	17
Proximity ratio	2.00	1.28	1.23	1.33	1.48	1.65	1.94
Within 1,000-yard buffer	20	50	63	58	39	53	31
Outside 1,000-yard buffer	9	36	46	34	23	24	14
Proximity ratio	2.22	1.39	1.37	1.71	1.70	2.21	2.21

Note: "In" records the percentage of populations below poverty inside a given buffer, while "out" records the percentage of populations below poverty outside the buffer.

Table 4–7 Differences in Proximity Ratios by Geodemographic Variables and Proximity Measures

Proximity Measure	Whites	African Americans	American Indians	Asians	Hispanics	Population Aged 0–5	Total
Block groups	1.98	1.07	1.22	1.15	1.80	1.46	1.72
100-yard buffer	1.83	1.27	1.13	1.26	1.66	1.48	1.78
500-yard buffer	2.00	1.28	1.23	1.33	1.48	1.65	1.94
1,000-yard buffer	2.22	1.39	1.37	1.71	1.70	2.21	2.21

times. For each random configuration, they used the spatial coincidence method, comparing populations within and outside block groups containing TRIs, and they used the buffering method, comparing populations within and outside buffers around each TRI. Repeating the process 1,500 times resulted in a simulated distribution of poverty rates for each race/ethnic population. Investigators chose 1,500 repetitions because it took this number before the mean poverty rate in each subpopulation closely approached its citywide mean. Then they looked at where the actual, observed rates fell within the distributions for the total population and each subpopulation.

Figure 4–27 is a histogram showing the distribution of the percentage of people living below poverty for one subpopulation, the white population, living within a 100-yard buffer of the 1,500 simulated locations of TRI facilities. The numbers in Table 4–8 indicate where the *observed* poverty rate

values for proximate populations fall in comparison to the simulated distribution of poverty rate values for proximate populations for the total population and all population subgroups. The histogram (Figure 4–27) shows that the observed poverty rate for the white population living within 100-yard buffers around TRI facilities exceeds that for all 1,500 random simulations. Table 4–6 reveals that this is also true for white populations living within block groups containing TRIs (spatial coincidence method) and for white populations living within 500- and 1,000-yard buffers around TRIs. Investigators recorded these observed values as lying in the 99.9th percentile because they exceeded more than 99.9 percent of the values resulting from the 1,500 random simulations. Following statistical convention, such results could be considered as significant enough to reject the null hypothesis of no relationship between proximity to TRI site and the percentage of population living below the poverty line.[30]

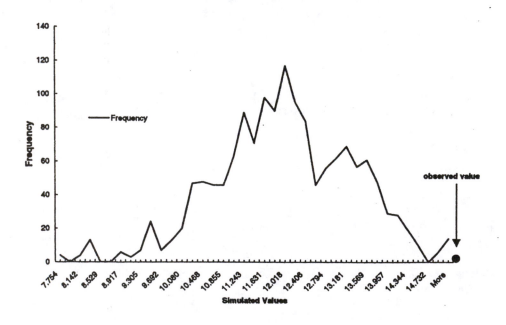

Figure 4–27 Histogram of percentage of whites in poverty within 100 yards of randomly simulated TRI sites

For all populations in Minneapolis, including racial/ethnic minorities and young children, the results in Table 4–8 suggest that the association between proximity to TRI site and the percentage below poverty is greater than chance once distances reach 1,000 yards. In other words, the study indicates that people living within 1,000 yards of a TRI facility are more likely to be poor compared to those living further away. One factor that could have affected these results is that the spatial randomization test did not account for all available information related to possible TRI sites. Although the test constrained the possible location of TRI facilities to all areas within the city, the city allows them only in areas zoned for industrial and commercial activities. If low-income populations are more likely to reside in areas zoned for such activities, the zoning itself could serve as a confounding variable. Future spatial randomization tests could adjust for this by constraining the randomization process to areas zoned for TRI-type facilities.[30]

An additional lesson learned from the study is that proximity measures are not consonant with significance. Inspection of Tables 4–6 and 4–7 reveals no relationship between proximity ratio size and significance. For example, the proximity ratio for Hispanic American population based on spatial coincidence within block groups (1.80) was nearly identical to the proximity ratio for whites at the 100-yard buffer (1.83), yet only the latter ratio was significant. In addition, the proximity ratio for Hispanic Americans at the 1,000-yard buffer was significant but smaller than the nonsignificant proximity ratio at the block group level. Clearly, standard tests of significance may be unreliable in studies of environmental equity.[30] No matter what measure of proximity they choose, future environmental equity investigations will need to be careful in how they evaluate the significance of observed differences in proximate and nonproximate populations.

Besides differences in resolution and scale, differences in how environmental equity studies measure or estimate exposure can lead to different results. One problem with the previously described simple approaches is that they use proximity as a surrogate measure of exposure and thus may inaccurately reflect the degree of actual human exposure to the environmental hazard. For example, the size and shape of buffers and the methodology used to create buffers can affect study results. The Minneapolis study shown in Figures 4–24 through 4–27 and Tables 4–5 through 4–8 used predetermined, arbitrary circular buffers that did not account for other factors that could influence exposure to airborne toxins, such as wind speed and wind direction.[30] Although the study did not prove that low-income people suffer from disproportionate exposure to toxins, they may have a disproportionate *potential* exposure based on proximity.

Future studies could help evaluate this by using methods of evaluating exposure superior to mere proximity measures. For example, investigators could perform the same study with randomization tests using buffers of any shape or size, including those based on plume dispersion models. GIS technology can help improve the measures of exposure by incorporating other databases (such as climatic information) to create such plume dispersion models. A 1994 study in Des Moines, Iowa, compared two types of buffers in evaluating potential exposure to industrial polluters in the TRI database. Compared to circular buffers around the industries, buffers constructed on the basis of likely plumes revealed a higher proportion of minorities and low-income populations within the buffered area.[30] Even these models may not be sufficient because the data sets they use may contain simple, summary data, such as average wind speed or direction, rather than the actual conditions over short time periods. In addition, models take more time to develop and apply than the simpler proximity models.[30]

Data quality and data quantity can also influence study outcomes. Studies based only on a single environmental database, such as the TRI data, may fail to account for other environmental hazards. TRI facilities are not the only emitters of environmental toxins, and not all toxics are reportable.[41] Communities contain many other emission sources

Table 4–8 Minneapolis: Observed Poverty Levels as Percentiles of the Simulated Distribution for Populations Near TRI Sites, 1995

Proximity Measure	Whites (%)	African Americans (%)	American Indians (%)	Asians (%)	Hispanics (%)	Population Aged 0–5(%)	Total (%)
Block groups	99.9*	86.8	87.1	73.1	80.1	97.9	99.9
100-yard buffer	99.9	95.5	78.8	86.4	94.1	97.8	99.9
500-yard buffer	99.9	98.8	96.6	88.8	94.5	99.9	99.9
1,000-yard buffer	99.9	99.9	99.9	99.9	99.9	99.9	99.9

*Observed value greater than 1,500 simulated values.

besides TRI facilities, such as motor vehicle emissions, lead paint, and household waste products. The EPA began collecting TRI data in 1987, so the database fails to account for historical releases that may persist in the environment. In addition, the TRI database relies on self-reporting and omits hundreds of potentially hazardous substances. To account for these omissions, investigators should consider adding additional data sets, including those provided by municipalities, such as recycling sites and the location of pollution permit holders.[30]

An additional, serious problem with the TRI database is that it measures emissions in total pounds, without regard to the degree of toxicity of specific compounds or how they persist in the environment.[41,42] Not all released toxins are equally harmful to human health, and environmental equity investigators should consider the toxicity of specific chemicals in addition to the quantity released in their analysis. For instance, releases of thousands of pounds of a chemical with relatively small toxicity could pose less of a threat than release of a few pounds of a highly toxic chemical. One method that can account for both mass and toxicity is the chronic index (CI), developed by the EPA's Region III Air, Radiation and Toxics Division. The CI combines TRI release data and data sets containing chronic oral toxicity factors to create a better measure of the potential health risk from chemical releases into the environment.

Two databases, the EPA's Integrated Risk Information System (IRIS) and the Health Effects Assessment Summary Tables (HEAST), provide the oral toxicity data required to calculate the CI. IRIS, available through the National Library of Medicine's TOXNET system or from the EPA, contains quantitative estimates for carcinogens and noncarcinogens. The EPA periodically updates both data sets, subjecting them to extensive peer review. Calculating the CI takes three steps. The first step, accounting for the relative hazard of the chemical, calculates the human risk, using different equations for carcinogens and noncarcinogens. For carcinogens, the calculation takes high-dose data from animal and epidemiologic studies and EPA-derived weight of evidence classifications for carcinogenicity and uses mathematical models to project the risk at low doses. For noncarcinogens, the calculation considers the dose for which humans could be exposed during a lifetime, or part of a lifetime, and incorporates a margin of safety. Specific equations for the calculation of the hazard dose are available from the EPA and from Neumann et al.[43] The second step, determining the theoretical exposure dose, accounts for the size of the release in pounds per year. The final step, calculating the CI, is a simple equation dividing the theoretical exposure dose by the hazard dose:

$$CI = \frac{\text{Theoretical Exposure Dose (mg/day)}}{\text{Hazard Dose (mg/day)}}$$

Table 4–9 compares the potential hazards of TRI chemical releases in Oregon in 1992 based on mass alone (the typical measure) with the same hazards based on the CI. If only TRI data are used, methanol tops the list because TRI facilities reported releasing more methanol by weight that year than any other chemical. When accounting for toxicity of specific chemicals as well as release in pounds, however, glycol ether moved from 18th to the top of the list, because, pound for pound, it is more toxic for human health than methanol.[42]

Because the CI expresses relative hazard and is not expressed in units, it can also account for aggregated exposures to more than one TRI facility and more than one chemical. Figure 4–28 is a choropleth map of North Portland, Oregon, showing the proximity between African American populations and hazardous releases from TRIs based on the CI. Census block polygon shades represent the percentage of population within each block that is African American. Symbols represent TRI facilities, and their shades represent the CI for each facility. The map includes 1-mile buffers around each TRI facility, many of which overlap. Some blocks are located within buffers around multiple TRI facilities.

Table 4–9 Ranking of TRI Chemical Releases in Oregon

Top 20 by Total Mass	Top 20 by Chronic Index
Methanol	Glycol ether
Nickel	Nickel
Ammonia	Trichloroethylene
Acetone	Chloroform
Toluene	Manganese
Methyl ethyl ketone	Dichloromethane
Formaldehyde	2-Methoxyethanol
Xylene	Acetone
Hydrochloric acid	Hexachlorethane
Methyl isobutyl ketone	Chromium
Trichloroethylene	Arsenic
1,1,1-Trichloroethane	Methanol
Chloroform	Methyl isobutyl ketone
Styrene	Toluene
Dichloromethane	1,1,1-Trichloroethane
Freon 113	Formaldehyde
Manganese compounds	Naphthalene
Glycol ethers	Epichlorhydrin
Chlorine	Methyl ethyl ketone
Sulfuric acid	Styrene

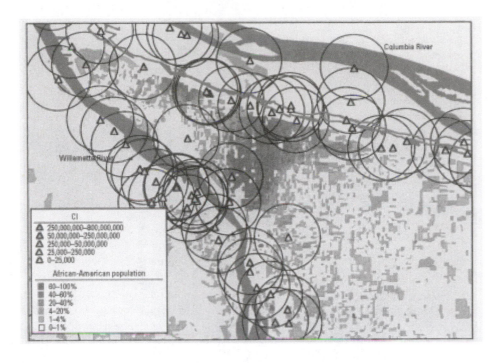

Figure 4–28 Bivariate mapping of total on-site chronic toxicity index (CI) and percent black population. This is a map of North Portland, Oregon, showing census-block boundaries. Circle radii around each Toxic Chemical Release Inventory (TRI) facility are one mile.

Table 4–10 shows the demographics of populations within 1-mile buffers around the top 10 facilities based on CI and compares these with the county demographics. Compared to buffers around all 254 sites within the state, percentages of Asian Americans and Hispanic Americans within one mile of these 10 facilities are 1.5 times and 0.5 times respectively. Investigators found no differences in the percentages of African American and Native American populations around these sites compared to all TRI sites. However, Table 4–11, showing census block groups with the highest aggregated total CI based on overlapping buffers, tells a somewhat different story. Many of the blocks included in this table are located in dense urban areas with multiple TRI facilities. The percentage of ethnic and racial minorities in some of these blocks is more than three times the percentage within the entire counties containing the TRIs. However, increasing buffer sizes masked the contributions of blocks with higher proportions of minorities.[43]

Although environmental equity analyses based on measures like the CI, which account for toxicity, may be an improvement over studies based only on mass of chemicals re-

leased, they have some significant limitations, including but not limited to the following:

- *Lack of toxicity data*: Toxicity data are not available for many TRI chemicals. In the Oregon study, investigators could rank only 67 percent of the chemicals for which they had toxicity data.
- *Inability to account for multiple routes of exposure*: Because the CI uses oral toxicity measures, it cannot account for toxicity from inhalation, the route of many chemical exposures from TRIs and other potentially hazardous facilities.
- *Inability to account for ongoing contamination*: The CI does not account for the ability of some chemicals to persist in the environment, resulting in prolonged exposure.
- *Lack of consideration of acute toxicity*: In some instances, acute toxicity poses the greatest risk following industrial accidents and certainly should be considered in studies of environmental equity. For example, 50 years ago in Japan, a vinyl chloride producer discharged mer-

Table 4–10 Demographics within 1.0 Mile of Top 10 Toxic Chemical Release Inventory (TRI) Facilities (Rank Based on Total Chronic Index [CI]) Compared with Those of the County Populations in Which Facility is Located

Site Number[a]	CI × 1,000[b]	Total Population Near Site[c]	White		Black		Native American[d]		Asian or Pacific Islander[e]		Other		Hispanic[e]	
			Site[f]	County[g]	Site[f]	County[g]	Site[f]	County[g]	Site[f]	County[g]	Site[f]	County[g]	Site[f]	County[g]
1	1,792,688	8	100	96.9	0.0	0.2	0.0	1.6	0.0	0.7	0.0	0.7	0.0	2.4
6	1,558,296	27	100	96.4	0.0	0.3	0.0	1.1	0.0	1.3	0.0	0.8	0.0	1.9
37	909,200	6,669	85.2	87.0	6.5	6.0	2.7[h]	1.2[h]	7.0	4.7	2.4[h]	1.2[h]	4.7	3.1
19	886,239	9,920	76.5	87.0	11.8[h]	6.0[h]	2.6[h]	1.2[h]	7.0	4.7	2.1	1.2[h]	4.7	3.1
26	697,195	8,925	85.5	92.0	1.7	0.9	0.9	0.8	10.5[h]	5.5[h]	1.4	0.9	3.2	2.5
5	494,634	2,472	95.8	97.3	0.2	0.1	1.8	1.4	1.5	0.8	0.7	0.5	2.6[h]	1.0[h]
63	407,788	8,925	85.5	92.0	1.7	0.9	0.9	0.8	10.5[h]	5.5[h]	1.4	0.9	3.2	2.5
27	392,672	16,567	94.7	87.0	0.7	6.0	0.7	1.2	3.1	4.7	0.7	1.2	2.0	3.1
10	386,701	6	100	96.9	0.0	0.2	0.0	1.2	0.0	0.9	0.0	0.9	0.0	2.4
67	374,101	2,925	96.2	93.35	0.2	0.3	1.3	1.5	0.7	1.4	1.5	3.5	2.8	5.7

[a]Site numbering is based on pounds of chemicals released on site.

[b]Total CIs are computed for each TRI facility and include air, water, and land emissions for all chemicals reported.

[c]Total population living within 1.0 mile of the TRI site. Data are from the U.S. Bureau of the Census (24).

[d]Native American includes American Indian, Eskimo, and Aleut.

[e]Hispanics are an ethnic population, not a race, and are counted separately by the census; therefore, a white Hispanic person can be identified and counted as both white and Hispanic.

[f]Percentage of race or ethnic population living within 1.0 mile of the TRI site; the percentage is based on count of race or ethnic population divided by total population living within 1.0 mile of site.

[g]Percentage of race or ethnic population living within the county in which the TRI facility is located; the percentage is based on count of race or ethnic population in the entire county divided by the total population in the same county.

[h]Sites whose racial and ethnic populations within 1.0 mile of the facility are greater than twice that found in the county in which the facility is located.

Table 4–11 Areas with Highest Aggregated Total Chronic Index (CI)

No. Census Blocks	Total Population[a]	Total CI[b]	No. TRI Sites[c]	Percent Minority Population[d]
28	1,653	1,795,439,348	4	20
2	8	1,792,668,159	1	0
3	27	1,598,286,051	1	0
101	6,903	1,105,144,828	3	15
20	1,412	1,104,983,950	2	15
26	1,731	$9.1–9.2 \times 10^8$	4	16
93	3,285	$9.0–9.1 \times 10^8$	3	12
167	8,267	886,239,094	1	24
1	2	623,492,097	6	0
51	2,455	494,634,769	1	4
133	6,889	$4.0–4.9 \times 10^8$	6	6

Note: TRI, Toxic Chemical Release Inventory.

[a]Total population living in selected census blocks (1990 U.S. Bureau of the Census block-level data) within one mile of TRI site(s) with same total aggregated CI.
[b]Sum of total on-site chronic indices for all TRI facilities within one mile of census blocks.
[c]Number of TRI sites within one mile of census block.
[d]Percent minority population including black; Asian or Pacific Islander; American Indian, Eskimo, or Aleut; and other nonwhite races.

cury into Minamata Bay. Acute mercury poisoning resulting from the discharge caused 41 deaths and 30 cases of cerebral palsy in children.[41]

- *Basis on toxicological data for adults only*: CI calculations are based on toxicity studies from adults and may not accurately reflect the toxic potential for children.
- *Limitations in measuring total potential risk*: Aggregating CIs for populations within overlapping buffers may not adequately measure total potential risk because adverse health effects from different chemicals are not necessarily additive.
- *Inability to account for sources of environmental contamination other than the TRI facilities.*

These data limitations provide useful lessons for data producers, such as the EPA, and these agencies are responding. Recently, the EPA has developed a chemical indexing methodology that accounts for environmental persistence and acute toxicity. The EPA is also modifying the CI approach so that it can account for the health effects of chemicals lacking oral toxicity data.[43]

In spite of limitations in data and technology, some local health departments are already using GIS to engage their communities in activities aimed at reducing adverse environmental health impacts. Frequently, they have access to additional sources of data, available from other local and state agencies, that can be helpful in performing GIS environmental equity assessments.[23] Lancaster County, Nebraska,

with over 230,000 residents, is mostly rural but contains an urban center, the city of Lincoln, home to 90 percent of the county's population. The agency responsible for public health activities, the Lincoln-Lancaster County Health Department (LLCHD), began using GIS technology in 1996 for drinking-water pollution prevention, starting with the creation of a geographic groundwater database. In 1998, the EPA gave the LLCHD and a partner, the University of Nebraska, an Environmental Justice through Pollution Prevention grant, allowing them to demonstrate the use of GIS technology in evaluating the impact of environmental pollution on minority populations.

Responding to the grant objectives, the University of Nebraska conducted the Health Hazard Risks in the Minority Community Survey. The purpose of the survey was to identify the perceptions, knowledge, and beliefs of Lincoln minority populations regarding community environmental health hazards. In partnership with the university, the LLCHD used survey results to map community perceptions in comparison to the location of facilities storing potentially hazardous chemicals. Figure 4–29, a choropleth map of census tracts within Lincoln, Nebraska, containing the highest percentages of minorities, shows the results. Polygon shades represent the percentage of minority population within these census tracts. Symbol shapes represent survey responses by where responders lived: squares are those responders concerned about hazardous chemicals in their neighborhood, and triangles represent unconcerned resident responders. Overlaying these are the locations of Tier II sites, businesses storing hazardous chemicals, with a 0.2-mile buffer around each one, representing their "vulnerable zones," based on the U.S. Department of Transportation's *North American Emergency*

Response Guidebook. Not included in Figure 4–29 but studied by the Lancaster County Health Department are other sources of easily mapped environmental contamination, such as Title V sites, businesses that emit air pollutants, and spe-

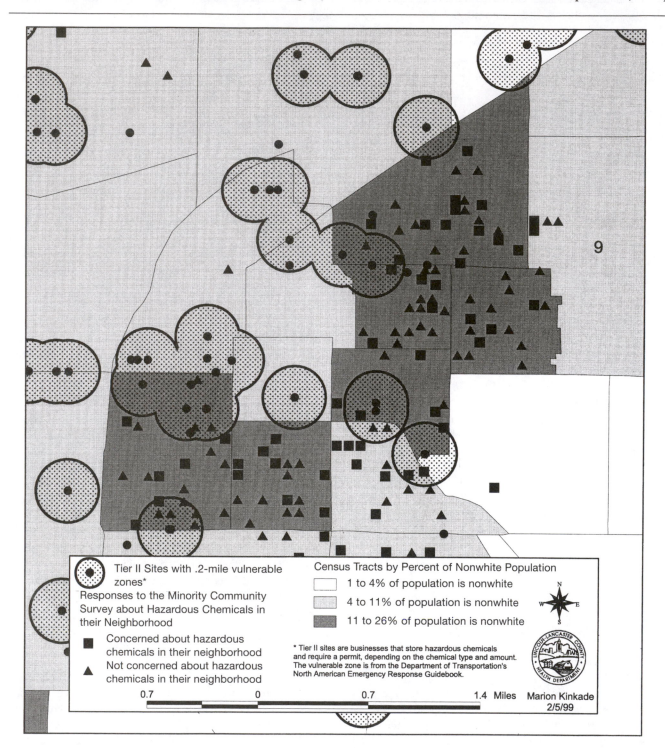

Figure 4–29 Responses to the survey of environmental health hazard risks in the minority community, in relation to the primary minority census tracts and the evacuation zones for Tier II sites in Lincoln, Nebraska, February 1999

cial waste sites, businesses requiring permits to dispose of nonhazardous "special" wastes. The LLCHD can also map the location of vulnerable populations, such as schools, nursing homes, and child care providers, and community assets, such as libraries, clinics, and community centers.

To successfully develop and enter the multiple layers of attribute data, the LLCHD collaborated with several governmental, academic, and community-based organizations, including minority organizations. Governmental agencies involved at the local level were the Lincoln Water System and the Lincoln Planning Department. The Lincoln Planning Department provided the spatial database, which included streets, aerial photos, and the water system. The EPA supplied data on Tier II sites. At the state level, collaborating agencies were the Nebraska Department of Environmental Quality and the Nebraska Game and Parks Commission. Participating community organizations included the Asian Center, the Malone Center (serving the African American community), the Hispanic Center, and the Indian Center.

Costs for the project were[23]

- $6,000 for a Compaq Professional Workstation 5100, which included a computer (Pentium II 300 MHz, with sufficient memory), Windows NT software, and a 21-inch monitor
- $4,190 for GIS software
- Additional software, X-tools, and Project_o1, available free as downloads from the Oregon Department of Forestry Web site <www.odf.state.or.us/StateForests/sfgis/default.htm>

(See Chapter 10 for a description of basic hardware and software requirements for most GIS applications.)

The LLCHD presented the results of its analysis, including maps, to the Lincoln City Council and, through a series of public meetings, to minority communities. Besides serving the purpose of community education, the information was useful to the mayor and city council for making planning decisions, and it helped focus the efforts of the health department's Pollution Prevention Technical Assistance Program.[23] Additionally, the data will help in development of the county's emergency response plan.

We have pointed out some current applications for GIS technology in environmental equity analysis. Clearly, the technology has great promise, but researchers and other GIS users will have to address several design and methodological issues, some of which we will discuss further in Chapter 9. In spite of the methodological problems, the preponderance of published studies suggests that low-income and minority communities are more likely to suffer from exposure to environmental hazards than the general population.[35] If so, these populations are then more likely to suffer the con-sequences of this exposure, which may account for at least part of the disparities in health status we see in the United States.

Given the ramifications of these findings, future environmental equity analyses will have to address questions raised by these early GIS studies:

- *Which came first*: Were environmental hazards preferentially placed in poor and minority neighborhoods, or did low-income people, including minorities, move into areas with already existing environmental hazards?[41] One argument in favor of the "causal" hypothesis, that government and business specifically target poor and minority areas with hazardous industrial facilities, is that these areas contain cheaper land and the residents are less likely to offer resistance. The opposite argument, in favor of the "drift" hypothesis, is that minorities and low-income people move into areas with hazardous facilities because of low housing costs or racist real estate and lending practices.[41] Although both scenarios can result in differential exposure to hazardous facilities, policy implications (and resulting remedies) differ. Most likely, both factors are at work. Fortunately, GIS technology can help evaluate these hypotheses because it can link population data (migration data) with environmental data.[41] In addition, GIS technology can help evaluate the spatial relationships over time with spatio-temporal statistics (see Chapter 3).
- *Data quality*: We have already discussed the need to develop better methods of estimating exposure from individual and multiple sources and from different exposure pathways (e.g., inhalation vs. ingestion). Future studies will also need to address duration of exposure. In addition, many currently available attribute databases lack information on socioeconomic status, such as income level and occupation, another source of potential exposure.
- *Definition of community*: The discussions on the effect of buffer size lead to an obvious question for investigations of environmental equity: How should each study define a community? Is it a geographic area, and if so, how large? What role do potentially affected study subjects play in defining their community?
- *Outcomes*: Besides differential exposure, and the incidence/prevalence of acute and chronic illness, what other end points should investigators use in evaluating environmental equity? Does the presence of hazardous facilities in neighborhoods lead to other adverse outcomes, such as lowered property values, inferior schools, increased crime, and other adverse social outcomes?[41] Many public health professionals consider such outcomes as health related. Fortunately, the inte-

grative capacity of GIS technology makes it useful in evaluating such outcomes, as long as the data are available.

- *The potential for misinterpretation of results*: Although many studies suggest a relationship between the location of hazardous facilities and low-income and minority populations, current scientific data cannot reliably characterize how this relationship affects health status and health outcomes.[35] As mentioned in Chapter 1, most health determinants—age, ethnicity, socioeconomic status, and education being only the most common examples—cluster geographically. Most GIS analyses assessing whether there is an association between geography and a health outcome will find one.[1] In studies of environmental equity, some health outcomes could cluster geographically because of underlying population characteristics, not because of the proximity of hazardous facilities. Experienced public health professionals

can facilitate the study of environmental equity by using epidemiologic methods to identify associations between exposures and disease and, by doing so, can determine whether and how these associations are due to cause and effect.

We still know little about how environmental hazards differentially affect the health status of low income and minority populations. Considering the multitude of potentially confounding variables involved, such as housing, land use, access to care, and employment, the integrative capacities of GIS could be particularly helpful in increasing our knowledge in this area. Chapter 7 will give some examples of how GIS can evaluate the association between some of these conditions and chronic disease outcomes. Although GIS technology may not necessarily provide all the answers, it has raised and will continue to raise appropriate questions for further study.

CHAPTER   REVIEW

1. GIS are tools that can help us
   - Understand the risks of disease related to environmental exposures
   - Target public health interventions based on these risks
2. Gathering accurate exposure information usually is the most difficult, expensive, and time-intensive component of any study. Before the development of modern GIS technology, studies relied on indirect or surrogate measures of exposure. With available GIS technology, epidemiologists can combine existing databases, including environmental data, to make better estimates of exposure levels.
   - Historically, most environmental epidemiological studies relied on case-control designs to evaluate the association between rare cancers and nonionizing radiation exposures. Because these case-control studies selected subjects on the basis of disease and not exposure to nonionizing radiation, they were limited in accurately characterizing exposures and in evaluating unusually high levels of exposure. GIS technology now provides the means for identifying individuals exposed to high residential levels of nonionizing radiation for cohort studies by easily locating and characterizing these cohorts on the basis of potentially confounding socioeconomic variables.

   - GIS models can identify at-risk populations for health screening, such as those living downwind from a nuclear power plant release of radioactive iodine or children at risk of lead exposure from multiple sources.
   - GIS technology's capacity to integrate several data sets can help us gain a new understanding of the relationships between environment and disease (such as exposure to automobile exhaust and asthma) while raising questions for further study.
3. Health officials can use GIS technology to prevent exposure to pollution in a couple of ways:
   - GIS overlays of environmental, health, and demographic data can identify persons and communities at risk of environmental exposure from industry. Public health officials can share this information with businesses to encourage them to use less toxic chemicals.
   - GIS technology can help officials identify and characterize many non–manufacturing-related potential sources of drinking-water pollution, such as sewers, landfills, underground storage tanks, and chemical storage facilities. Using GIS mapping technology, public health officials can evaluate groundwater quality and define populations at risk for exposure—for example, when an industrial plant releases

a plume of hazardous materials into the groundwater supply.

4. During the past two decades, the publication of studies identifying an unequal distribution of environmental hazards across racial, ethnic, and socioeconomic groups has led to nationwide concerns about environmental inequity. GIS technology has helped federal, state, and local agencies and academic institutions investigate potential environmental inequities because questions about whether minorities suffer disproportionately from exposure to environmental hazards are inherently spatial. While some GIS studies have found that racial/ethnic minorities and low-income populations suffer disproportionately from exposure to environmental toxins, others have found no associations, and some have even found that white and higher-income communities suffer more. These inconsistencies have several probable causes, including

- The spatial resolution and scale of the geographic area studied
- The type/quality of data used (e.g., accurate address information)
- The measures of exposure

In spite of the methodological problems, the preponderance of published studies suggests that low-income and minority communities are more likely to suffer from exposure to environmental hazards than the general population. Future studies must address spatial relationships over time, data quality, community definitions, health outcomes, and the risk of misinterpreting study results. We still know little about how environmental hazards differentially affect the health status of low income and minority populations. Although GIS technology may not necessarily provide all the answers, it has raised and will continue to raise appropriate questions for further study.

REFERENCES

1. A.L. Melnick and D.W. Fleming. "Modern Geographic Information Systems: Promise and Pitfalls." *Journal of Public Health Management and Practice* 5, no. 2 (1999): viii–x.

2. U.S. Tim. "The Application of GIS in Environmental Health Sciences: Opportunities and Limitations." *Environmental Research* 71 (1995): 75–88.

3. M. Vine et al. "Geographic Information Systems: Their Use in Environmental Epidemiologic Research." *Environmental Health Perspectives* 105 (1997): 598–605.

4. C.M. Croner et al. "Geographic Information Systems (GIS): New Perspectives in Understanding Human Health and Environmental Relationships." *Statistics in Medicine* 15 (1996): 1961–1977.

5. D. Wartenberg et al. "Identification and Characterization of Populations Living Near High-Voltage Transmission Lines: A Pilot Study." *Environmental Health Perspectives* 101 (1993): 626–632.

6. N. Wertheimer and E. Leeper. "Electric Wiring Configuration and Childhood Cancer." *American Journal of Epidemiology* 109 (1979): 273–284.

7. W.D. Henriques and R.F. Spengler. "Locations around the Hanford Nuclear Facility Where Average Milk Consumption by Children in 1945 Would Have Resulted in an Estimated Median Iodine-131 Dose to the Thyroid of 10 Rad or Higher, Washington." *Journal of Public Health Management and Practice* 5, no. 2 (1999): 35–36.

8. Centers for Disease Control and Prevention. "Asthma Mortality and Hospitalization among Children and Young Adults: United States 1980–1993." *Morbidity and Mortality Weekly Report* 45 (1996): 350–353.

9. Committee of the Environmental and Occupational Health Assembly, American Thoracic Society. "Health Effects of Outdoor Air Pollution." *American Journal of Respiratory and Critical Care Medicine* 153, no. 1 (1996): 3–50.

10. P. English et al. "Examining Associations between Childhood Asthma and Traffic Flow Using a Geographic Information System." *Environmental Health Perspectives* 107 (1999): 761–767.

11. Centers for Disease Control and Prevention. "Targeted Screening for Childhood Lead Exposure in a Low Prevalence Area, Salt Lake County, Utah, 1995–1996." *Morbidity and Mortality Weekly Report* 46, no. 10 (1997): 213–217.

12. Centers for Disease Control and Prevention. *Preventing Lead Poisoning in Young Children.* Atlanta, Georgia: U.S. Department of Health and Human Services, Public Health Service, 1991.

13. D. Wartenberg. "Screening for Lead Exposure Using a Geographic Information System." *Environmental Research* 59 (1992): 310–317.

14. W.G. Guthe et al. "Reassessment of Lead Exposure in New Jersey Using GIS Technology." *Environmental Research* 59 (1992): 318–325.

15. Centers for Disease Control and Prevention. *Screening Young Children for Lead Poisoning: Guidance for State and Local Public Health Officials.* Atlanta, GA: CDC, 1997.

16. C.L. Hanchette. "GIS and Decision Making for Public Health Agencies: Childhood Lead Poisoning and Welfare Reform." *Journal of Public Health Management and Practice* 5, no. 4 (1999): 41–47.

17. C. Duclos et al. "Development of Childhood Blood Lead Screening Guidelines, Duval County, Florida, 1998." *Journal of Public Health Management and Practice* 5, no. 2 (1999): 9–10.

18. S. Wilkinson et al. "Lead Hot Zones and Childhood Lead Poisoning Cases, Santa Clara County, California, 1995." *Journal of Public Health Management and Practice* 5, no. 2 (1999): 11–12.

19. R. Rao et al. "Geographic Distribution of Mean Blood Lead Levels by Year in Children Residing in Communities Near the Bunker Hill Lead Smelter Site, 1974–1983." *Journal of Public Health Management and Practice* 5, no. 2 (1999): 13–14.

20. Environmental Protection Agency. Record of Decision (ROD) Abstract. *Site:* Bunker Hill Mining & Metallurgical. *Location:* Kellogg, ID. *EPA ID Number:* IDD048340921. ROD Number: EPA/AMD/R10–96/146 ROD Date: 09/09/96 <www.epa.gov/superfund/sites/query/rods/a1096146.htm>.

21. Agency for Toxic Substances and Disease Registry. *Study of Former Female Workers at a Lead Smelter: An Examination of the Possible*

Association of Lead Exposure with Decreased Bone Density and Other Health Outcomes. Atlanta, GA: ATSDR, 1997.

22. Agency for Toxic Substances and Disease Registry. *A Cohort Study of Current and Previous Residents of the Silver Valley: Assessment of Lead Exposure and Health Outcomes.* Atlanta, GA: ATSDR, 1997.

23. P.B. Bouton and M. Fraser. "Local Health Departments and GIS: The Prospective of the National Association of County and City Health Officials." *Journal of Public Health Management and Practice* 5, no. 4 (1999): 33–41.

24. M. Ralston. "Elevated Nitrate Levels in Relation to Bedrock Depth, Linn County, Iowa, 1991–1996." *Journal of Public Health Management and Practice* 5, no. 2 (1999): 39–40.

25. W. Boria et al. "Public Notification to Families with Newborns at Risk of Methemoglobinemia from Drinking Water Exposure, Clymer, New York, 1996–1998." *Journal of Public Health Management and Practice* 5, no. 2 (1999): 37–38.

26. Centers for Disease Control and Prevention. "Continued Use of Drinking Water Wells Contaminated with Hazardous Chemical Substances: Virgin Islands and Minnesota, 1981–1993." *Morbidity and Mortality Weekly Report* 43, no. 5 (1994): 89–91.

27. Agency for Toxic Substances and Disease Registry. *Public Health Assessment Guidance Manual.* Atlanta, GA: U.S. Department of Health and Human Services, Public Health Service, Agency for Toxic Substances and Disease Registry, 1992.

28. J. Pruitt. "Monitoring Volatile Organic Compounds in Private Wells Near a Community Landfill by Tax Parcel, Harford County, Maryland, 1986–1998." *Journal of Public Health Management and Practice* 5, no. 2 (1999): 41–42.

29. D.L. Partridge and M.D. Mathews. "A Computer Simulation of Groundwater Withdrawal Patterns for Public Water Supply Wells, Hutchinson, Kansas, 1998–2003." *Journal of Public Health Management and Practice* 5, no. 2 (1999): 43–44.

30. E. Sheppard et al. "GIS-Based Measures of Environmental Equity: Exploring Their Sensitivity and Significance." *Journal of Exposure Analysis and Environmental Epidemiology* 9 (1999): 18–28.

31. U.S. Department of Health and Human Services. *Healthy People 2010* (conference edition, 2 vols.). Washington, DC: USDHHS, 2000.

32. D.L. Anderton et al. "Environmental Equity: The Demographics of Dumping." *Demography* 3, no. 2 (1994): 229–248.

33. United Church of Christ, Commission for Racial Justice. *Toxic Wastes and Race in the United States: A National Report on the Racial and Socioeconomic Characteristics of Communities with Hazardous Waste Sites.* New York: UCC, 1987.

34. W. Clinton. Executive Order No. 12898. Federal actions to address environmental justice in minority populations and low-income populations. Section 1-101. Washington DC. The White House. February 11, 1994; <http://www.epa.gov/swerosps/ej/html-doc/execordr.htm>.

35. K. Sexton and J.L. Adgate. "Looking at Environmental Justice from an Environmental Health Perspective." *Journal of Exposure Analysis and Environmental Epidemiology* 9 (1999): 18–28.

36. U.S. Environmental Protection Agency. "1998 Environmental Justice Biennial Report: June 1999." <http://es.epa.gov/oeca/main/ej/98biennial.pdf>.

37. S. Cutter et al. "The Role of Geographic Scale in Monitoring Environmental Justice." *Risk Analysis* 16 (1996): 517–526.

38. T.S. Glickman. "Measuring Environmental Equity with Geographic Information Systems." *Renewable Resources Journal* 12, no. 3 (1994): 17–21.

39. R. McMaster et al. "GIS-Based Environmental Equity and Risk Assessment: Methodological Problems and Prospects." *Cartography and Geographic Information Systems* 24, no. 3 (1997): 172–189.

40. W.M. Bowen et al. "Toward Environmental Justice: Spatial Equity in Ohio and Cleveland." *Annals of the Association of American Geographers* 85 (1995): 641–663.

41. P. Brown. "Race, Class and Environmental Health: A Review and Systemization of the Literature." *Environmental Research* 69 (1995): 15–30.

42. C.M. Neumann. "Improving the U.S. EPA Toxic Release Inventory Database for Environmental Health Research." *Journal of Toxicology and Environmental Health*, part B, no. 1 (1998): 259–270.

43. C.M. Neumann et al. "Hazard Screening of Chemical Releases and Environmental Equity Analysis of Populations Proximate to Toxic Release Inventory Facilities in Oregon." *Environmental Health Perspectives* 106 (1998): 217–226.

Public Health GIS Applications: Communicable-Disease Prevention and Control

Many diseases not caused directly by environmental exposures still cluster geographically.[1] Besides time and person, knowledge of the spatial distribution of communicable-disease cases is essential in understanding disease transmission.[2] John Snow's cholera study served as a good example of how geographic mapping could provide new insights into communicable-disease etiology and intervention, helping disease control efforts. Although his map alone did not determine the cause of the 1854 cholera epidemic, it served as a useful tool to summarize his data and convince his contemporaries of his conclusions.[2] The integrative features of modern GIS technology are incredibly helpful in summarizing the complex relationships between communicable-disease pathogens, associated vectors and reservoirs, the environment, and human populations.[2] In this way, GIS mapping can provide new insights into both communicable-disease etiology and appropriate interventions, enhancing our ability to prevent and control communicable disease and to evaluate the effectiveness of our efforts.

VACCINE-PREVENTABLE DISEASES

Targeting Immunization Programs

Although school exclusion laws have ensured adequate vaccination of school-aged children, immunization rates for younger children are still suboptimal. For example, in 1998 only 79 percent of children 19 to 35 months of age had received a complete series of the required vaccines. Compared to other children, low-income and minority children are at greater risk for underimmunization. "Pockets of need," defined by the Centers for Disease Control and Prevention (CDC) as specific geographic areas containing large numbers of underimmunized children,[3] still exist within our nation's inner cities. These areas have the highest risk of vaccine-preventable disease for children.[3] Additionally, improvements in childhood immunization rates have lessened. Between 1996 and 1998, immunization rates improved only for hepatitis B and varicella. It is easier to increase immunization levels from 55 to 65 percent than from 75 to 85 percent because as programs approach desired outcome goals, each increment of improvement is increasingly difficult to achieve. As we approach our national immunization goals, we will need new, more effective immunization strategies.[4] Such strategies must increase immunization levels using the least expenditures because public health departments will be facing resource constraints. A Florida study illustrates how local immunization programs, using models developed with GIS technology, can efficiently identify and target "pockets of need" to raise immunization levels.[3]

Figure 5–1, a choropleth map of Hillsborough County, Florida, shows census block groups predicted to have the greatest density of underimmunized children.[3] The shading of each block group polygon is proportional to the number of children per square mile predicted to be underimmunized at age 24 months. Darkest shades represent census block groups with at least 50 children per square mile predicted to be underimmunized at 24 months. Intermediate-shaded census block groups have between 25 and 50 children per square mile predicted to be underimmunized, while unshaded block groups have 25 or fewer predicted underimmunized children. The Florida Bureau of Immunization produced similar maps for each Florida county to help local health departments identify pockets of need so that they could target their immunization outreach efforts more efficiently.

All GIS maps represent the accumulation of data from several sources. For example, in creating the Hillsborough

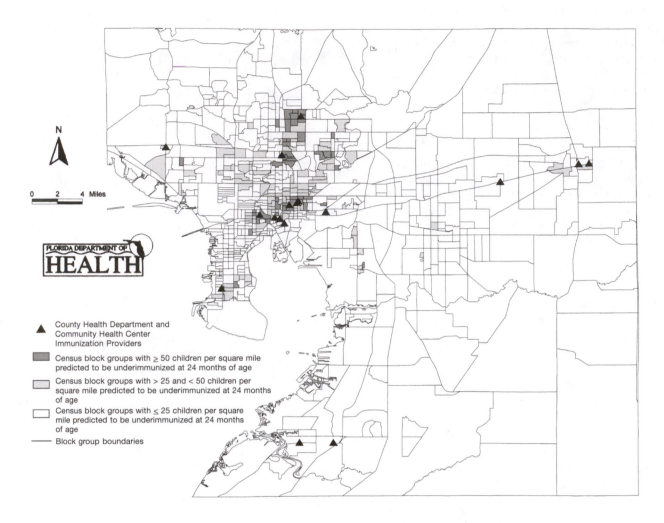

Figure 5–1 Identifying predicted immunization "pockets of need," Hillsborough County, Florida, 1996–1997

County maps, the Bureau of Immunization staff combined three years of data from the annual Florida survey of two-year-olds' immunization levels with birth certificate and census data. Using GIS software, they geocoded each survey response and assigned it to the appropriate census block group, making it possible to include individual and community characteristics in the analysis. Then, using logistic regression, they developed a model predicting the probability that a child had received appropriate immunizations by age two. Once they developed the model, they applied it to predict the level of immunizations of current two-year-old children. First, they geocoded the birth database for resident children born in 1996 and 1997 (these children would be two years old at the time of the analysis). Next, they assigned the probability of being underimmunized, based on the predicted model, to each child in the database. They then geographically aggregated these data by assigning each case to

the appropriate census block group, giving them a predicted number of underimmunized children for each block group. Finally, using the spatial data incorporated into their GIS, they created the map (Figure 5–1) with predicted density (number per square mile) of underimmunized children.[3] Future immunization surveys must be done to assess whether the model accurately predicted areas with immunization needs. Several states have enacted legislation creating immunization registries. In these states, immunization administration is reportable, and the reports include residence address of the child receiving the immunization. Immunization registry data obviate the need to use survey-based models because health departments can incorporate the registry data directly into the GIS application.

Such maps are useful in identifying and predicting pockets of immunization need, enabling health departments to direct their programs to the highest-priority areas. Additionally, the overlay capability of GIS technology allows health departments to add map layers containing the location of public vaccine providers, helping direct and, if necessary, reallocate resources to these pockets of need.[3] Maps created in subsequent years can help immunization program staff evaluate the outcome of their targeted efforts.

Hepatitis A and Pertussis

As we discussed in Chapter 2, in most states, vaccine-preventable diseases are reportable, and the disease reports include a residence address. By combining disease report data with population data, health departments can use GIS to map incidence rates for vaccine-preventable disease. In addition, states with immunization registries can provide data on im-

munization rates for children. We will use the examples of hepatitis A and pertussis to illustrate how health departments, using GIS technology, can target and evaluate their efforts directed at controlling these diseases. Similar methods would be helpful in controlling other vaccine-preventable diseases.

Hepatitis A

A Salt Lake County, Utah, study of hepatitis A illustrates the potential of GIS technology to help local (and state) health departments target their communicable-disease control efforts. Like other reportable diseases, hepatitis A reports include the address of each case, allowing for geographic analysis. Figure 5–2 is a choropleth map of hepatitis A incidence by ZIP codes in Salt Lake County, Utah. During a five-year period from 1992 to 1996, the hepatitis A rate in Salt Lake

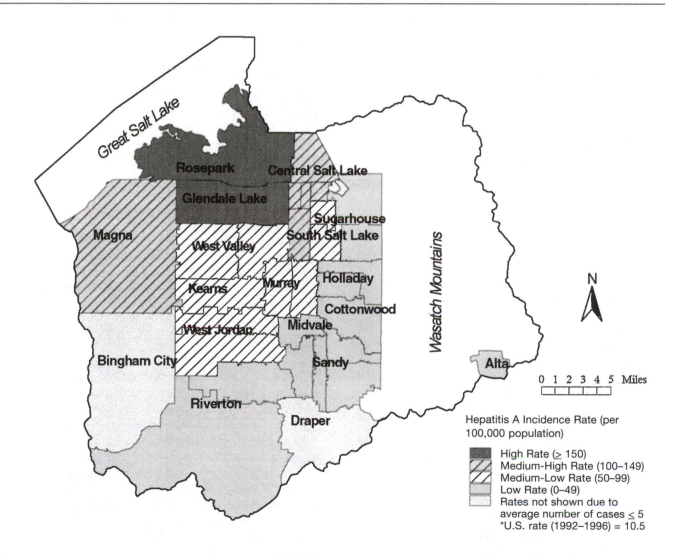

Figure 5–2 Incidence rates of hepatitis A by ZIP code area, Salt Lake County, Utah, 1992–1996

County was six times the national rate.[5] In this case, the local health department determined that preschool-aged children were at highest risk for acquiring and spreading hepatitis A. Figure 5–2 illustrates that the hepatitis A incidence rates were highest in two ZIP code areas in the northern part of the county. Consequently, the health department targeted its hepatitis A immunization program to children aged two through six who were living in these two most affected ZIP codes.

This study also illustrates how GIS technology can help health departments evaluate the effectiveness of their interventions. In this case, the health department can use GIS to continue to monitor and map incidence rates in years following its stepped-up efforts. Monitoring changes in incidence rates in the target area and surrounding ZIP codes will also provide information on the effect of herd immunity. For example, GIS monitoring can help tell if adequate immunization of children in one geographic area will protect children that they may have contact with in other areas. In addition, lessons learned from these evaluations may help other health departments determine how to target their own immunization efforts most effectively.[5]

Pertussis

Although an effective vaccine for pertussis, a bacterial infection, is widely available (and usually required for school entry), some communities continue to experience outbreaks, resulting in significant morbidity and cost.[6] A Denver study demonstrates how GIS technology could help public health departments control and prevent future pertussis outbreaks by identifying risk factors in communities where these outbreaks are likely to occur.

The study used an ecologic design to evaluate the association between factors such as poverty, race/ethnicity, the proportion of infants and children, population density, population mobility, and pertussis incidence.[6] The first source of attribute data included January 1, 1986, through December 31, 1994, reported pertussis cases in Denver residents that met the case definition established by the CDC. Typically, because of underreporting, grossly incomplete data limit the accuracy of communicable-disease analyses, including those for pertussis. This study illustrates how the integrative capabilities of GIS technology can reduce this problem. Investigators easily supplemented outpatient reported pertussis data with cases that they identified through the Colorado Hospital Association Discharge Database and confirmed by either chart review or ICD-9 coding.

For socioeconomic and denominator data, investigators added another attribute data layer, the 1990 U.S. census database. The outcome measure was the age-adjusted incidence rate of pertussis for each census tract in Denver. Because

case reports included an address, investigators were able to use GIS software (MapInfo) to geocode cases and assign each case to a census tract. Using the direct method, they calculated the age-adjusted rate for each census tract. To improve the detection of spatial patterns irrespective of political boundaries, they calculated smoothed rates. They then used statistical methods to confirm whether observed clusters were statistically significant.[6]

Figure 5–3 is a map illustrating smoothed age-adjusted pertussis rates in Denver County for 1986 through 1994.[6] The map clearly shows that the northwestern and western areas of Denver contained the highest density of pertussis cases over this time period. Elevated pertussis rates were also associated with increased poverty and decreased mobility (based on increased proportions of residents living in the same house for at least five years).

Like other ecologic studies, this particular study led to additional questions. For example, was increased incidence associated with reduced access to preventive care, including pertussis immunizations? Previous studies had found higher rates of preventable mortality in this geographic region, including deaths due to diabetes, HIV infection, homicide, and unintentional injury.[6] In addition, this area of Denver contains most of Denver's minority population and has higher rates of unemployment.[6]

The investigators tried to answer this question by examining immunization levels for individual cases. For the case patients with available immunization information, 50 percent of children younger than 6 months of age had no immunizations, and 78 percent of children between 6 months and five years were underimmunized, suggesting that improved access to immunizations might help.[6] Combined with the geographic analysis, such information could help the local health department target its immunization efforts. Additionally, future geographic analysis could help determine whether these targeted efforts had any benefit.

Animal Rabies

Two studies illustrate the effectiveness of GIS technology in helping health departments target their rabies control efforts. Figure 5–4 is an incidence map showing the location of reported animal rabies cases during a five-year period from 1994 to 1998 in Central Palm Beach County, Florida. Although most of the cases were in wild animals, where the disease is endemic in the county, the map highlights two cases occurring in domestic cats in 1994. These cases occurred in a residential area where abandoned cats and dogs were running free. Because of this map, the county health department declared a rabies alert for the area, cautioning residents to stay away from stray animals and high-risk wildlife.

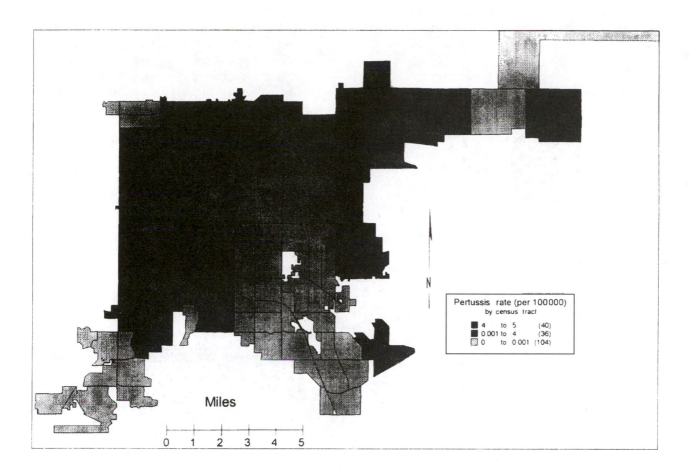

Figure 5–3 Smoothed age-adjusted pertussis rates, Denver County, 1986 through 1994

In addition, the county launched low-cost rabies vaccination clinics and removed feral dogs and cats from the area. The map suggests that the intervention may have been effective, in that the health department received no reports of domestic rabies cases in the subsequent four years.[7]

In 1997, migrating rabid raccoons carried rabies westward from Pennsylvania into Ohio. Figure 5–5 is an incidence map documenting this movement of raccoon-strain rabies into Mahong County, Ohio.[8] In this example, investigators used hand-held global positioning satellite (GPS) units to mark the location where they found each rabid animal. Information on this map helped the district health department determine where to conduct active surveillance for the disease (where to find additional animals for testing). In addition, the map helped the health department determine the most effective locations for placing oral vaccine bait to reduce the number of raccoons with rabies. Subsequent maps could be helpful in evaluating the effectiveness of the oral vaccine–baiting program.

VECTOR-BORNE AND PARASITIC COMMUNICABLE DISEASES: USING GIS TO TARGET COMMUNITIES FOR INTERVENTIONS

Targeting interventions toward vector control and educating the public on how best to avoid contact with vectors can prevent many diseases transmitted by arthropod vectors. The risk of disease transmission is often associated with specific environmental conditions that support vector populations. The overlay feature of GIS technology facilitates the identification of many of these factors, including climate, vegetation type, soil pattern, and the size of insect, human, and animal reservoir populations, to explain and predict disease transmission and distribution. GIS can help us consider questions such as: Where do emerging diseases arise? What determines the geographic distribution of disease? How do we determine the local and regional risk of disease transmission?[9] Answers to these questions are critical for developing the most efficient and effective methods to protect

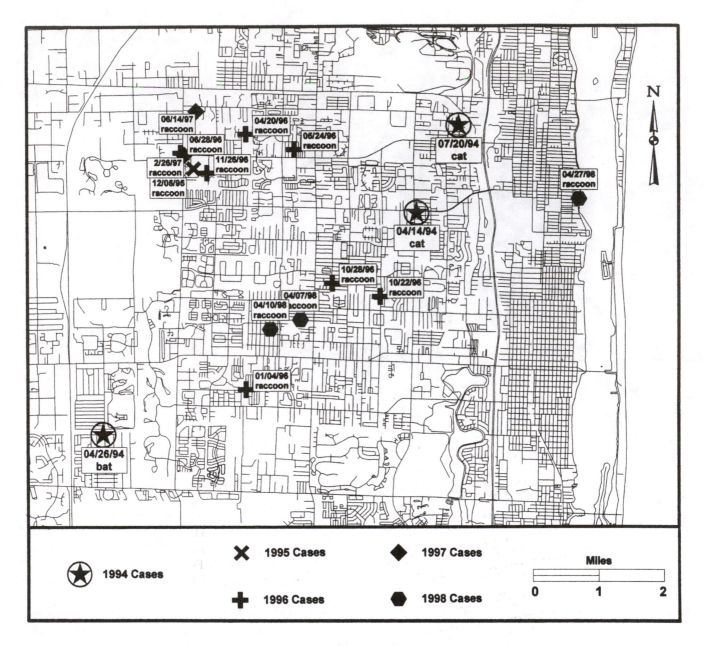

Figure 5–4 Animal rabies cases in central Palm Beach County, Florida, 1994–1998

communities from these diseases. We will provide a few examples.

Malaria

Malaria, a parasitic disease transmitted through mosquito vectors, is a major cause of illness in many tropical and subtropical areas. Worldwide, over two billion people are at risk for contracting malaria.[10] A study in Israel illustrates the use of GIS technology in helping target malarial control efforts on the basis of the location of reported human cases and the location of potential malarial vectors.[11] Although at the time of the study, malaria was not endemic in Israel, the existence of malaria in immigrant populations in proximity to mosquito breeding areas could present a risk for disease transmission. This study used a vector format for its spatial foundation database, including all settlements, roads, and administrative boundaries in Israel. Attribute data included laboratory malarial blood smear results from people emigrating from Ethiopia, a population most often associated with ma-

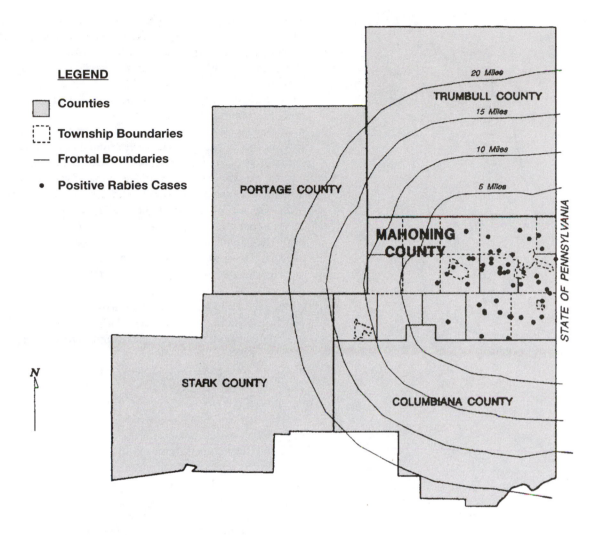

Figure 5–5 Positive raccoon-strain rabies cases in Mahoning County, Ohio, 1997

laria. The Israeli Ministry of the Environment provided mosquito surveillance data obtained from reports by regional mosquito control inspectors. Figure 5–6 is an event map, based on 1992 data, showing mosquito breeding sites and location of diagnosed imported malarial cases in Israel. Because different mosquito vectors have different flight ranges, similar maps can show breeding sites for each mosquito species. Such easy-to-create maps proved useful in targeting vector control effort by giving highest priority to breeding sites within flight distance of malarial cases.[11] Such cheap and efficient methodology should be helpful in developing countries with minimal resources and high endemic malaria rates.

Before the development of GIS technology, the only way to assess human risk was to manually monitor larval and adult mosquito populations. Such time-consuming fieldwork has been costly and frequently impractical in countries with fewer resources than Israel. In many areas, public health authorities either have not conducted vector control activities or have been unable to target their efforts to areas with the greatest risk.[10] In addition, many developing countries have not conducted surveillance for malaria, preventing them from identifying and targeting affected human populations.

The location of mosquitoes is associated with environmental factors, such as elevation, temperature, precipitation, and humidity. In addition, these environmental factors are associated with the type and distribution of vegetation, which can also influence mosquito populations. For example, in Chiapas, Mexico, field studies have shown that flooded pastures and transitional swamps (seasonally flooded scrub/shrub

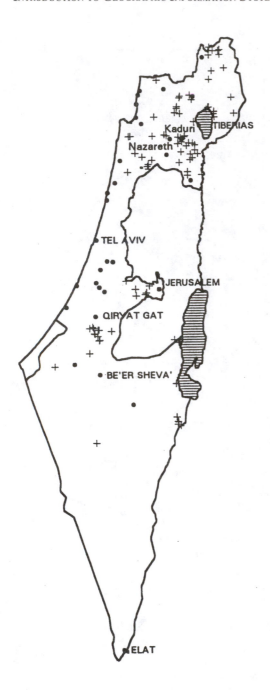

Figure 5–6 Imported malaria cases (•) and *Anopheles* breeding sites (+) in Israel, 1992

A study examined how GIS technology could help identify likely mosquito habitats near human populations for targeting. Remotely sensed data, in raster format, over a 1,270 km² area in southern Mexico served as the spatial database. Spatial data included two digital LANDSAT Thematic Mapper I satellite scenes, from wet and dry seasons, with each pixel representing a 28.5 × 28.5 m ground area. The Thematic Mapper data identified several different landscape elements, including mangrove forest, transitional swamp, secondary forest, riparian vegetation, managed and unmanaged pasture, annual crop, banana plantation, burned fields, and urban and inland water. Investigators then selected 40 villages within the study area and, using ultraviolet mosquito traps, measured the abundance of mosquitoes in each village. They divided villages into high or low categories based on measured mosquito abundance. Next, investigators created one km buffer zones around each village, based on the typical mosquito flight range, and overlaid these buffers on the landscape map to calculate percentage of area occupied by each landscape element within each buffer. They then used statistical methods to identify landscape variables contributing most to the separation of villages with the highest mosquito abundance from those with the lowest abundance. They also used linear regression to create a model predicting mosquito abundance in these villages.

The study results demonstrated that GIS technology could help predict which villages in the area were likely to have small or large numbers of mosquito vectors present. Villages within buffer zones containing larger proportions of two landscape elements identified by remotely sensed data, transitional swamp and unmanaged pasture, were more likely to contain larger numbers of mosquitoes. Although the threshold of mosquito abundance for efficient malarial disease transmission was unknown, people living in villages with the greatest densities of mosquitoes should be at higher risk of malaria if the parasite were present in the mosquito vector. Clearly, if we understand what landscape elements are related to mosquito survival, and if remote-sensing data containing these elements are available in digital format, GIS can help identify human populations at increased risk for disease transmission. This approach can help target malarial vector control much more cheaply and efficiently than older manual field methodologies.[10] A subsequent study in another area of Mexico did show that GIS methodology using remotely sensed data could be helpful elsewhere.[12]

A recent study in Trinidad showed how GIS technology, using a combination of GPS data and remote-sensing data, could help vector control programs efficiently allocate resources for malarial surveillance and control.[13] Although Trinidad successfully eradicated malaria in 1965, environmental conditions supporting vector habitat still exist on the island, and it is susceptible to sea and air importation of the

open forests) are preferred breeding habitats for *Anopheles albimananus*, the local mosquito vector. Consequently, if digital landscape data were available, GIS technology could help target control efforts by identifying these mosquito habitats[10] without the need to send inspectors into the field for manual testing.

malaria parasite. If this were to occur, the parasite could establish itself on the island and infect susceptible populations. For example, in 1991, an outbreak did occur in Icacos, a small town on the island, 19 km from Venezuela. The index case, an adult male, became infected in Venezuela, and mosquitoes transmitted the disease to nine other people living near the Icacos swamp. Clearly, the island is at risk for redevelopment of malaria, given the favorable vector habitat, the importation of cases from endemic areas on the mainland, and the lack of immunity of the local population.[13] By incorporating GPS data, GIS can precisely locate and map malaria cases and associate these with remote-sensing data that identify the location of vector habitats.

In Trinidad, four mosquito vector species inhabit four different environments, including *Anopheles aquasalis* in coastal swamps, *Anopheles bellator* in bromeliad vegetation, *Anopheles albitarsis* in rice fields, and *Anopheles oswaldoi* in small running streams. Since 1965, the Insect Vector Control Division (IVCD) of the Trinidad Ministry of Health has routinely conducted surveillance for imported cases of malaria. The IVCD requires hospitals and physicians to report patients with a febrile illness and a history of travel or residence to countries endemic for malaria. Additionally, the IVCD stations malaria evaluators at health centers. The evaluators collect blood samples on suspected patients and send the samples to the IVCD for malaria examination. Whenever a testing identifies malaria, the IVCD performs a thorough investigation to classify the case and determine whether any transmission occurred. Classifications include imported cases, introduced cases, and cryptic cases. Imported cases acquired their infection in another country, while introduced cases acquired their malaria infection by mosquito transmission from an imported case. The IVCD defined cryptic cases as isolated cases not associated with introduced cases. As part of the investigation, after enough time has elapsed for extrinsic incubation, the IVCD conducts active surveillance. The active surveillance includes deploying malaria evaluators to conduct mass malarial blood smear surveys and placing all health care providers and hospitals on alert for febrile illnesses. Because drugs for self-treatment are unavailable in Trinidad, the surveillance system probably identifies all clinical cases of malaria.[13]

After the Ministry of Health supplied the surveillance data, the Trinidad GIS study used a GPS to determine the geographic location of every case and entered the precise geographic coordinates into GIS software.[13] The study identified cases by parasite species, year, and origin. Some cases involved mixed infections with two parasites. Mixed infections counted twice when considering parasite species and once otherwise. Investigators performed a "*k*–nearest neighbor test" to evaluate the likelihood of spatial clustering (see Chapter 3). Of the 213 cases reported between 1968 and 1997, more than 40 percent (89) were *P. falciparum*, 30 percent (64) were *P. vivax*, and 25 percent (54) were *P. malariae*. One hundred and sixty-four cases were imported, and 49 were either cryptic or introduced. Of the imported cases, almost half (80) acquired the infection in Africa, while South America (45) and Asia (39) split the rest equally. Most of the African cases were *P. falciparum*, most of the Asian cases were *P. vivax*, and South America contributed equal proportions of *P. vivax* and *P. falciparum*. Table 5–1 reveals that the number of cases nearly tripled in the period from 1988 to 1997 compared to the period from 1968 to 1977.

Figure 5–7 is a map showing the spatial and temporal distribution of malaria cases in Trinidad.[13] The map displays the concentration of imported malaria near the port cities of Port of Spain and San Fernando on the west coast. However, cases reported most recently, between 1990 and 1997, were concentrated inland. Further geographic analysis by parasite species revealed a concentration of *P. malariae* cases in

---

Table 5–1 Imported Malaria Cases in Trinidad by Continent of Origin, and All Malaria Cases by *Plasmodium* Species, 1968–1997

Years	Continent of Origin			Parasite Species		
	Africa	Asia	South America	*P. vivax*	*P. malariae*	*P. falciparum*
1968–1972	10	1	0	1	6	8
1973–1977	5	3	2	3	6	6
1978–1982	11	8	1	8	4	8
1983–1987	26	14	9	15	7	29
1988–1992	17	9	8	25	9	17
1993–1997	11	4	25	17	25	23
Total	80	39	45	69	57	91

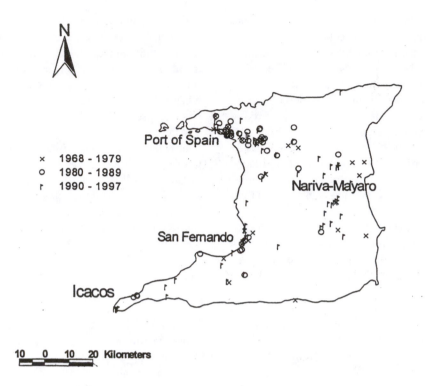

Figure 5–7 Spatial distribution of malaria cases in Trinidad, 1968–1997, according to decade

the center of the island, in the area around Nariva-Mayaro, and a small concentration of *P. vivax* near Icacos, at the southwest tip of the island (see Figure 5–8). Spatial analysis, using the *k*–nearest neighbor statistic, indicated that the *P. malariae* and *P. vivax* clusterings were significant, consistent with local transmission of cases. In contrast, *P. falciparum* cases did not cluster significantly, indicating that these cases were imported and not involved in the local transmission. The *P. vivax* cluster was associated with 1991 outbreak discussed earlier.

The results of this GIS analysis are useful for developing efficient malarial control programs in countries with limited resources. The study demonstrated that nearly all infections involving two parasite species, *P. falciparum* and *P. vivax*, were imported, most involving foreigners or Trinidad citizens infected while visiting another country. Not surprisingly, these cases were concentrated in the large port cities. These cases did not result in any local transmission. Even the Icacos *P. vivax* cluster, with its nine locally transmitted cases, was originally due to an imported index case. On the other hand, in the central part of the island, *P. malariae* cases were mostly due to local transmission associated with bromeliad malaria vectors. In this area, the Immortelle tree is a favored host for

bromeliad plants, which provide the breeding habitat for two species of malaria mosquito vectors, *Anopheles bellator* and *Anopheles homunculus*. These mosquito vectors can effectively transmit *P. malariae* to humans.

What does this mean for malaria control programs? The GIS study revealed that local transmission was associated with parasite species and index case location. Most cases of *P. vivax* and *P. falciparum* malaria occurring in urban areas were unlikely to result in further local transmission. On the other hand, cases of *P. malariae* detected in areas where a specific vector, *Anopheles bellator*, was common, were much more likely to result in further local transmission. On the basis of this analysis, the IVCD could safely change its policy of intensive follow-up active surveillance and control for every case. Such follow-up is incredibly expensive, averaging $100,000 U.S. for each case. Instead, the IVCD could adopt a policy of active surveillance and control only for *P. malariae* cases in rural areas and in coastal areas with marshes located near human dwellings. For imported cases, mostly *P. falciparum* and *P. vivax* detected in cities, case treatment and cheaper passive surveillance would be effective, especially in the dry season, when the probability of transmission is low.[13]

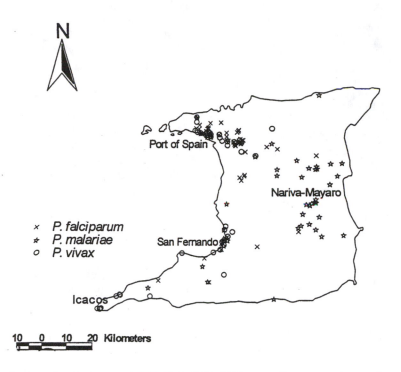

Figure 5–8 Spatial distribution of malaria cases in Trinidad, 1968–1997, according to parasite species

LaCrosse Encephalitis

GIS technology may prove helpful in helping target control efforts for mosquito-borne arboviral diseases, such as LaCrosse encephalitis.[14] Although most cases of this viral disease are asymptomatic, children younger than 15 years of age have the greatest risk for severe symptoms, including seizures. In most states, infectious encephalitis cases are reportable, and the reports include address information, making geographic analysis possible. An Illinois study used the U.S. Bureau of the Census as a source for spatial data, obtaining latitude and longitude data for the centroids of each Illinois city and county. The same source provided denominator population data, while the Illinois Department of Health provided data on location, age, gender, and month of onset of reported LaCrosse encephalitis cases for the period from 1988 to 1994. Investigators used these data sets to calculate incidence rates at the town and county levels and, using GIS technology, created maps showing cases, incidence rates, and clustering. They used spatial statistical methods to identify "hot spots" of encephalitis transmission and to measure the extent of clustering.

Figures 5–9 and 5–10 show the distribution of encephalitis in Illinois by county. Figure 5–9 is a choropleth map

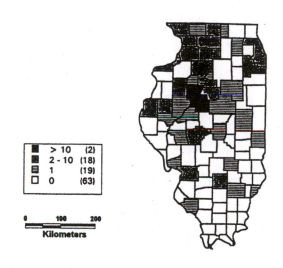

Figure 5–9 Distribution of LaCrosse encephalitis in Illinois by county, 1966–1995, total number of cases

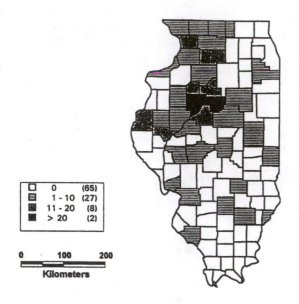

Figure 5–10 Distribution of LaCrosse encephalitis in Illinois by county, 1966–1995, incidence (per 100,000) of cases (county population densities based on 1990 census data)

with county shading based on numbers of cases, while Figure 5–10 is a choropleth map with shading based on incidence rate (cases per 100,000 population).[14] Over 50 percent of the reported cases were located in three counties in central Illinois, with two of them having the highest cumulative incidence of the disease. Peoria, the third largest city in the state, appeared to be the center of LaCrosse encephalitis endemicity in Illinois.[14] Within this region, an event map showed that one-third of all reported cases were from Peoria and two of its suburbs, East Peoria and Bartonville (see Figure 5–11). Spatial statistical analysis revealed several significant clusters of cases[14] (see Figure 5–12).

Clusters of encephalitis cases, as seen in this study, may be associated with the presence of factors known to support breeding and biting activities of the LaCrosse encephalitis mosquito vector, including forested areas, tree holes, and discarded tires and containers.[14] Such conditions are common in the Peoria region. A GIS analysis like this can help local health departments target vector control activities, such as community education and removal of discarded tires and containers. Follow-up studies can help evaluate the effectiveness of vector control efforts.

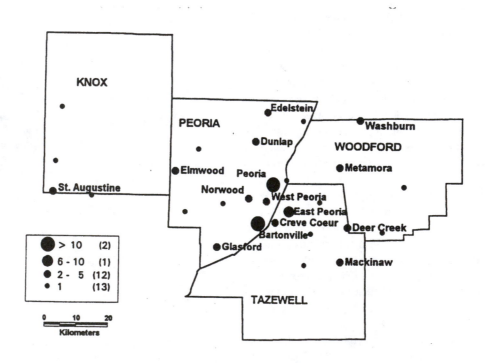

Figure 5–11 Distribution of LaCrosse encephalitis cases by town in the Peoria region, 1966–1995, number of cases

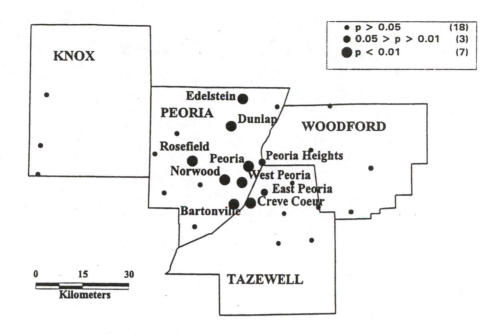

Figure 5–12 Distribution of LaCrosse encephalitis cases by town in the Peoria region, 1966–1995, significance level clustering of cases as measured by the $G_i(d)$ local spatial statistic over a distance of 10 km around each town

Onchocerciasis

Onchocerciasis, a filarial worm infection transmitted by the bite of a black fly vector, and a major cause of blindness in Guatemala,[15] provides another example of the usefulness of GIS technology in targeting public health measures. Drug treatment with Ivermectin, requiring only a single oral dose once or twice each year, is safe and effective enough to prevent blindness in entire populations of at-risk communities.[15] GIS technology can identify these communities because the risk of infection is associated with altitude. Below an elevation of 500 m, hot temperatures suppress the fly vector. Above 1,500 m, cooler temperatures suppress fly biting and reduce development of the parasite. To determine communities suitable for public health intervention, investigators entered into their GIS the names, elevations, and longitude/latitude coordinates of nearly 3,000 communities located in onchocerciasis endemic areas of the country. Then they stratified the communities by elevation, producing a map with communities specifically located between 500 and 1,500 m elevation (see Figure 5–13). Figure 5–14 is a map of a zoomed-in area, clearly showing communities appropriate for targeted treatment. Added overlays could include roads, road conditions, rivers, streams, demographic data, and other information potentially useful in targeting interventions.

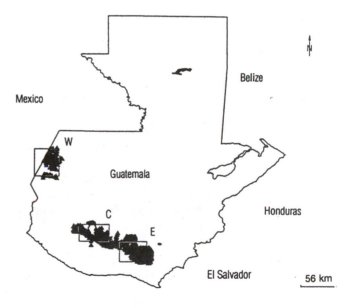

Figure 5–13 A total of 1,228 triangles are plotted on the map of Guatemala, these representing communities located between 500 and 1,500 m elevation, most of them within or bordering the western (W), central (C), and eastern (E) zones of endemic onchocerciasis in Guatemala

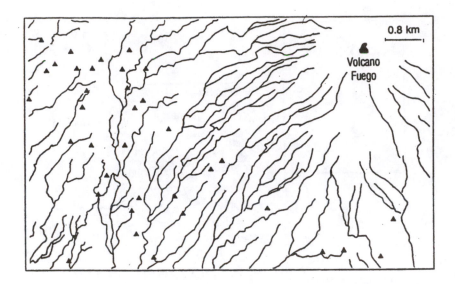

Figure 5–14 This more detailed map provides zoom magnification of a portion of Figure 5–13. That portion, considerably smaller than any of the rectangles in Figure 5–13, comes from a part of the central (C) zone on the slopes of the volcano Fuego. The communities targeted for potential treatment are again represented by triangles, and the thin lines show rivers and streams. These thin lines terminate near the western and eastern edges of the chart, where map digitization has not yet been completed. The crater of the volcano Fuego is shown in the upper right corner of the map.

Lyme Disease

Lyme disease, caused by the tick-borne spirochete *Borrelia burgdorferi*, is the most frequent vector-borne disease in the United States.[16,17] Epidemiologists consider geographic areas providing habitat for the tick vector and animal hosts as high-risk areas for disease transmission.[17] Environmental factors that may be important include tick habitat suitability, size, and access to human dwellings. Suitable habitats consist of areas with mixtures of hardwood and conifer trees with layers of shrubby vegetation, such as forest edges. Some studies have associated tick quantities with climatic factors such as humidity and temperature and other factors such as landscape slope, forested areas with sandy soils, and density of human residential development.[17] In several states, increases in reported Lyme disease cases in one year, 1996, were limited to certain counties, consistent with differences in the distribution and density of the tick vector.[16]

A few studies have recognized home residence as a risk factor for the disease, and investigators have used expensive techniques, such as surveying tick vectors and estimating the number of nearby animal host populations, to identify high-risk residential areas.[17] As with other vector-transmitted diseases, GIS technology may provide a cheaper and more efficient way for health departments to identify and target high-risk areas for prevention efforts by incorporating and displaying easily identified environmental factors associated with vector and host populations. Data sets containing detailed information on many of these factors are now available from several federal, state, and local agencies (see Chapter 2). An example from Maryland shows how GIS technology can integrate these data sets to develop Lyme disease risk models, useful for health departments for public education and disease control efforts.[17]

The Baltimore County, Maryland, study used cases and controls in developing the risk model. Cases, based on reports to the Maryland State Health Department during 1989 and 1990, met the CDC case definition of Lyme disease. The Baltimore County Department of Environmental Protection and Resource Development supplied the residence database for the randomly selected controls. Investigators added information on the geographic location where the tick bite occurred. For 6 of the 48 cases, the bite occurred at a location away from the residence.

Next, the investigators incorporated six environmental databases supplied by the Baltimore County Department of Environmental Protection and Resource Management and the Department of Geography, Towson State University. These databases contained information on land use/land cover, forest distributions, soils, elevation, geology, and watershed. All of these had a 400 foot × 500 foot (121.9 m × 152.4 m) resolution, resulting in a county grid map with 164,248 cells for each variable.[17]

The land use/land cover database, in raster format, was a composite derived from two sources of data: a 1990 LANDSAT Thematic Mapper satellite image and planimetric maps of the urban portions of the county. The land use/land cover database contained three categories of residential property, six categories of urban property, three categories of zoned but undeveloped residential land, four categories of zoned but undeveloped urban property, and one category each of agricultural land, recreational land, forested land, and water.

The LANDSAT image also helped generate the forest distribution database. Investigators classified cells as forest if more than half of the cell contained forest. In contrast to the land use/land cover database, the forest distribution database classified some recreational areas, agricultural areas, and low-density residential areas as forest if cells within them were more than half forested.

The U.S. Department of Agriculture supplied the soil survey database for Baltimore County. This database, with a 1-acre (0.004 km^2) resolution, contained 61 soil series recognized in the county. To incorporate geology data, the investigators digitized 1:63,360–scale Maryland Geological Survey maps. This database contained the 30 rock formations within the county. Similarly, the investigators digitized 1:63,360–scale maps provided by the Baltimore City Department of Public Works to incorporate data containing the distribution of the 15 watersheds in the county.[17]

After incorporating all the environmental data sets, the investigators extracted 127 study variables. In keeping with their case-control design, they evaluated each of these variables at the residence of each case patient and control subject. After using stratified analysis and logistic regression to control for confounders and identify significant variables, the investigators used a logistic regression equation to generate a map predicting areas of the county where people were at risk for Lyme disease. Although 6 of the 48 cases suffered their tick bite away from their residence, results were similar whether or not these six cases were included in the analysis. They validated their predictive model by using statistical methods (the Hosmer-Lemeshow goodness-of-fit statistic) and by comparing the model's predicted risks, based on 1989–90 data, with the following year's (1991) actual incidence data.

The final logistic regression model included five variables. Increased risk for Lyme disease was associated with residence in two combined watersheds, in forested areas, in some specific underlying geological formations, and on deep, loamy soils in a specific area, the Piedmont. Residence in highly developed areas was a protective factor. The presence of loamy soils and forest around residential areas interacted to increase the risk for Lyme disease. Figure 5–15 is a map predicting Lyme disease risk based on the final logistic regression model.[17] Table 5–2 categorizes risk for areas of the county by quartile.[17] Total county land area is 1,560 km^2. Of this area, 486 km^2, or 31.2 percent of the county, was in the lowest-risk quartile, while 19.0 percent of the county, a 296 km^2 area, was in the highest-risk quartile. Incidence of Lyme disease in 1991, the following year, validated the predicted risk model. In 1991, the gradient of risk across the three highest quartiles increased exponentially compared to that of the lowest-risk areas (see Table 5–2).[17] Residence in the highest-risk areas was associated with the greatest increase in the odds of infection in 1991 compared to residence in the lowest-risk areas. Specifically, the 1991 incidence rate was 72 per 100,000 in the predicted high-risk areas compared to 4.35 per 100,000 in the predicted lowest-risk areas.

This Lyme disease study further illustrates the potential of GIS technology in helping public health agencies to identify environmental factors associated with vector-borne diseases and, in turn, to identify human populations at risk. Residential developments continue to move into and change vector and animal-reservoir habitat areas. GIS analysis may be critical in evaluating the effects of these landscape changes, the presence of humans, and the resulting changes in transmission opportunities of vector-borne pathogens on the emergence of new diseases and the resurgence of old ones.[9] In addition to Lyme disease, GIS technology could be useful in identifying human populations at risk for other tick-borne infections, such as babesiosis, ehrlichiosis, and Rocky Mountain spotted fever. Health departments could then use this information to protect the public in several ways. For example, they could target educational messages to people living in identified high-risk areas. These messages could include instructions on wearing light-colored clothing (to more readily detect ticks), tucking long pants into socks, using insect repellents and acaricides according to label directions, and performing tick checks at least daily.[16] Health departments could target health care providers in high-risk areas with information on how to recognize the disease and on drugs of choice for their infected patients. Once vaccines for Lyme disease and other vector-borne diseases become available, health departments could use the GIS-developed risk models to target populations for immunization programs. Finally, the risk models could help target environmental interventions for residential properties in high-risk areas. Such interventions could include the application of insecticides, the use of deer fencing, and removal of leaf litter[16] or even zoning changes to prevent development in high-risk areas. Follow-up incidence studies using GIS in subsequent

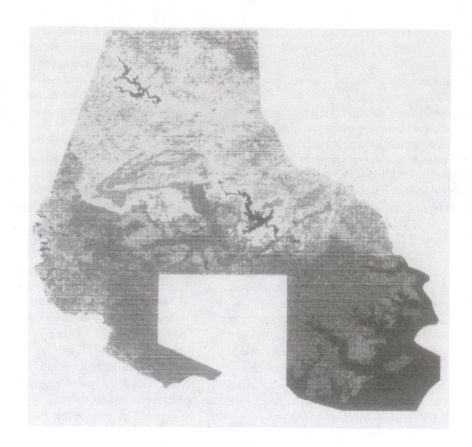

Figure 5–15 Lyme disease—risk density map from logistic regression model that used environmental variables in Baltimore County, Maryland, 1989 through 1990

Table 5–2 Linear Trends for the Association of Lyme Disease in 1991 with Lyme Disease Risk at the Place of Residence in 1989 through 1990, the Areal Extent of Baltimore County in Each Category, and the Estimated Incidence of Disease

Risk Category 1989 through 1990[a]	OR (95% CI)	Area, km²	1991 Incidence (per 100,000)
Lowest[b]	1.0	486	4.35
Low	2.2 (1.0, 4.8)	403	9.54
Moderate	3.2 (1.2, 8.6)	374	13.91
High	16.4 (4.7, 58.5)	296	71.52

[a]Test for linear trend for association: $\chi^2 = 29.10$; $P < .00001$.
[b]Reference category.

years could help evaluate the effectiveness of these interventions.

Schistosomiasis

Schistosoma mansoni, a parasite that causes schistosomiasis, is transmitted to humans through contact with several species of an intermediate host, *Biomphalaria*, a freshwater snail. Schistosomiasis has become a significant threat to health in northeastern Brazil, where the disease is now endemic. The likelihood of disease transmission is associated with ecologic factors favoring snail habitat and concentrations of susceptible human populations. Studies have shown that the volume, distribution, and rate of infection of the snail population and contact with domestic water are important factors associated with the risk of human infection. In addition, snail populations vary with seasonal rainfall, with larger numbers found during rainy periods and smaller numbers in drought months.[18] High altitude, low human population density, high-quality sanitation, and limited numbers of snail breeding sites are other factors associated with lower rates of human infection.[18] Consequently, GIS technology, with its ability to integrate landscape, climatic, demographic, and disease report data sets, is especially suited as a tool for identifying areas and populations at risk for this disease, enabling public health authorities to target preventive interventions, such as suppression of the snail population with molluscides, efficiently and effectively. A study from Bahia, Brazil, shows how this might be successful.

Bahia, a state in northern Brazil, contains over 12 million people in 415 municipalities. Investigators selected 270 municipalities for the study. The Brazil Ministry of Health Schistosomiasis Control Program, conducted from 1991 through 1993, had provided standard chemotherapy and snail control interventions for these municipalities and had maintained records on them. To obtain prevalence data, investigators used a sample of school children aged 7 to 14 years, born and living in one of 30 municipalities randomly selected for the study. They screened children for infection using the Kato-Katz technique, a way of measuring *S. mansoni* eggs in feces.[18] Investigators selected the 30 municipalities using a random-sample scheme after they ranked all 270 municipalities by prevalence on the basis of Ministry of Health Data. They selected 10 municipalities each from three prevalence groups and assigned municipalities with prevalence rates of 0.1 to 4.9 percent to the low-prevalence group, those with rates of 6.3 to 18.0 percent to the medium-prevalence group, and those with prevalence rates of 21 to 61 percent to the high-prevalence group. The Brazilian Foundation Institute of Geography and Statistics supplied the census data for each municipality, which contained population density (people per square kilometer) information. Investigators obtained spatial data, with municipality borders at a 1:1,000,000 scale, from the Digital Chart of the World (DCW; 1993. Defense Mapping Agency, MIL-D-89009, Philadelphia, PA).

Investigators next created four categories of snail distribution, based on the presence of distinct snail species, for each municipality. They defined category A as municipalities containing *B. glabrata*, category B as municipalities containing *B. straminia*, category C as municipalities with *B. tenagophila*, and category F as municipalities free of all *Biomphalaria* species. Category A + B included municipalities containing two species, *B. glabrata* and *B. straminia*. Investigators digitized snail distribution data from a 1:12,000,000–scale map. They then incorporated four environmental databases: elevation, climatic variables, soil type, and vegetation type. The DCW supplied elevation data. The investigators used cartographic maps, at a 1:5,000,000 scale, to create climatic variables for the study. Climatic variables contained 30-year average climate data for each municipality, including maximum rainfall, mean number of dry months during the year, mean maximum temperature, mean minimum temperature, mean rainfall in three consecutive months, temperature difference, and mean monthly maximum and minimum temperatures during the year. Maps of vegetation and soils, at a 1:10,000,000 scale, provided the soil and vegetation data.

Figure 5–16 shows the structure of the GIS application used in the study. Investigators used several techniques to incorporate data in different formats and scales and to develop their GIS application. These techniques, using GIS software, included digitizing hard-copy maps, transforming different map projections, matching edges of adjacent maps, assigning attribute data to spatial features, and constructing spatial queries. They created several layers of data, including variables for climate, soil type, vegetation, elevation, municipal boundaries, disease prevalence, snail distribution, and population. Finally, they georeferenced the digitized maps to the 1:1,000,000–scale DCW base maps.

Spatial analysis revealed a significant association between prevalence group with two variables, length of dry period and population density, and showed that one snail species, *B. glabrata*, was the chief species of snail found in high-prevalence areas. Figure 5–17, a choropleth map of Bahia, illustrates the relationship between dry periods, snail species, and municipal prevalence of schistosomiasis. Municipalities with high schistosomiasis prevalence tended to have shorter dry periods and higher population densities. One snail species, *B. glabrata*, was found in 100 percent of municipalities with high prevalence rates. The presence of a high proportion of one soil type, latossolo, and transitional vegetation were also associated with high disease prevalence,

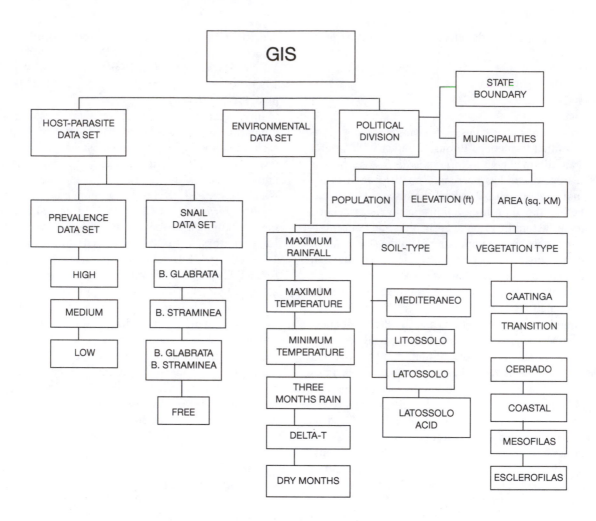

Figure 5–16 Computer graphic representation of the GIS constructed for schistosomiasis in Bahia, Brazil. B. = *Biomphalaria;* DELTA-T = diurnal temperature difference

while litossolo soil was present only in areas with low disease prevalence.

What does this mean for schistosomiasis control programs? The map clearly indicates areas of high prevalence for targeting control efforts. Results of the study also suggest that public health authorities might want to begin chemotherapy at the end of the dry season to diminish the level of infection in the water. Additionally, public health authorities might consider using molluscide agents to kill the snails at the beginning of the rainy season, when they are beginning to recover from aestivation during the drought.[18]

SEXUALLY TRANSMITTED DISEASE: GONORRHEA

As with other reportable diseases in the United States, gonorrhea reports include case addresses, making the disease suitable for GIS analysis. In the United States and other developed countries, gonorrhea incidence tends to cluster in core areas.[19] Before the development of GIS technology, most public health departments could only analyze and report county or statewide rates of gonorrhea. This was a serious limitation, especially in urban areas with significant ethnic,

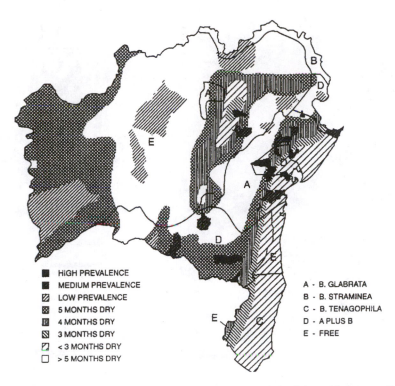

Figure 5–17 Map of GIS feature overlays showing the spatial distribution of 30 municipalities with low, medium, and high prevalence, boundaries of snail host distribution, and length of the dry period in Bahia, Brazil. B. = *Biomphalaria*

racial, and socioeconomic diversity. By identifying core areas within jurisdictions and depicting them on a map, GIS technology can help with disease control efforts. In addition, because gonorrhea has a short incubation period, can recur, and is easy to diagnose and treat, GIS technology can help health departments evaluate the short-term effectiveness of targeted disease control programs by depicting changes in local incidence.[19]

Figure 5–18 is a choropleth map, with census tracts shaded on the basis of case counts for each census tract in Baltimore, Maryland. A commercial source supplied the digital spatial data, including street addresses, streets, ZIP codes, and census tracts for Baltimore. Attribute data included demographic data by census tract and gonorrhea case reports. The same commercial source supplied the demographic data, which provided population denominators for calculating incidence rates. The Baltimore City Health Department and the Maryland State Health Department provided gonorrhea report data. The Baltimore City data included disease reports from Baltimore public and private providers. The state data provided case reports for Baltimore residents seen by providers outside the city limits. Figure 5–19 is an incidence map, showing actual location of each reported case.

Figures 5–20 and 5–21 show the value of GIS technology in integrating census data and disease report data in depicting incidence rates. Although two census tracts in northwestern Baltimore had large numbers of cases, these areas also had large underlying populations of individuals aged 15 to 39 years, the age group at highest risk for gonorrhea. Consequently, incidence rates were relatively low in these areas, as shown in Figure 5–21, a choropleth map of incidence rate. This map also illustrates the core distribution of gonorrhea in central Baltimore. Although the map, based on an ecologic analysis, does not explain the reason for this distribution, it can help the local health department in its disease control efforts. For example, because of the disease distribution, sexual contacts living within the core area may be more likely to be infected and may be a higher priority for targeted screening and treatment.[19] Follow-up geographic analysis of incidence rates in the core can help evaluate the effectiveness of these targeted interventions.

Besides helping target gonorrhea prevention efforts, the GIS analyses provided additional "quality control" information helpful to the health department in improving health care delivery in Baltimore.[2] Specifically, the analyses revealed that private health care providers failed to report ra-

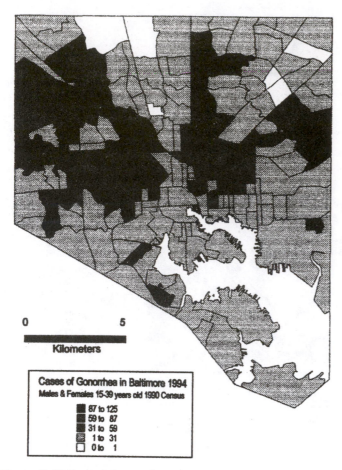

Figure 5–18 Reported gonorrhea case counts by census tract for persons aged 15–39 years (1990 census), Baltimore City, Maryland

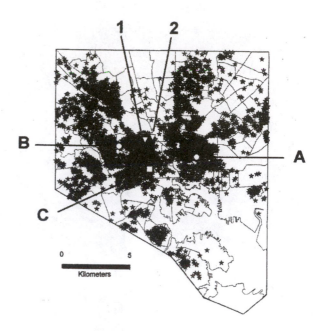

Figure 5–19 Dot map of reported gonorrhea for cases with valid residential addresses ($n = 6,831$), Baltimore City, Maryland, 1994. The Baltimore City Health Department sexually transmitted disease (STD) program operates two STD clinics located within high incidence areas (A & B). Point C represents the geographic centroid of the city. Point 1 represents the mean vector of private sector cases from the geographic centroid; point 2 represents the mean vector of public sector cases. The scalar distance between point 1 and point 2 is 299 m

cial data on 28 percent of their cases, compared to a 1 percent failure rate for public clinics. In addition, the analyses revealed that some of the patients with sexually transmitted diseases visited private offices and public clinics on the same day. Previous studies had failed to identify this because private providers and public clinics used different identification numbers. The GIS software was able to identify these duplicate visits because it identified cases by specific demographic information and residence address. Follow-up inspection of confidential information by health department staff revealed that private providers did not treat these individuals, instead sending them to public clinics for treatment.[2]

Another ecologic GIS analysis of gonorrhea, this time in New Orleans, illustrates the use of overlays in generating questions about a disease for further study. In this study, compared to the Baltimore study, investigators overlaid an additional layer of attribute data, the location of retail alcohol outlets.[20] The Louisiana Office of Alcoholic Beverage Control (ABC) provided the alcohol outlet license data, which included the address of all retail outlets. The ABC classified alcohol outlets as "on premises" where alcohol was consumed on site, such as bars and restaurants, and "off premises" where alcohol was purchased for later consumption, such as liquor stores, grocery stores, and convenience stores.[20] A commercial source, the Claritas Corporation, supplied the population denominator data (based on 1994 projections of census data) and sociodemographic data, and the Louisiana Health Department supplied the gonorrhea report data. TIGER served as the spatial database foundation. Investigators calculated alcohol outlet density in two ways. First, they divided the number of outlets in each census tract by the census tract population. Second, they divided the number of outlets in each census tract by the census tract size in square miles. Because the investigators were interested in studying the relationship between gonorrhea incidence and alcohol outlets in urban residential neighborhoods, they eliminated rural, commercial, and tourist census tracts from the study.

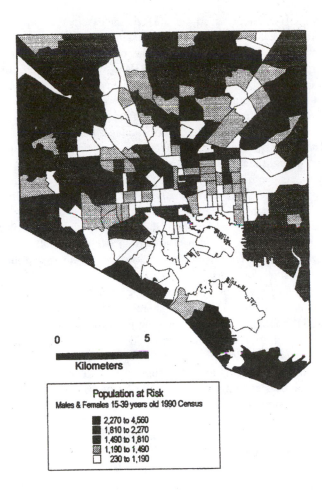

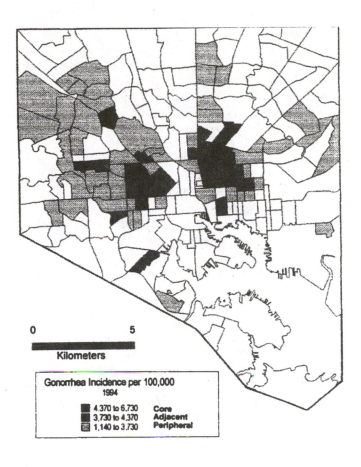

Figure 5–20 Population density of census tracts for persons aged 15–39 years (1990 census), Baltimore City, Maryland. Note that the population in the northwest quadrant of the city is denser than the population in the inner-city areas adjacent to the sexually transmitted diseases clinics

Figure 5–21 Gonorrhea incidence per 100,000 by census tract, for census tracts with >30 cases (1990 census), Baltimore City, Maryland, 1994. Note that when rates are calculated, disease density is highest in the inner-city core areas, in contrast to Figure 5–18

The result is a choropleth map of alcohol outlet density per 10,000 population by census tract, with an overlay of gonorrhea incidence. The map illustrates that gonorrhea cases are concentrated in areas of high outlet density. After accounting for sociodemographic variables, such as race and employment, alcohol outlet density by population and by square mile was still statistically associated with gonorrhea incidence. The relationship was stronger for off-premise outlets and for outlet density per square mile.

Like other ecologic analyses, the map does not address the cause of gonorrhea, but it does raise questions for further analyses based on individual exposure measures. For example, does alcohol consumption promote high-risk sexual behavior? Alternatively, is alcohol consumption a marker for individuals with risk-taking behaviors? Certainly, studies of

individual behaviors and exposures are necessary to answer many of these questions. Besides raising hypotheses, the map provides opportunities for evaluation of neighborhood-level interventions. For example, some neighborhoods are voting to remove alcohol outlets. Subsequent geographic studies can evaluate whether gonorrhea incidence rates change after these interventions.[20]

TUBERCULOSIS

Tuberculosis is a major worldwide cause of communicable disease death for adults.[21] Between 19 and 43 percent of the world's population is infected with *Mycobacterium tuberculosis*, the organism that causes the disease. Once an individual is infected, the organism usually remains dormant in the body. In about 10 percent of infected people, the organism eventually begins replicating, leading to active disease that can result in transmission of the organism to others. The World Health Organization (WHO) estimates that more than eight million of those infected, including children, develop active tuberculosis and that approximately three million die from the disease each year.[22,23] Within the United States, the CDC estimates that tuberculosis infects 15 million people, who provide a reservoir for potentially future active cases.

Once someone is diagnosed with active tuberculosis, treatment to eradicate the infection requires the administration of several medications for a minimum of six months. Like many other communicable diseases, tuberculosis has social determinants, occurring disproportionately in the homeless and other socioeconomically deprived, hard-to-reach populations.[22] Failure to complete the required course of treatment can lead to disease recurrence with the added risk of drug resistance. Consequently, to ensure completion of therapy and protect communities, the CDC has recommended treating all active cases with directly observed therapy (DOT).[24] With DOT, a health care provider or other responsible person, such as an outreach worker, observes the patient swallowing each dose of tuberculosis medication. This can occur in any office or clinic, at the patient's home, work site, school, or any other place agreed to by the patient and outreach worker. In specific cases, corrections staff, drug treatment providers, community volunteers, or family members can assist with DOT.[24]

In several developing countries with huge increases in tuberculosis incidence, traditional treatment strategies based on prolonged hospitalization are not economically feasible. As a result, WHO has recently promoted community-based outpatient strategies employing DOT,[21] similar to strategies used in the United States. A study in South Africa illustrates the use of GIS technology in supporting these strategies by helping health officials locate target populations and available resources.[21] Results from this study have applications for health officials interested in efficiently targeting their DOT programs in the United States and elsewhere.

The HIV epidemic has greatly increased problems with tuberculosis for the population of 210,000 in the Hlabisa Health District, located in northern KwaZulu/Natal, South Africa. Between 1993 and 1997, HIV prevalence among adults with tuberculosis increased from 36 to 67 percent, resulting in significant increases to the health district's tuberculosis caseload. The tuberculosis program treats all patients for the first two to three weeks in the hospital and uses community-based DOT to treat 90 percent of the patients for the remaining five and a half months after they leave the hospital. The other 10 percent of patients are too ill for discharge. When the health district began the program in 1991, available village clinic nurses and community health workers (CHWs) supervised the DOT. As the caseload grew, program directors realized that the distance to the village clinics was too great for many of the patients and that many areas within the district lacked CHWs. As a result, program managers recruited volunteer DOT supervisors, including storekeepers and school and church personnel. Because the program maintained a computerized database of demographic, clinical, and program management information, including type and location of supervisors, program managers thought that a GIS approach might be helpful in linking patients geographically with DOT supervisory resources.

To perform their GIS analysis, program managers first created a spatial database in raster format by digitizing a series of geographic layers of the district (including magisterial and nature reserve boundaries) from 1:50,000 topographic maps. They used two methods to map the geographical position of every homestead within the district. Using GPS, they positioned the location of 16,583 homesteads. To position the other 7,741 homesteads, they digitized 1:10,000 aerial photographs. After locating the residences of potential patients, program managers added an attribute database containing the location of DOT supervision sites and the number of patients annually supervised at each site. They created raster images (at a resolution of 20 m) containing supervision sites in 1991 and 1996 and potential supervision sites, including clinics, CHW homes, shops, churches, schools, and the local hospital. Next, program managers compared the number of patients and the geographic distribution of DOT supervision sites in 1991 against 1996. The analysis included the distance of each homestead to the nearest DOT supervision site by category of site and the average distance of homesteads to each DOT supervision site in use in 1991 and 1996, as well as potential DOT supervision sites in 1998.

Figures 5–22 and 5–23 show that the proportion of patients treated in the hospital significantly decreased from 1991 to 1996 (50/268 to 100/773, $p = 0.01$), despite the large increase in caseload. During the same time, the number of community DOT sites increased from 37 to 147. As further evidence of the changes to a community-based system, the proportion of patients supervised by volunteers and CHWs increased significantly (16 to 41 percent, $p < 0.0001$), while the proportion supervised at clinic sites significantly decreased (56 to 24 percent, $p < 0.0001$). Figures 5–22 and 5–23 and Table 5–3 show that the average distance from homestead to DOT supervisor fell from 2.3 km in 1991 to 1.5 km in 1996. Table 5–3 also shows that adding community-based DOT sites, such as clinics, CHWs, and volunteers, in 1991 and 1996 enhanced geographic access for patients. As the program added these sites, the distance from home to DOT diminished from 29.7 to 2.3 km in 1991 and

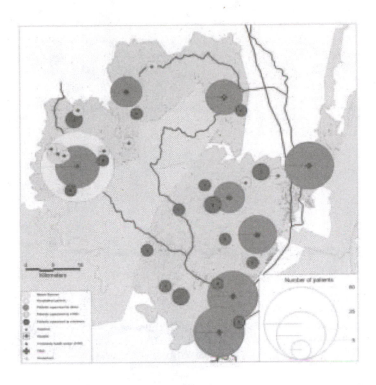

Figure 5–22 Treatment and supervision of tuberculosis patients in Hlabisa district, 1991

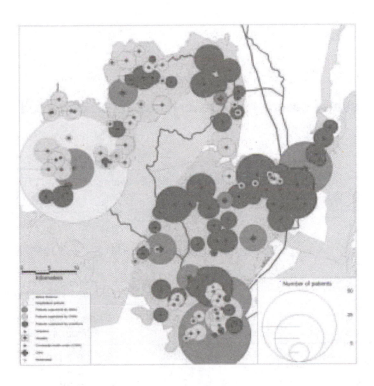

Figure 5–23 Treatment and supervision of tuberculosis patients in Hlabisa district, 1996

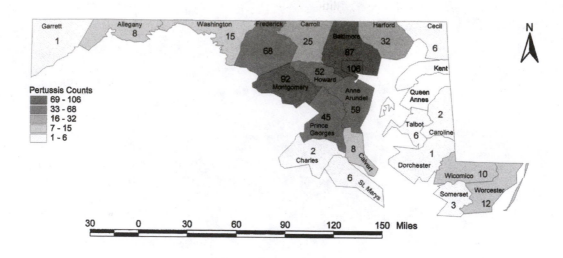

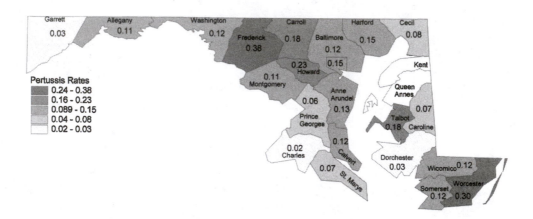

Note: Counties rates based on 5 or fewer cases should be viewed as statistically unstable

Figure 5–24 Numbers of pertussis cases and rates per 1,000 population by county, Maryland, 1997

Table 5–3 Mean (SD) Distance (km) from Homestead to Nearest Actual (1991 and 1996) and Potential Tuberculosis Treatment Point

	Distance to Tuberculosis Treatment Point (Mean, SD)		
	Actual Supervision Points 1991	Actual Supervision Points 1996	Potential Supervision Points
Hospital	29.7 (17.4	29.7 (17.4)	29.7 (17.4)
Hospital and clinics	5.5 (3.7)	4.6 (2.7)	4.2 (2.7)
Hospital, clinics, and CHWs	4.7 (3.7)	2.7 (2.2)	2.0 (1.8)
Hospital, clinics, CHW, and volunteers	2.3 (1.7)	1.5 (1.0)	0.8 (0.6)

from 29.7 to 1.5 km in 1996. The addition of additional potential supervision sites could decrease the distance further to 0.8 km.

This study illustrates the potential use of GIS in helping health departments enhance access to DOT for their patients with active tuberculosis. The technology is as applicable in the United States as South Africa. The South Africa study analyzed the distance between all residences and DOT resources. A future study hopes to analyze the distance for actual patients to DOT supervision sites.[21] Most large local health departments in the United States already have electronic databases containing information on the residence of individual tuberculosis patients. These local health departments could use GIS to identify the location of potential DOT supervision, including volunteer resources, in proximity to patients with active tuberculosis. Additionally, health departments could evaluate the most cost-efficient way to deploy their own DOT resources, such as nurses and CHWs. Further studies could address the relationship between patient geographic access to DOT supervision by type of supervision (e.g., volunteer or nurse), patient demographics, and successful treatment completion, helping local health departments design more effective tuberculosis treatment programs.

PUTTING IT ALL TOGETHER: AN AUTOMATED COMMUNICABLE DISEASE SURVEILLANCE SYSTEM

The Maryland Department of Health and Mental Hygiene is developing a GIS application that will automatically collect, analyze, and map all reportable communicable diseases.[25] The system will incorporate five sources of attribute data:

1. Routine mandated disease reports to local health departments, including communicable disease
2. Special communicable-disease studies, such as active surveillance by hospitals for nosocomial infections
3. Results of active surveillance for sentinel infections, such as drug-resistant infections in hospitalized patients
4. Data produced by collaborative research between public health agencies and the private sector, including managed care organizations
5. Other sources of communicable-disease data, such as Medicaid billing data

Local health departments in Maryland already have electronic access to the first two sources of data and software applications through either wide-area networks (WANs) or dial-up connections. The Maryland Department of Health and Mental Hygiene GIS application, called YourData, will work through either type of connection. Using YourData, local health departments can map communicable-disease events and rates, odds ratios, and relative risks by county, ZIP code, and census tract boundaries. Local health department staff without database management skills can use the application because it automates GIS database management operations such as importing and integrating data tables with a map.[25]

The maps in Figure 5–24 show how the application can map pertussis cases and rates by county in several easy steps. First, working off-line, state staff used standard spreadsheet software to create a table containing four variables (see Table 5–4):

1. A county Federal Information Processing (FIPS) geographic identifier code
2. Numbers of pertussis cases by county in 1997
3. The county population
4. Pertussis rates per county (column 3 divided by column 4 and multiplied by 1,000)

Table 5–4 Numbers of Pertussis Cases and Rates per 1,000 Population by County, Maryland, 1997

County FIPS Identifier Code	Numbers of Cases	Population	Rate per 1,000 Population*
24001	8	74,924	0.11
24003	59	463,199	0.13
24005	87	713,527	0.12
24009	8	66,203	0.12
24011	2	29,321	0.07
24013	25	140,660	0.18
24015	6	79,362	0.08
24017	2	114,925	0.02
24019	1	30,414	0.03
24021	68	180,204	0.38
24023	1	29,735	0.03
24025	32	212,165	0.15
24027	52	223,167	0.23
24031	92	816,985	0.11
24033	45	778,139	0.06
24037	6	82,282	0.07
24039	3	24,529	0.12
24041	6	32,759	0.18
24043	15	128,126	0.12
24045	10	80,232	0.12
24047	12	40,389	0.30
24510	106	691,465	0.15

*Rates based on small numbers (less than five cases) may be statistically unreliable.

The application can accommodate other variables of interest, such as race and gender, as long as the incorporated population data include denominator data for these populations.

Next, still working off-line, state staff store the table data on the computer network as a database [dBase (*.dbf)] file, a common database format.

The third step occurs automatically. When a user starts the YourData application, an automatic prompt appears directing the application to the dBase file on the computer network system. YourData then automatically joins the database (*.dbf) file to the spatial database on the basis of the common FIPS identifier field. (The application can produce maps by smaller geographic areas, such as census tracts, if the attribute database file and the spatial database both include the same information at the smaller geographic level.)

Using the YourData graphical interface (containing customized buttons and menus), local health departments can then create maps of communicable-disease counts and rates by county, such as the maps of pertussis in Figure 5–24. For presentations, the maps are exportable as Windows metafiles (*.wmf) to the computer network system. With little training, staff can import the metafiles onto a slide within a slide presentation program. To create the maps in Figure 5–24, the authors printed the slide in black and white, using a 600 dots-per-inch laser printer. They recommend using a color printer with higher resolution to illustrate contrasting polygon colors, especially if the analysis involves smaller geographical units, such as census tracts or census block groups.

The creators of YourData are developing training sessions to help local health department staff learn to use the application. They are planning future versions to include a module to geocode street addresses, allowing the user to perform additional analytical tests, such as spatial scan statistics and cluster analysis. For more information, and for downloading program source codes, those interested should contact the Web site at <www.digizen.net/member/jayanthd/gis.html>.

CHAPTER   REVIEW

1. Knowledge of the spatial distribution of communicable-disease cases is essential in understanding disease transmission. The integrative features of modern GIS technology are incredibly helpful in summarizing the complex relationships between communicable-disease pathogens, associated disease vectors and reservoirs, the environment, and human populations. GIS mapping can provide new insights into both communicable-disease etiology and appropriate interventions, enhancing our ability to prevent and control communicable disease and to evaluate the effectiveness of our efforts.

2. Public health officials can use GIS technology to prevent and control vaccine-preventable communicable disease by
   - Targeting immunization efforts to geographic areas ("pockets of need") containing large numbers of underimmunized children
   - Targeting immunization efforts to geographic areas with high incidence rates for vaccine-preventable diseases, such as hepatitis A and pertussis
   - Targeting rabies control efforts to geographic areas with reported rabies cases

3. For communicable diseases transmitted by arthropod (insect) vectors, the risk of disease transmission is often associated with specific environmental conditions that support vector populations. The overlay fea-

ture of GIS technology facilitates the identification of many of these factors, including climate, vegetation type, soil pattern, and the size of insect, human, and animal reservoir populations. By using this information to explain and predict disease transmission and distribution, health officials can develop improved methods for preventing arthropod-borne diseases such as malaria, LaCrosse encephalitis, onchocerciasis, and Lyme disease.

4. Before the development of GIS technology, most public health departments could only analyze and report county or statewide rates of sexually transmitted diseases such as gonorrhea. This was a serious limitation, especially in urban areas with significant ethnic, racial, and socioeconomic diversity. By identifying core areas within jurisdictions and depicting them on a map, GIS technology can help with disease control efforts. In addition, because gonorrhea has a short incubation period, can recur, and is easy to diagnose and treat, GIS technology can help health departments evaluate the short-term effectiveness of targeted disease control programs by depicting changes in local incidence.

5. Health officials can use GIS technology to improve the efficiency of their tuberculosis treatment programs. The CDC has recommended treating all active tuberculosis cases with directly observed therapy

(DOT). With DOT, a health care provider or other responsible person, such as an outreach worker, observes the patient swallowing each dose of tuberculosis medication at home, work, school, or any other place agreed to by the patient and outreach worker. Local health departments could use GIS to identify the location of potential DOT supervision, including volunteer resources, in proximity to patients with active tuberculosis. Further studies could address the relationship between patient geographic access to DOT supervision by type of supervision (e.g., volunteer or nurse), patient demographics, and successful treatment completion, helping local health departments design more effective tuberculosis treatment programs.

6. Automated GIS that collect, analyze, and map all reportable communicable diseases promise to improve the efficiency of disease control efforts. Such systems can incorporate multiple sources of data, such as

- Routine mandated disease reports to local health departments
- Special communicable-disease studies, such as active surveillance by hospitals for nosocomial infections
- Results of active surveillance for sentinel infections, such as drug-resistant infections in hospitalized patients
- Data produced by collaborative research between public health agencies and the private sector, including managed care organizations
- Other sources of communicable disease data, such as Medicaid billing data

REFERENCES

1. A.L. Melnick and D.W. Fleming. "Modern Geographic Information Systems: Promise and Pitfalls." *Journal of Public Health Management and Practice* 5, no. 2 (1999): viii–x.

2. G.E. Glass. "Geographic Information Systems," in *Infectious Disease Epidemiology: Theory and Practice,* eds. K.E. Nelson et al. Gaithersburg, MD: Aspen Publishers, Inc., 2000: 231–252.

3. J. Devine et al. "Identifying Predicted Immunization 'Pockets of Need,' Hillsborough County, Florida, 1996–1997." *Journal of Public Health Management and Practice* 5, no. 2 (1999): 15–16.

4. Public Health Foundation. "Immunization Strategies for Health Care Practices and Providers." Ch. 3 in *The Pink Book: Epidemiology and Prevention of Vaccine-Preventable Diseases*, 6th ed. (Training and Education Branch, Immunization Services Division, National Immunization Program, Centers for Disease Control and Prevention, 2000); http://www.cdc.gov/nip/publications/pink/: 27–44.

5. T.L. Schlenker et al. "Incidence Rates of Hepatitis A by ZIP Code Area, Salt Lake County, Utah, 1992–1996." *Journal of Public Health Management and Practice* 5, no. 2 (1999): 17–18.

6. C. Siegel et al. "Geographic Analysis of Pertussis Infection in an Urban Area: A Tool for Health Services Planning." *American Journal of Public Health* 87 (1997): 2022–2026.

7. R.H. Jenks and J.W. Jollye. "Animal Rabies Cases in Central Palm Beach County, Florida, 1994–1998." *Journal of Public Health Management and Practice* 5, no. 2 (1999): 31–32.

8. M. Stefanak et al. "Positive Raccoon-Strain Rabies Cases in Mahoning County, Ohio, 1997." *Journal of Public Health Management and Practice* 5, no. 2 (1999): 33–34.

9. U. Kitron. "Landscape Ecology and Epidemiology of Vector-Borne Diseases: Tools for Spatial Analysis." *Journal of Medical Entomology* 35 (1998): 435–445.

10. L.R. Beck et al. "Remote Sensing as a Landscape Epidemiologic Tool To Identify Villages at High Risk for Malaria Transmission." *American Journal of Tropical Medicine and Hygiene* 51 (1994): 271–280.

11. U. Kitron et al. "Geographic Information System in Malaria Surveillance: Mosquito Breeding and Imported Cases in Israel, 1992." *American Journal of Tropical Medicine and Hygiene* 50 (1994): 550–556.

12. L.R. Beck et al. "Assessment of a Remote Sensing-Based Model for Predicting Malaria Transmission Risk in Villages of Chiapas, Mexico." *American Journal of Tropical Medicine and Hygiene* 56 (1997): 99–106.

13. D.D. Chadee and U. Kitron. "Spatial and Temporal Patterns of Imported Malaria Cases and Local Transmission in Trinidad." *American Journal of Tropical Medicine and Hygiene* 61 (1999): 513–517.

14. U. Kitron et al. "Spatial Analysis of the Distribution of LaCrosse Encephalitis in Illinois, Using a Geographic Information System and Local and Global Spatial Statistics." *American Journal of Tropical Medicine and Hygiene* 57 (1997): 469–475.

15. F.O. Richards. "Use of Geographic Information Systems in Control Programs for Onchocerciasis in Guatemala." *Bulletin of Pan American Health Organization* 27, no. 1 (1993): 52–55.

16. Centers for Disease Control and Prevention. "Lyme Disease: United States, 1996." *Morbidity and Mortality Weekly Report* 46, no. 23 (1997): 531–535.

17. G.E. Glass et al. "Environmental Risk Factors for Lyme Disease Identified with Geographic Information Systems." *American Journal of Public Health* 85 (1995): 944–948.

18. M.E. Bavia et al. "Geographic Information Systems and the Environmental Risk of Schistosomiasis in Bahia, Brazil." *American Journal of Tropical Medicine and Hygiene* 60 (1999): 566–572.

19. K.M. Becker et al. "Geographic Epidemiology of Gonorrhea in Baltimore, Maryland, Using a Geographic Information System." *American Journal of Epidemiology* 147 (1998): 709–716.

20. R.A. Scribner et al. "A Geographic Relation between Alcohol Availability and Gonorrhea Rates." *Sexually Transmitted Diseases* 25 (1998): 544–548.

21. F. Tanser and D. Wilkinson. "Spatial Implications of the Tuberculosis DOTS Strategy in Rural South Africa: A Novel Application of Geographic Information System and Global Positioning System

Technologies." *Tropical Medicine and International Health* 4 (1999): 634–638.

22. American Thoracic Society. "Diagnostic Standards and Classification of Tuberculosis in Adults and Children." *American Journal of Respiratory and Critical Care Medicine* 161 (2000): 1376–1395.

23. World Health Organization. *Groups at Risk: WHO Report on the Tuberculosis Epidemic*. Geneva, Switzerland: WHO, 1996.

24. Centers for Disease Control and Prevention. "Essential Components of a Tuberculosis Prevention and Control Program: Recommendations of the Advisory Council for the Elimination of Tuberculosis. Advisory Council for the Elimination of Tuberculosis January 1995." *Morbidity and Mortality Weekly Report* 44, no. RR-11 (September 8, 1995): 1–16.

25. J.K. Devasundaram. "An Automated Geographic Information System for Local Health Departments." *Journal of Public Health Management and Practice* 5, no. 2 (1999): 70–72.

CHAPTER 6

Public Health GIS Applications: Injuries

The integrative and overlay capacities of GIS technology are particularly helpful in examining the epidemiology of injuries. In contrast to communicable disease, injuries are usually not reportable to local public health departments. Instead, injury data often reside in non–public health agencies, such as law enforcement or transportation departments. Public health practitioners can encourage these agencies to share these data by showing them how an epidemiological approach using GIS technology can help them understand the etiology of these events and prevent future occurrences.

UNINTENTIONAL INJURIES

Each year in the United States, unintentional injuries are responsible for nearly 70,000 deaths and millions of hospitalizations. For young people, aged 1 to 44, unintentional injuries are the leading cause of death. The leading causes of death from unintentional injuries are motor vehicle crashes, fires, falls, drownings, and poisonings, with motor vehicle crashes causing the most deaths for people aged 1 to 24.[1,2] For every injury death, there are about 19 hospitalizations, 233 emergency department visits, and 450 office-based physician visits for injuries.[3]

Injuries Associated with Motor Vehicles

In a Hartford, Connecticut, study, investigators used attribute data obtained from the state department of transportation to evaluate child pedestrian injuries. These data contained information on all motor vehicle accidents involving pedestrians younger than 20 years of age that had been reported to the Hartford, Connecticut, police department over a three-year period from January 1, 1988, to December 31,

1990. The data included date and time of the collision, collision location, environmental conditions at the time of the collision, vehicle type, pedestrian/vehicle maneuvers, contributing factors, pedestrian and driver age and gender, pedestrian residence, and injury severity.[4] For incidence rate determination, investigators added the 1990 census population as another attribute data layer. The 1990 TIGER line files for Hartford County served as the spatial database. Investigators used a commercial GIS, TransCad, to geocode the location of collisions and the residence of pedestrian involved by matching the police department data with the TIGER data. The GIS also calculated the distance from residence to the site of each collision.[4]

Figure 6–1 is an event map of motor vehicle collisions with child pedestrians.[4] The map clearly illustrates the uneven distribution of the collisions, with several areas having concentrations of collisions. Figure 6–2 depicts two of these high-frequency areas, accounting for 30 percent of all motor vehicle/child pedestrian collisions. One of the areas, Albany Avenue, is a major commuting road with an average daily traffic flow or volume (ADT) of 10,000 to 25,000 motor vehicles. The other area, Park Street, is a collector road, with an ADT of 3,000 to 10,000. Both areas have high population densities, with mixed residential and commercial use. Figure 6–3 is a map of the residencies of the children involved in the collisions depicted in the high-frequency areas of Figure 6–2.

Like other GIS analyses, these maps raised additional questions related to potential causes of the collisions. Fortunately, investigators had information on the time of each collision, the environmental conditions associated with each collision, and the drivers and pedestrians involved in each collision. Children involved in collisions on Albany Avenue, the main commuting thoroughfare, tended to be older, more seriously

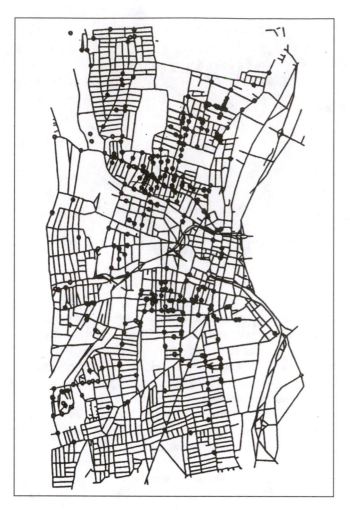

Figure 6–1 Child pedestrian–motor vehicle collision sites: Hartford, Connecticut, 1988 through 1990

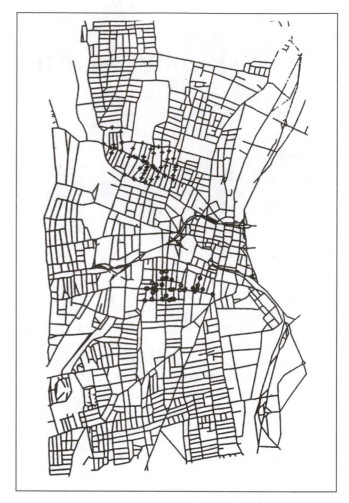

Figure 6–2 Albany Avenue (+) and Park Street (open circles) area collision sites, 1998 through 1990

injured, and further away from their residence than children involved in collisions on the smaller road, Park Street. Collisions on Albany Avenue were more often due to driver error, while collisions on the smaller street were more likely to occur at intersections without traffic signals. In addition, collisions on Park Street were more likely to occur after school dismissal, on weekends, and during the summer.

Such analyses have significant implications for communities trying to reduce the rate of childhood pedestrian injuries. In this case, authorities might want to tailor their interventions on the basis of pedestrian, driver, and environmental conditions associated with collisions. For example, on Albany Street, the larger arterial, interventions might include education aimed at older children, street modifications to reduce traffic flow and speed, and increased police enforcement of speed limits and traffic signals. In contrast, on Park Street, appropriate interventions might include education directed at preschoolers and parents, more warning signs and

traffic signals, and more off-street playground areas.[4] Subsequent GIS analyses looking at the frequency, time of occurrence, and geographic distribution of injuries and the associated driver, pedestrian, and environmental conditions would be helpful in evaluating the effectiveness of these interventions.

Another study, in Ventura County, California, used Emergency Medical Service transport data to illustrate the locations of serious injuries involving teenage pedestrians.[5] Figure 6–4 shows that injuries were located near high schools. In this study, the three largest concentrations of injuries were located near the three largest high schools. These data will be useful to the county in targeting education and prevention efforts.[5] Future studies will help the county evaluate the effectiveness of these efforts.

The DeKalb County Board of Health (DCBOH), in Decatur, Georgia, a suburb of Atlanta, used GIS technology to compare fatal and nonfatal motor vehicle crashes.[6] In-

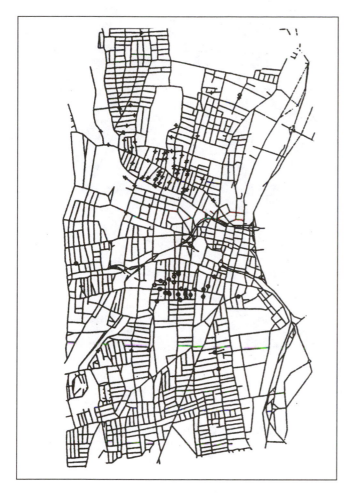

Figure 6–3 Residential locations of children involved in pedestrian collisions in the Albany Avenue (+) and Park Street (open circles) areas, 1988 through 1990

stead of using TIGER as its spatial database, the DCBOH used a locally developed spatial database, the Economic Development Information System (EDIS) CD-ROM street file. The Atlanta Regional Commission (ARC), the official planning agency for the 10-county Atlanta metropolitan area, prepares the EDIS CD-ROM street file every year and sells it for about $245. The file includes streets, census tracts, and ZIP codes for the entire 10-county region. Compared with a match rate of 60 percent using TIGER files, the board of health achieved a match rate of 85 percent with the EDIS CD-ROM street file. The board of health further increased its match rate to 95 percent by referring to hard-copy city maps obtained annually from a commercial source.

Attribute databases for the DeKalb County Board of Health project came from two sources. The DeKalb County Medical Examiner's Office provided data on motor vehicle fatali-

ties. DeKalb County Public Safety supplied data on 32,808 motor vehicle accidents, including site and type of roadway, for 1995 in unincorporated DeKalb County. Of these, the board of health selected a 20 percent random sample for geocoding and analysis. Figure 6–5 is a map showing the location of motor vehicle crashes in unincorporated DeKalb County. Most of the crashes occurred on interstates and highways, roads with high volumes of traffic. In contrast, as portrayed in Figure 6–6, nearly 80 percent of crashes resulting in fatalities occurred on less traveled surface streets. Board of health staff have used these maps in presentations to local health and public safety officials and civic groups. The maps have helped the board of health recruit community members and agencies in its efforts to find ways to reduce motor vehicle accidents and fatalities in their community.[6]

Studies like these illustrate how GIS technology can help local health departments develop partnerships with other agencies to reduce morbidity and mortality from unintentional injuries. For example, health departments could use GIS to identify neighborhoods where transportation safety agencies could efficiently target driver education and pedestrian safety programs.[6] Well-designed maps created with GIS provide information in a format that is easy for the public to understand, and they can be useful in enlisting businesses, consumers, and other agencies in efforts to reduce unintentional injuries.

Injuries Resulting in Hospitalization

Because injuries are a major cause of hospitalization, analysis of hospital discharge data with GIS can provide information helpful to communities and public health agencies in targeting injury prevention programs. Figure 6–7 is a choropleth map displaying rates of hospitalization for adults aged 25 to 44 by ZIP code in Boston, Massachusetts, from 1994 to 1996.[7] During those years, injury was the fifth leading cause of hospitalization for Boston adults in this age group. To create the map, Boston Public Health Commission staff integrated two attribute databases. The first database, supplied by the Massachusetts Health Data Consortium, contained hospital discharge data with causes of hospitalization aggregated by diagnosis-related groupings (DRGs). These groupings included traumatic injury, poisoning and toxic effects of drugs, burns, multiple significant trauma, and trauma to skin and tissue under the skin and breast (open wounds and contusions).[7] Unfortunately, the data set did not contain information on the nature and cause of the injury, and, unlike mortality data, it did not distinguish between intentional and unintentional injuries. A commercial source, the Codman Research Group, provided the second database containing ZIP code population information.

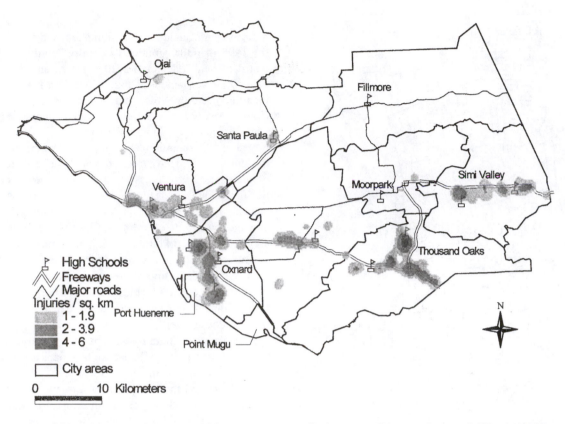

Figure 6–4 Automobile accidents to teenagers requiring emergency medical transport, Ventura County, California, 1996

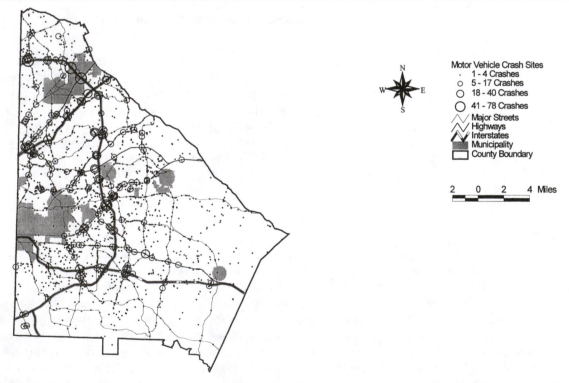

Figure 6–5 Location of motor vehicle crashes (based on a 20% sample of 32,808 crashes included in county public safety records) in DeKalb County, Georgia, 1995

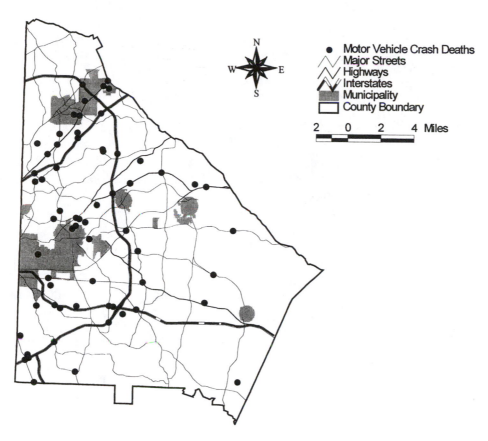

Figure 6–6 Location of motor vehicle crash fatalities (based on county medical examiner reports) in DeKalb County, Georgia, 1995

Although the Boston area contains 28 ZIP code areas, the map contains only 21 polygons. The analysis revealed that residents from 7 of the 28 ZIP code areas accounted for fewer than 20 hospital discharges over the three-year period. As we discussed in Chapter 3, such small numerator numbers can lead to unreliable rates. To avoid this problem, the Boston Public Health Commission investigators aggregated these seven ZIP code areas with adjacent ZIP code areas, resulting in the 21 ZIP code "units" (17 single ZIP code areas and 4 areas of aggregated ZIP codes) in Figure 6–7. In making decisions on how best to aggregate the areas, investigators relied on local, subjective knowledge of community neighborhoods.[7] They chose polygon shades and patterns based on the midpoints between rated clusters observed in a table of rank-ordered rates.[7]

The map in Figure 6–7 reveals a "corridor" of high rates of injury hospitalizations for residents in the central portion of Boston. Rates tended to be lower for ZIP code units progressively further from the city center. The Boston Public Health Commission created this and other maps for its annual publication, *The Health of Boston*. The other maps display injury rates for other age groups and maps on other public health indicators within Boston, allowing for comparisons. These maps have proven useful for local and state governmental and nonprofit agencies and universities in several ways, including community development planning, resource allocation, and grant writing.[7]

Earthquakes

While uncommon, large earthquakes have caused significant numbers of injuries and fatalities. As populations grow and move into areas at risk for earthquakes, the risk for future extensive morbidity and mortality increases. Many factors are associated with the risk of injury from earthquakes. These factors include the extent of ground shaking, which in turn is associated with earthquake magnitude, geographic distance from the epicenter, and depth and radius of the fault activity. Other factors associated with injury are the victim's behavior at the time of the earthquake, personal factors (such as age) associated with vulnerability to injury, housing contents, and building damage.[8] Although we have not yet learned

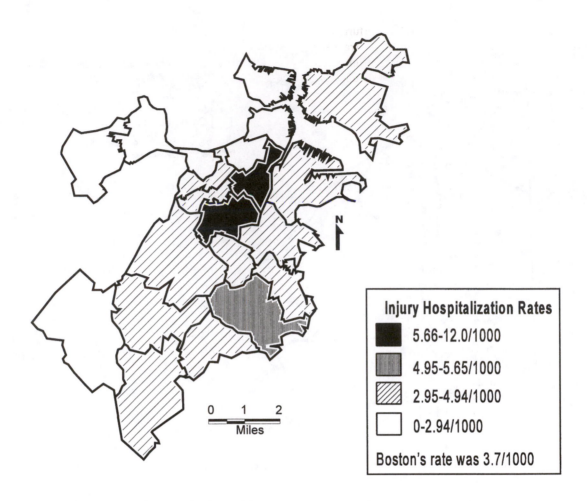

Figure 6–7 Hospitalizations for all injuries, average annual rates per 1,000 adults ages 25–44 by ZIP code, Boston, Massachusetts, 1994–1996

---

how to prevent earthquakes, models predicting the boundaries for severe injuries following earthquakes can help target search and rescue efforts and help local hospitals prepare to treat injured patients.[8] By incorporating multiple data sets containing risk factors associated with earthquake injuries, GIS technology can help health officials develop such models and display them on an easy-to-understand map.

For example, investigators used GIS to map earthquake-related deaths and hospital admissions from the 1994 earthquake in Northridge, California.[8] The U.S. Bureau of the Census provided the spatial foundation database. Attribute data came from several sources. The Los Angeles County Coroner's Office supplied data on earthquake-related deaths.

Investigators surveyed 78 hospitals within the county for data on earthquake-related injury hospitalizations and identified injured patients from 16 of the hospitals. Next, they reviewed each medical record for injury admissions from January 17, 1994, through January 31, 1994, to determine whether the injury was due to the earthquake. They identified 171 injuries meeting these criteria, resulting in 33 traumatic deaths and 138 hospitalizations. Investigators included only injuries and deaths due to physical injury, excluding patients who suffered heart attacks or other stress-related illness following the earthquake. They defined physical injuries as earthquake related if they were due directly or indirectly to ground shaking and categorized these injuries as direct or indirect.

Examples of direct injuries were those due to structural failure, resulting from dislodged objects hitting or trapping people, or to a fall during the quake. Indirect injuries resulted from events following earthquake-related damage, such as fires, traffic accidents, and injuries suffered during cleanup activities.[8] The 1990 U.S. Census of Population and Housing provided population by ZIP code, and the U.S. Geological Survey supplied the coordinates for the epicenter of the Northridge earthquake.[8]

The GIS database for fatal and nonfatal injuries included injury diagnoses, cause and address of each injury, hospital course, and demographic information. Investigators coded injury diagnoses according to the Abbreviated Injury Severity Scale and calculated Injury Severity Scores (ISS) for each victim. The ISS is a measure of injury severity and ranges from 1 to 76. ISS scores of 1 to 24 represent mild and moderate injuries, scores of 25 to 75 are severe, and injuries with a score of 76 are invariably fatal.[8,9] In geocoding the address of each injury, investigators successfully matched 133 of the 171 injuries, a match rate of 77.8 percent. Of the 38 unmatched records, 35 had unrecognizable or unknown locations, and three had occurred on undetermined areas on freeways. For the 133 matched records, investigators then used the GIS to measure the distance from injury location to the earthquake epicenter and calculated the mean, median, and range of these distances.

The mean distance was the arithmetic average of all distances associated with injuries, and the range was the difference between the smallest distance and the greatest distance of injury from the epicenter. The median distance was the distance dividing 50 percent of the injuries: half occurred within this distance, and half occurred beyond this distance. In comparing distances, investigators chose to use the median because the distribution of distances was not normal and had wide variation. In other words, a few distances, either very large or very small, could affect the mean in such a way that it would be less useful as a measure of distances associated with injuries. For example, if most injuries occurred within a few miles but a few occurred at great distances, the mean would be greater than the distance associated with most of the injuries, while the median would still be the dividing line between half of them.

In performing the analysis, the investigators created a new measure, the median distance ratio (MDR), for comparing several variables of interest. These variables included fatal/nonfatal outcome, injury severity, injury cause, structural damage as a contributor to injury, and direct/nondirect injury. For each variable, the MDR was equal to the median distance from the epicenter for that variable divided by the median distance for an assigned reference. Consequently, an MDR greater than one meant that the median distance from

the epicenter for the variable of interest was greater than the median distance for the reference.

As a measure of ground shaking, investigators used the Modified Mercalli Intensity (MMI) scale and measure of peak ground acceleration (PGA). The MMI scale has 12 contiguous categories, with XII representing the strongest activity, equivalent to near-complete destruction. In Los Angeles County, the Northridge earthquake ranged from I to IX (Table 6–1). Categories of V or less are associated with minimal damage, and investigators combined these in their analysis. Level VI indicates shaking felt by all persons, the movement of heavy objects, and the possibility of cracked walls. Level VII refers to considerable damage to weak structures and broken chimneys. Level VIII refers to fallen chimneys, deformed walls, and heavy damage to weak structures, and Level IX implies the deformation of well-built structures, shifting of building frames, and breaking of underground pipes. PGA is equivalent to the maximum acceleration of ground motion detected by instruments throughout the county, expressed in terms of the gravity constant (g).

Using published maps, a commercial vendor, EQE International, and the California Office of Emergency Services summarized both of the ground-shaking measures for ZIP codes in Los Angeles County and calculated average values for each ZIP code area. The U.S. Geological Service MMI map supplied the MMI estimates, and a GIS overlay was used to determine the distribution of MMIs within each ZIP code. EQE and the Office of Emergency Services computed the area within each ZIP code falling into the following categories of MMI: lower than V, VI, VII, VIII, and IX. Because these areas varied in size, investigators weighted each severity level by its area in determining an average MMI for each entire ZIP code area. Similarly, using a map of Log(PGA) that they created, EQE and the Office of Emergency Services calculated average PGA for each ZIP code area.

For measures of building structure and integrity, investigators used postearthquake inspection data obtained from the City of Los Angeles Department of Building and Safety. They determined the proportion of damaged buildings in each ZIP code by dividing the number of buildings inspected and damaged by the total number of inventoried buildings in each ZIP code. Investigators considered only residential buildings because the inventory was incomplete for nonresidential buildings and most injured victims were at home at the time of the earthquake. Finally, they used linear regression models to determine the association between injury rates and MMI, PGA, and the proportion of damaged buildings for each ZIP code.

Figure 6–8 is an event map showing injuries by severity in relation to the earthquake epicenter. Map symbol shapes re-

Table 6–1 Modified Mercalli Intensity (MMI) Scale Levels of Ground Shaking Associated with the Northridge Earthquake

MMI	Amount of Damage
I-V	Minimal damage
VI	Shaking felt by all persons, movement of heavy objects, possible cracked walls
VII	Considerable damage to weak structures, broken chimneys
VIII	Fallen chimneys, deformed walls, heavy damage to weak structures
IX	Deformation of well-built structures, shifting of building frames, breaking of underground pipes

fer to the severity of the injury. Of the 133 successfully matched injuries, 98 were minor or moderate, 10 were severe, and 25 were not survivable. One hundred and sixteen of the injuries occurred at independent sites, 16 deaths occurred in one apartment complex, and two homes each had two injuries. Fatal injuries and injuries resulting in hospitalization extended far from the epicenter and were not symmetrically distributed. For example, although all 25 fatal injuries occurred within 20 km of the epicenter, 23 of them occurred more than 10 km away. Most of the injuries close to the epicenter, within 5 km, were mild or moderate. Although investigators did not perform spatial scan statistics or statistical tests for global clustering, there appears to be a cluster of lethal injuries to the southeast of the epicenter. Severe injuries were widespread, with only one severe injury near the epicenter.

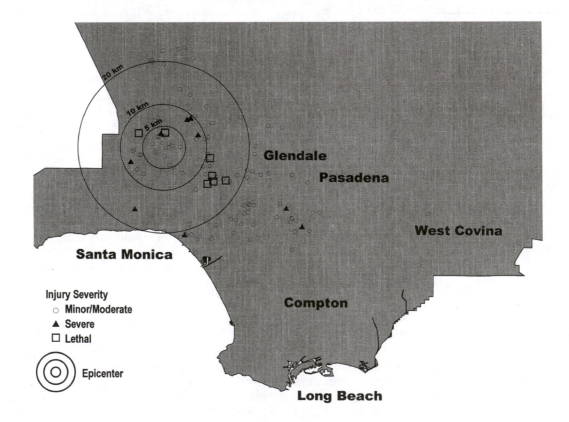

Figure 6–8 1994 Northridge earthquake injury locations by injury severity

MDR calculations revealed that nonfatal injuries requiring hospitalization were on the average 5.2 times further from the epicenter than fatal injuries (see Table 6–2). Analysis based on the ISS showed that injury severity decreased with increasing distance from the epicenter, although there was much overlap for the ranges of varying degrees of severity. Compared to lethal injuries, severe injuries were on the average 2.5 times further from the epicenter, and moderate and minor injuries were more than 5 times further. On the other hand, the injury closest to the epicenter was minor, and a nonsurvivable injury occurred over 14 km away from the epicenter.

Table 6–3 shows the relationship between external cause of injury and distance from the epicenter. In calculating the MDR, investigators used the median distance for all injuries as the reference. The external cause of injuries occurring closest to the epicenter was being hit or trapped by building parts. In addition, burns and trauma from household or other objects occurred closer to the epicenter than the average for all injuries. On the other hand, cutting and piercing injuries occurred farthest on average from the epicenter compared to all injuries. Injuries due to falls and motor vehicle injuries also occurred farther than average from the epicenter.

Table 6–3 also shows that injuries with concomitant structural damage occurred 5.6 times closer to the epicenter than injuries without associated structural damage. The range of distance for structurally related injuries was also smaller and closer to the epicenter compared to that for nonstructural

Table 6–2 Distance from Epicenter and Average Peak Ground Acceleration (PGA) by Fatal/Nonfatal Outcome and Injury Severity Score (ISS); Northridge Earthquake, California, 1994

	Number	*Median Distance in km (Range)*	*Median Distance Ratio*	*Average PGA (Range)*
Outcome				
Fatal	30	3.451 (3.332–32.396)	1.00 (ref.)	0.59 (0.19–0.73)
Nonfatal	103	17.899 (0.311–53.208)	5.19	0.42 (0.13–0.75)
Injury severity (ISS)				
Minor/moderate (0–24)	98	18.936 (0.311–53.208)	5.49	0.42 (0.13–0.75)
Severe (25–75)	10	8.489 (3.332–32.396)	2.46	0.57 (0.19–0.73)
Nonsurvivable (76)	25	3.451 (3.409–14.107)	1.00 (ref.)	0.70 (0.42–0.72)

Table 6–3 Distance from Epicenter and Average Peak Ground Acceleration (PGA) by Cause of Injury and Structural Damage; Northridge Earthquake, California, 1994

	Number	*Median Distance in km (Range)*	*Median Distance Ratio*	*Average PGA (Range)*
Total	133	12.442 (0.311–53.208)	1.00 (ref.)	0.46 (0.13–0.75)
Cause of injury				
Motor vehicle	3	13.873 (3.332–17.522)	1.12	0.53 (0.42–0.70)
Fall	65	19.505 (0.311–34.369)	1.57	0.39 (0.19–0.75)
Cutting/piercing	5	20.740 (9.731–25.611)	1.67	0.37 (0.24–0.48)
Hit/caught by building parts	31	3.451 (2.598–27.590)	0.28	0.58 (0.19–0.75)
Hit/caught by object	15	8.770 (1.081–29.916)	0.70	0.43 (0.19–0.70)
Burn	8	7.448 (5.034–20.932)	0.60	0.58 (0.42–0.75)
Other	6	18.804 (2.701–53.208)	1.51	0.49 (0.13–0.75)
Structural damage				
Yes	37	3.451 (2.598–25.916)	1.00 (ref.)	0.58 (0.23–0.75)
No	88	19.423 (0.311–53.208)	5.63	0.41 (0.13–0.75)
Unknown	8	13.795 (2.037–30.714)	N/A	0.42 (0.19–0.75)
Injury Type				
Direct	119	13.195 (0.311–53.208)	1.38	0.45 (0.13–0.75)
Indirect	14	10.067 (3.332–20.932)	1.00 (ref.)	0.52 (0.42–0.75)

injuries. On the other hand, injuries associated with ground shaking occurred further from the epicenter than injuries caused indirectly. While this may not make intuitive sense, most of the indirect injuries occurred during cleanup after the earthquake, and investigators postulated that building damage may have increased their risk.

Figure 6–9 is a choropleth map with aggregations of ZIP code polygons shaded on the basis of ground-shaking intensity, as measured by the MMI, with superimposed fatal and nonfatal injury events. The accompanying legend depicts injury rates derived from dividing the number of events by the population within each polygon. As ground-shaking intensity (MMI) increased, injury rates increased more than exponentially. Areas located further from the epicenter but with higher ground-shaking intensities had higher injury rates than areas closer to the epicenter with lower ground-shaking intensities. Figure 6–10 is a choropleth map with ZIP code polygons shaded on the basis of the percentage of residential buildings damaged within each ZIP code. The accompanying legend shows the distribution of ZIP codes by proportion of damaged buildings. Of the 271 county ZIP codes, 159 had no damage. Cartographers created three intervals of proportion of building damage that evenly distributed the remaining 112 ZIP codes. As the map shows, ZIP codes in the highest category of building damage were located closer to the epicenter, and injury rates (population as the denominator) were higher in ZIP codes with greater building damage. On the other hand, injury rates per residence (residence as the denominator) were lower in areas with greater degrees of building damage. Areas with the smallest percentage of buildings damaged and the lowest injury rates had the highest number of injuries per damaged building. As with other ecologic analyses, investigators needed to look further—for example, exploring the association between individual injuries and building damage—to explain these findings. Further study revealed that most damaged buildings were not associated with occupant injuries and that many of the injuries were not associated with building damage.

In developing their model, investigators assumed that earthquake intensity and building damage could predict the risk of individual injury. They cited earlier theoretical models showing that ground shaking was associated with build-

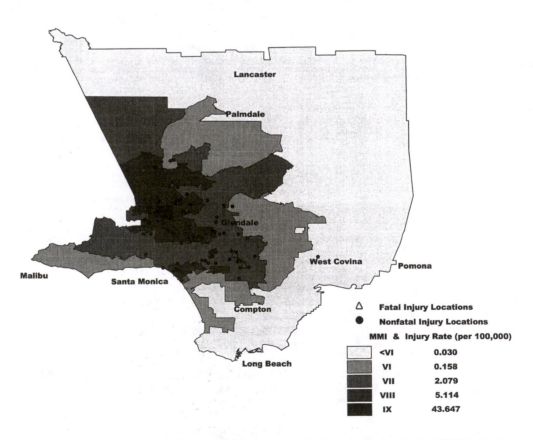

Figure 6–9 Modified Mercalli Index intensity regions and injury rates per 100,000 population in the 1994 Northridge earthquake

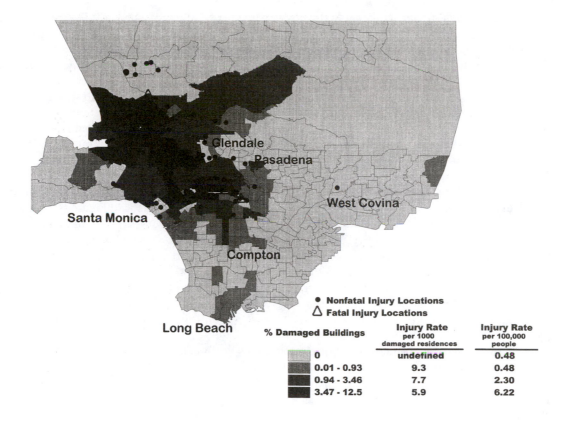

Figure 6–10 Proportion of damaged residential structures, injury rate per 1,000 damaged residences, and injury rate per 100,000 population in the 1994 Northridge earthquake

ing damage, increasing the risk of injury. In addition, investigators noted that previous studies, including a cohort study in Armenia, identified building structure, contents, and location as independent potential risk factors for earthquake-related injury.[8] This study's full model predicting injury rates included the percentage of buildings damaged and the two measures of earthquake intensity, the MMI and PGA. In a linear regression analysis, only the MMI was significantly associated with injury rates, and the three independent variables accounted for only 17.4 percent of the variation in injury rates. Obviously, investigators will need to evaluate and include other potentially related predictive factors in future models.

In the meantime, this study has implications for public health and public safety officials interested in minimizing the human costs of future earthquake disasters. Investigators showed (at least for Northridge) that although severe and fatal injuries concentrate near an earthquake epicenter, the area containing significant injuries can be quite large

and does not radiate out from the epicenter in a simple, regular, concentric pattern.[8] Public safety and emergency management agencies will need to be prepared to respond to such an irregular area, much larger than they might expect. Future GIS models could include other predictive factors, such as demographic characteristics, and emergency resources, such as hospital and ambulance locations, in communities at risk for earthquakes. Data sets containing information with these factors could be entered and ready for analysis in case of an earthquake. When the earthquake occurred, officials could quickly input earthquake data, such as epicenter and ground shaking (PGA), obtained from already in-place accelerographs. The resulting map would help officials efficiently target search and rescue efforts and notify local hospitals to prepare for patients. Similar models using GIS technology could be valuable for other disasters, such as floods and storms. Following the Hurricane Andrew disaster, the Federal Emergency Management Agency (FEMA) began the development of a GIS to respond to the need for easily understood visual representations of the scope and nature of many types of disasters. Readers can find additional information on FEMA's GIS at their GIS Web site, <www.gismaps.fema.gov/index.htm>.

Fires

Injuries resulting from fires are a major cause of morbidity and mortality in the United States. Of all deaths due to fires, most (81 percent) occur at home, indicating that strategies aimed at residential fire injury prevention should have the greatest effect on fire-related mortality.[10] Within the United States, residential fires kill 3,000 to 5,000 people and injure over 15,000 people every year.[10, 11] Children under 5 years of age and adults over 65 years are particularly susceptible, with fire-related death rates two to six times higher than the national average for all ages. Because most deaths are due to inhalation of carbon monoxide and smoke, young children and the elderly with physical limitations can benefit from the early warning provided by smoke alarms.[10, 11] Not surprisingly, homes with smoke alarms have about half as many fire-related deaths as homes without smoke alarms.[10] The Centers for Disease Control and Prevention recommends that to reduce the risk for death or injury from fires, smoke alarms should be installed outside each sleeping area and on every habitable level of a home.[10]

Thanks in part to local public health and fire department smoke detector promotion, distribution, and installation programs, the prevalence of smoke alarms across the United States is high.[10] However, some areas, especially low-income areas, may still lack smoke detectors, and even when present, the smoke detectors may not be functional. The effectiveness of smoke alarms is dependent on correct installation and maintenance. Approximately 50 percent of smoke alarms are no longer functional 12 months after installation,[10] highlighting the need to continue public health programs targeting installation, testing, and maintenance.

In Chapter 4, we discussed the use of geographic information systems in targeting public health lead abatement programs to geographic areas where children are more likely to have an increased risk of lead exposure. The approach to smoke detector promotion campaigns, identifying local areas and their residences for smoke detector programs, is similar, as illustrated by a program in Hartford, Connecticut. The Hartford Fire Department provided attribute data, which included computerized incidence data for all residential fires from 1992 to 1994. This data set contained information about the date, time, and cause of each fire, the extent of flame and smoke damage, the type and street location of the residence, the room of origin, the injured persons, the method of alarm, the fire department response time, and the presence of func-

tionality of any smoke detector.[11] The 1990 census provided data on population, income, and housing by census tract. Investigators entered information on the street addresses of schools, firehouses, community centers, and churches that they obtained from a local telephone directory.

Figure 6–11 is a map of Hartford showing residential fires and population density. Census tract polygon shades indicate the population density by equal intervals, and each dot represents a residential fire. During the study period, there were 942 house fires causing 41 civilian injuries, 9 civilian deaths, and 282 firefighter injuries. Figure 6–12 identifies four census tracts with the highest frequency of fires in homes without smoke detectors, and Figure 6–13 identifies a census tract (census tract #10) with the highest frequency of house fires in homes with present but nonfunctional smoke detectors.[11] Clearly, the census tracts identified in Figures 6–11 and 6–12 are prime areas for targeting smoke detector installation, testing, and maintenance programs.

Besides identifying areas needing smoke detector promotion, the GIS project in Hartford identified resources and collaborators available to address these needs. Figure 6–14 shows community fire prevention resources available in census tract #10, the census tract with many nonfunctional smoke detectors and high frequency of residential fires. In November 1997, the information depicted on these easily understandable maps led to a specific targeted campaign involving many community organizations. Fire Station House #7 provided the central location for Project Get Alarmed. Working out of the fire station, firefighters, police officers, teenage volunteers from Explorer Posts from both departments, and volunteers from Connecticut Children's Medical Center, and Connecticut SAFEKIDS distributed 75 smoke detectors door to door. For homes with smoke detectors, volunteers tested the detectors, replaced batteries, or installed new ones for those beyond repair. In addition, the project reached other neighborhoods with extensive media coverage emphasizing the value of smoke detectors. The GIS maps will facilitate similar efforts in other high-risk areas of the city.

For additional information on the use of GIS for analyzing fire-related injuries, readers should consult the National Fire Administration Incident Reporting System Web site at <www.nfirs.fema.gov/news.htm>. The U.S. Fire Administration (USFA), an agency within FEMA, developed the system as a tool for fire departments to report and maintain computerized records of fires and other fire department incidents in a uniformed manner. The reporting system includes a GIS component and can examine fire incident trends on local, state, and national levels. The USFA believes that the resulting information will be helpful in reducing fire-related mortality and property loss throughout the United States.

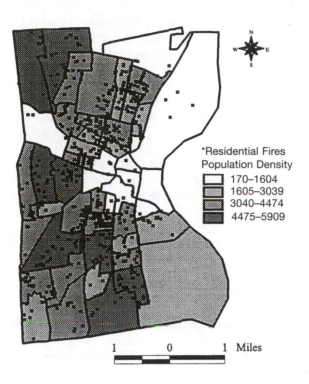

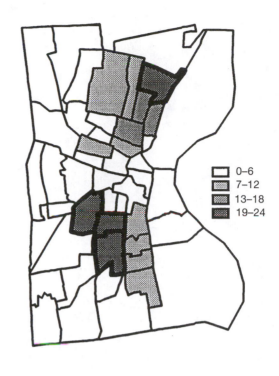

Figure 6–11 Residential fires, 1992–1994 (*n* = 942), and population density by census tract, Hartford, Connecticut

Figure 6–12 Residential fires, smoke detectors not present (*n* = 286), by frequency and census tract, Hartford, Connecticut

INTENTIONAL INJURIES: HOMICIDE

GIS technology is also helpful in evaluating intentional injuries, such as homicides and suicides. Homicide, a major public health problem, is the second leading cause of death for Americans between 15 and 24 years of age and is the leading cause of death for young African American males.[12,13] For young adults, aged 25 to 44, homicide remains the sixth leading cause of death.[12,13] Most homicides, including nearly all homicides involving teenagers, are committed with firearms.[12] Like other public health problems, homicide incidence is associated with multiple risk factors, including socioeconomic factors. A 1986 study concluded that geographic variation in crime incidence was associated with the physical and social environment at the subneighborhood level of street blocks and multiple dwellings.[12,14] GIS technology, with its capacity to incorporate multiple data sources, is particularly helpful to public health and law enforcement officials and their communities interested in targeting and evaluating

violence prevention interventions. Another study, in 1995, used GIS to analyze narcotics sales arrests, drug-related emergency calls, and narcotics tip line information in Jersey City, New Jersey.[12,15] Investigators determined that most of the drug activity in Jersey City was conducted at 14 percent of the city's intersections. Using this information, the Jersey City Police Department replaced its more random drug enforcement tactics with an experimental strategy targeting the high-risk intersections. Later evaluation showed that the GIS-based strategy was effective.[12,15]

Death certificate data, which included information on cause of death, served as source of attribute data for a Kansas City, Missouri, study of homicide. Investigators calculated age-adjusted homicide rates for Kansas City ZIP codes for the period from 1991 to 1995. Using ZIP code coordinate databases, they created a map of homicide rates (see Figure 6–15). The map illustrates homicide rates only for the 17 ZIP codes with six or more cases and divides these rates into quartiles. Three ZIP codes had the highest age-

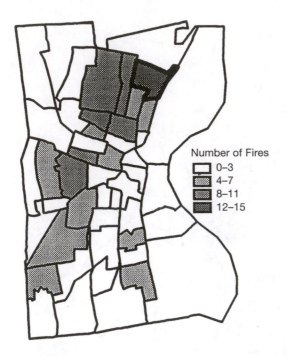

Figure 6–13 Residential fires, smoke detectors present but not working (*n* = 151), by frequency and census tract, Hartford, Connecticut

adjusted homicide rates, which were about three times higher than the rate for all ZIP codes in the Kansas City area. High age-adjusted homicide rates were statistically associated with low per capita income. The information depicted on this map has been useful for educating the community about the geographic distribution of homicides in Kansas City. Because more than 85 percent of the population of the three high-impact ZIP codes is African American, the Kansas City Black Health Care Coalition has been particularly interested in the data for their prevention efforts.[16]

A descriptive study, spurred on by community participants in Fulton County, Georgia, used several sources of data in a GIS analysis of firearm-associated homicides.[12] The Fulton County Medical Examiner (FCME) death records contained information on race, age, sex, and resident status of the victims. Emergency 911 computer-aided dispatch data (CAD) provided information on firearm-related emergency calls, including specific types of calls. Call type criteria included whether someone fired any shots, whether anyone was shot, and whether someone was armed. In addition, the data included incident location, time and date of the call, priority, zone, police beat, dispatch time, arrival time, call completion time, and event description. The firearm injury surveillance system developed by the investigators added data on nonfatal firearm injuries. The system brings together data

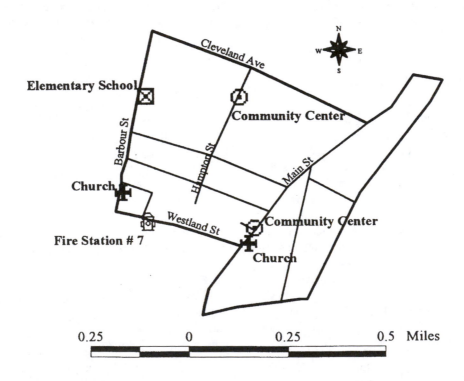

Figure 6–14 Potential collaborators for a targeted smoke detector campaign, census tract 10

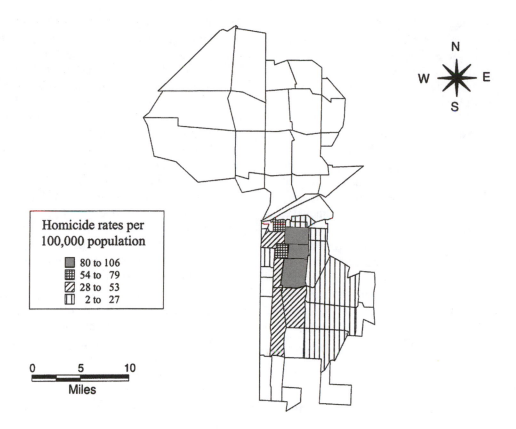

Figure 6–15 Age-adjusted homicide rates by ZIP codes, Kansas City, Missouri, 1991–1995. Rates are not shown for ZIP codes with five or fewer cases. The average age-adjusted homicide rate for all ZIP codes in the Kansas City area is 30 homicides per 100,000 population.

from police reports, emergency room records, and medical examiner records.[12]

On the basis of the GIS analysis of these data, investigators were able to identify geographic areas (by census tracts and at lower levels) with high frequencies of firearm activity, including homicides. Using overlays of data on homicides, assaults, and 911 calls, they identified "clusters" of activity in specific neighborhoods and streets and surrounding certain public housing units. These areas were also associated with indices of poverty, including high percentages of female-headed households, unemployment, and persons living below the poverty level. In addition, these areas were associated with high levels of illicit drug activity. Although investigators have not analyzed this information statistically, it has been useful for public health and law enforcement agencies as they target crime prevention interventions.[12]

CHAPTER REVIEW

1. Public health officials can use injury data found in non–public health agencies, such as law enforcement or transportation departments, to understand the etiology of injuries and prevent future occurrences.
2. Transportation data are helpful for GIS studies evaluating injuries associated with motor vehicles, including pedestrian injuries. GIS analysis of data containing information on the time of motor vehicle collisions, environmental conditions associated with each collision, and individuals, drivers, and pedestrians involved in each collision can help public health officials and their partners tailor preventive interventions. Subsequent GIS analyses, looking at the frequency, time of occurrence, and geographic distribution of

injuries and associated driver, pedestrian, and environmental conditions would be helpful in evaluating the effectiveness of these interventions.

3. Injuries are a major cause of hospitalization. Analysis of hospital discharge data with GIS can provide information helpful to communities and public health agencies in targeting injury prevention programs.

4. Many factors are associated with the risk of injury from earthquakes. These factors include the extent of ground shaking, earthquake magnitude, geographic distance from the epicenter, and depth and radius of the fault activity. Other factors associated with injury are the victim's behavior at the time of the earthquake, personal factors associated with vulnerability to injury, contents of buildings, and building damage. Health officials can use GIS technology to develop models based on these risk factors that predict the boundaries for severe injuries following earthquakes. Such models, displayed on a map, can help target search and rescue efforts and help local hospitals prepare to treat injured patients.

5. Public health officials can use GIS technology to prevent fire-related morbidity and mortality in the same way that they use it for communicable-disease prevention. Most fire-related deaths are preventable with smoke alarms. Using GIS technology and available fire department data, local health officials can target smoke alarm promotion programs to neighborhoods containing high proportions of homes without functioning smoke alarms.

6. GIS technology is helpful in evaluating intentional injuries, such as homicides and suicides. Most homicides, including nearly all homicides involving teenagers, are committed with firearms. Like other public health problems, homicide incidence is associated with multiple risk factors, including socioeconomic factors. GIS technology, with its capacity to incorporate multiple data sources, is particularly helpful to public health and law enforcement officials and their communities interested in targeting and evaluating violence prevention interventions in neighborhoods with high homicide rates.

REFERENCES

1. Centers for Disease Control and Prevention, National Center for Injury Prevention and Control, Division of Unintentional Injury Prevention. "Unintentional Injury Prevention." <www.cdc.gov/ncipc/duip/duip.htm>.

2. Centers for Disease Control and Prevention, National Center for Injury Prevention and Control. *Ten Leading Causes of Death Tables, 1994.* Atlanta, GA: CDC, 1996.

3. C.W. Burt. "Injury-Related Visits to Hospital Emergency Departments: United States, 1992." *Advance Data,* no. 261 (February 1, 1995). Hyattsville, MD: National Center for Health Statistics.

4. M. Braddock et al. "Using a Geographic Information System To Understand Child Pedestrian Injury." *American Journal of Public Health* 84 (1994): 1158–1161.

5. P. Van Zuyle. "Automobile Accidents to Teenagers Requiring Emergency Medical Transport, Ventura County, California, 1996." *Journal of Public Health Management and Practice* 5, no. 2 (1999): 25–26.

6. M.Y. Rogers. "Getting Started with Geographic Information Systems (GIS): A Local Health Department Perspective." *Journal of Public Health Management and Practice* 5, no. 4 (1999): 22–33.

7. J. Slosek et al. "Hospitalizations for All Injuries, Average Annual Rates per 1,000 Adults Ages 25–44 by ZIP Code, Boston, Massachusetts, 1994–1996." *Journal of Public Health Management and Practice* 5, no. 2 (1999): 29–30.

8. C. Peek-Saa et al. "GIS Mapping of Earthquake-Related Deaths and Hospital Admissions from the 1994 Northridge, California, Earthquake." *Annals of Epidemiology* 10, no. 1 (2000): 5–13.

9. Association for the Advancement of Automotive Medicine. *Abbreviated Injury Severity Scale: 1990 Revision.* Des Plaines, IL: 1990.

10. Centers for Disease Control and Prevention. "Deaths Resulting from Residential Fires and the Prevalence of Smoke Alarms: United States, 1991–1995." *Morbidity and Mortality Weekly Report* 47, no. 38 (1998): 803–806.

11. G. Lapidus et al. "Using a Geographic Information System To Guide a Community-Based Smoke Detector Campaign," in *Geographic Information Systems in Public Health: Proceedings from the Third National Conference,* eds. R.C. Williams et al. San Diego, CA: U.S. Department of Health and Human Services, Agency for Toxic Substances and Disease Registry, 1998: 103–108.

12. D.S. Fuqua-Whitely et al. "GIS Analysis of Firearm Morbidity and Mortality in Atlanta Georgia," in *Geographic Information Systems in Public Health: Proceedings from the Third National Conference,* eds. R.C. Williams et al. San Diego, CA: U.S. Department of Health and Human Services, Agency for Toxic Substances and Disease Registry, 1998: 561–569.

13. National Center for Health Statistics. "Deaths: Final Data for 1997." *National Vital Statistics Reports* 47, no. 19 (1999): 8, 9, 28.

14. R.B. Taylor and S. Gottfredson. "Environmental Design, Crime and Prevention: An Examination of Community Dynamics," in *Communities and Crime,* Vol. 8, eds. A.J. Reiss and M. Tonry. Chicago: University of Chicago Press, 1987: 387–416.

15. D. Weisburd and L. Green. "Policing Drug Hot Spots: The Jersey City Drug Market Analysis Experiment." *Justice Quarterly* 12 (1995): 711–735.

16. J. Cai and Q.B. Welch. "Age-Adjusted Homicide Rates by ZIP Codes, Kansas City, Missouri, 1991–1995." *Journal of Public Health Management and Practice* 5, no. 2 (1999): 27–28.

CHAPTER 7

Public Health GIS Applications: Chronic Disease Prevention

Chronic diseases—illness that are prolonged, do not resolve spontaneously, and are rarely completely cured—affect over 90 million Americans and account for 70 percent of all deaths in the United States.[1] These illnesses disproportionately affect women and minority populations. For example, the death rate from cervical cancer is more than twice as high for African American women as for white women, and the death rate from prostate cancer is twice as high for African American men as for white men. Although deaths due to breast cancer are decreasing for white women, they are not decreasing among African American women. Diabetes prevalence is nearly two times higher for African Americans and Hispanic Americans and almost three times higher for American Indians and Alaska Natives than it is for non-Hispanic white Americans of similar age.[1]

As states develop and publicize cancer and other chronic disease registries, many communities are becoming interested in how their chronic disease rates compare to others'.[2] Cancer registries, which require hospitals, other health care facilities, and health care providers to report newly diagnosed cases of cancer, provide a means for monitoring cancer incidence by factors such as age, race/ethnicity, and geography.[3,4] Studies based on registry data have revealed that incidence rates for specific cancers frequently vary by region. People living in areas with high cancer incidence rates are beginning to ask public health officials why[2] and are requesting assessments and, in some cases, interventions regarding perceived risk factors. Such requests are challenging for public health officials because it is difficult to evaluate and explain variations in cancer incidence, especially in small areas. Many communities are concerned about local environmental hazards, yet differences in rates of chronic disease, including cancer, have many additional determinants, such as the be-

havioral, genetic, and socioeconomic characteristics of underlying populations.

For several reasons, GIS technology is especially suited to help public health officials respond to the challenge of chronic disease in their communities. First, because determinants of chronic disease, including behaviors, healthy and unhealthy, tend to cluster in populations, GIS technology can help health officials target communities with relevant health education and health promotion messages. Currently available, effective preventive interventions include programs such as smoking cessation programs, diabetes education, mammography screening, and cervical cancer screening.[1] Second, GIS software can integrate multiple data sets and evaluate many potential risk factors simultaneously, enabling health officials to determine whether there are associations between socioeconomic, behavioral, environmental, and other factors and local chronic disease incidence. Third, the greatest strength of GIS is that its product is a picture.[5] It allows health officials to show quickly, clearly, and convincingly the results of a complex analysis to concerned residents. In this chapter, we will discuss two uses of GIS software, first as a health promotion tool and second as a tool to help health officials evaluate chronic disease incidence and prevalence in their communities.

HEALTH PROMOTION

Marketing Messages To Reduce Alcohol and Tobacco Use

Many private businesses use marketing information to locate their "best customers" and focus their advertising campaigns. For public health officials, these best customers are those for whom health promotion messages (public health advertising) could lead to healthier behaviors and improved community health outcomes. Private marketing data sets such as the Claritas PRIZM Lifestyle Clusters are helpful because people with similar demographics and behaviors tend to cluster in specific neighborhoods.[6,7] The definition of a cluster is a predominant trait within a specific geographical area; this trait can be behavioral, or it can be a health outcome, such as a cancer cluster.

In 1995, Claritas, Inc. based its lifestyle clusters on a national sample of 500,000 people. Claritas first matched census demographics with information from consumer preference surveys. Survey data sources included Simmons Market Research, Mediamark Research Inc., Nielsen Television, Arbitron Radio and Television, and the National Family Opinion Research Study. Using this information, Claritas Inc. grouped the entire U.S. population into 62 lifestyle clusters. This information has been incredibly useful for businesses interested in deciding where to market their products. For example, the tobacco industry could use the data set to decide where to sell cigarettes. Likewise, public health officials could use the same data set to decide where and how to best target their smoking prevention and cessation campaigns.

Figure 7–1 is a choropleth map of census tracts along the Buford Highway Corridor in DeKalb County, Georgia. Census tract polygons are shaded and patterned on the basis of Claritas PRIZM lifestyle cluster groups. In the accompanying legend, the rows represent cluster groups and the columns represent traits. The higher the score for each trait, the more likely the cluster group was to have that particular trait. For each trait, the U.S. population average has an index score of 100.

In the Buford Highway corridor, the highest propensity to use tobacco, based on smoking more than 40 cigarettes daily or smoking in the past year, was associated with the Low-Income Hispanic Families cluster. Because the top media for this cluster was nostalgia TV, public health officials might want to use nostalgia TV programming to target this population with smoking prevention campaigns. In addition, because this cluster was more likely to use Medicaid for health insurance, the state Medicaid agency might be interested in providing and marketing smoking cessation programs, if they were not already doing so. On the other hand, the cluster with the greatest tendency to drink domestic beer was the Young Mobile City Singles, who were more likely to watch TV between 12:30 and 1:00 AM Monday through Friday. Early-morning TV messages promoting alcohol prevention and treatment might be successful in reaching this population.

Public health officials need to be careful with the use of marketing data. Unlike many other data sets discussed in Chapter 2, private marketing data sets are not created by rigorous epidemiologic methods. Marketers need only a "best guess" rather than exact knowledge about consumer behaviors to sell their products. Additionally, like other ecologic information, the lifestyle cluster says nothing about individual behaviors within an assigned cluster. Individuals within each cluster do not necessarily have all the characteristics of their cluster.[6] For example, many people living within the Low-Income Hispanic Families cluster in the Buford Highway corridor are probably nonsmokers, and many are probably single. Finally, although private industry finds marketing information useful, we do not know if public health interventions based on marketing data lead to improved community health outcomes. For example, future research studies might question whether public health interventions based on marketing during specific television programming are effective and whether lifestyle cluster information adds any useful information beyond that already obtained through the Centers for Disease Control and Prevention (CDC) Behavioral Risk Factor Surveillance Survey (BRFSS) data set.

Identifying Tobacco Billboard Locations

Although the 1999 settlement between states attorneys general and the tobacco industry removed all outdoor billboard tobacco advertising, the historic location of tobacco billboards, as determined by a St. Louis, Missouri, study using GIS technology, illustrates how the tobacco industry markets its products toward specific populations.[8] This information has implications for health officials interested in reducing the adverse health impact of tobacco and other unhealthy products.

The study objectives were to define the characteristics of tobacco billboard advertising in St. Louis and to determine whether the billboards were targeting specific vulnerable populations. Investigators defined billboards as outdoor stationary structures containing advertising or public service announcements. Billboards included elevated signs and signs attached to the sides of buildings but excluded ads on buses, highway department signs, bus shelter advertisements, banners, posters, and advertisements painted on the sides of buildings. The study was limited to St. Louis City and St. Louis County, with a combined population of 1,345,500. The demographics of the city and county were different. Within St. Louis City, 50.9 percent of the population was white and 47.5 percent was African American. Within the county, contiguous but separate from the city, 84 percent of the population was white while 14 percent was African American. Median household incomes were also different, with a 1993 median household income of $21,441 for the city and $42,328 for the county. Twenty-four percent of the city popu-

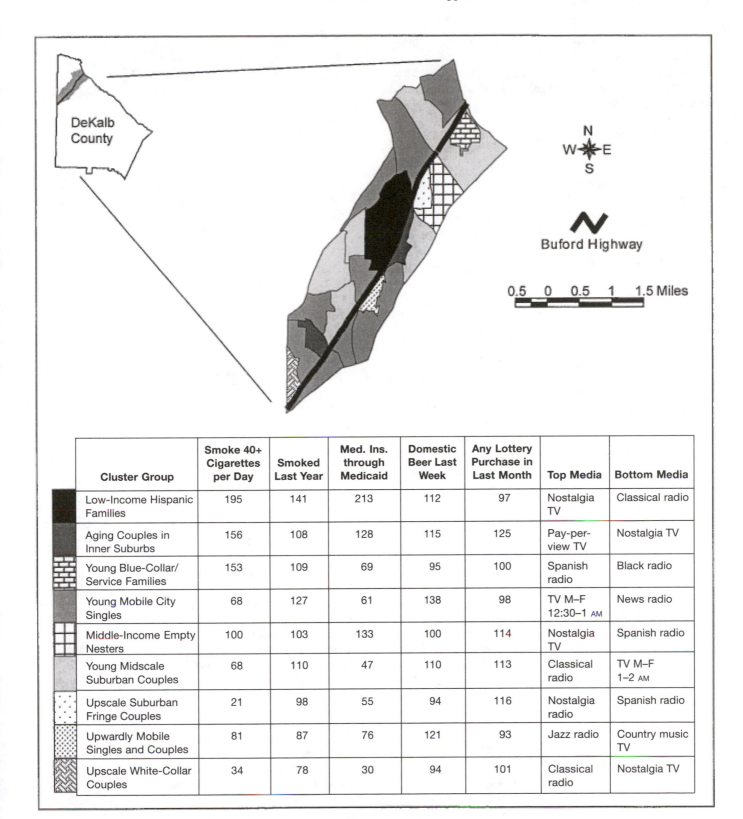

Cluster Group	Smoke 40+ Cigarettes per Day	Smoked Last Year	Med. Ins. through Medicaid	Domestic Beer Last Week	Any Lottery Purchase in Last Month	Top Media	Bottom Media
Low-Income Hispanic Families	195	141	213	112	97	Nostalgia TV	Classical radio
Aging Couples in Inner Suburbs	156	108	128	115	125	Pay-per-view TV	Nostalgia TV
Young Blue-Collar/ Service Families	153	109	69	95	100	Spanish radio	Black radio
Young Mobile City Singles	68	127	61	138	98	TV M–F 12:30–1 AM	News radio
Middle-Income Empty Nesters	100	103	133	100	114	Nostalgia TV	Spanish radio
Young Midscale Suburban Couples	68	110	47	110	113	Classical radio	TV M–F 1–2 AM
Upscale Suburban Fringe Couples	21	98	55	94	116	Nostalgia radio	Spanish radio
Upwardly Mobile Singles and Couples	81	87	76	121	93	Jazz radio	Country music TV
Upscale White-Collar Couples	34	78	30	94	101	Classical radio	Nostalgia TV

Figure 7–1 Using marketing information to focus smoking cessation programs in specific census block groups along the Buford Highway Corridor, DeKalb County, Georgia, 1996

lation was below the poverty line compared to 5 percent for the county (see Table 7–1).[8]

To prepare for the study, the research team identified that more than 99 percent of the billboards in the metropolitan area were on highways and major arterials. Consequently, they decided to collect data on four types of highways as defined by the National Department of Transportation. These included (1) divided highways with controlled access, (2) divided highways with uncontrolled access, (3) primary state undivided highways, and (4) secondary state undivided highways and primary arterials. They excluded secondary arterials and streets. As a result, the study included all commercial and industrial areas while excluding residential areas.

Next, the research team created a user-friendly data collection instrument, the Billboard Observation Form (BOF). The BOF included variables on billboard category, such as tobacco or alcohol, the brand of the product or advertising organization, the type of figure (gender, group, or animal), the style (text or picture), and whether the billboard had a standard rectangular shape. Investigators assigned drivers and observers to specific routes for data collection. While driving, they filmed billboards with a video camera and recorded verbal information with a data recorder. Once the drivers and observers completed several routes, they used the BOF form to record visual and verbal data. They also recorded each billboard location on a detailed St. Louis area map. Other attribute data for the study included population data obtained from the 1990 U.S. census and the addresses for 103 K–12 public schools in St. Louis City. 1995 TIGER files contained the spatial data for the study. Investigators geocoded the location of each billboard and drew ½-mile buffers around each public school.

The 1998 study identified and collected data on 1,309 billboards in the region. Of these, the research team excluded 70 because they were blank. Although they also excluded billboards on secondary arterials and residential streets, this probably did not affect the study results because pilot observations failed to find any billboards on these streets. Figure 7–2 shows the distribution of categories of advertising found on the 1,239 nonblank billboards. Tobacco adver-

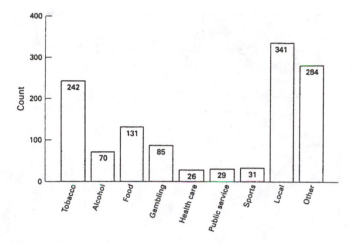

Figure 7–2 Billboard product category frequencies, St. Louis

tisements represented the largest category, at 19.5 percent, followed by food (10.6 percent), gambling (6.9 percent), and alcohol (5.6 percent). Table 7–2 shows how individual tobacco brands dominate billboard advertising in the area.

Table 7–2 Most Frequently Advertised Brands on Billboards in St. Louis

Brand	Product Category	Frequency
Newport	Tobacco	62
Kool	Tobacco	45
Dodge	Automobile	37
Basic	Tobacco	33
GPC	Tobacco	29
American Family	Other	23
Benson & Hedges	Tobacco	20
Dean's Milk	Food	18
Milk	Food	18
Arch Madness	Sports	16
E-file	Other	15
Chrysler	Automobile	15
Chuck Norman	Local	15
Marlboro	Tobacco	15
Pick 3 Lotto	Gambling	14
Copenhagen	Tobacco	14
Station Casino	Gambling	13
Canadian Mist	Alcohol	13
Crown Royal	Alcohol	12
Winston	Tobacco	12
Camel	Tobacco	12
Steak n Shake	Food	12
	Total	463

Table 7–1 Selected Population Characteristics of St. Louis City and St. Louis County, 1997

	St. Louis City	St. Louis County
White population	59.0%	84%
African American population	47.5%	14%
1993 median household income	$21,441	$42,328
Population below poverty line	24%	5%

Tobacco brands made up four of the top 5 and nine of the top 22 advertised brands of products.

Figure 7–3 shows the location of tobacco billboards within the region. On this map, polygon shades represent median family income for census block groups, with stars representing the tobacco billboards. It is easy to see that the tobacco billboards are located in less affluent areas of the region, although a similar map with all billboard categories shows the same pattern. No billboards of any type were located in the affluent "central corridor" of the county. Further analysis showed that a significantly larger proportion of tobacco billboards were located in the city compared to the county and that the density of tobacco billboards in the city compared to the county was 1½ times that for nontobacco billboards (see Table 7–3).

GIS technology allowed the research team to combine billboard data with census data to examine the relationship between tobacco advertising and sociodemographic factors. A

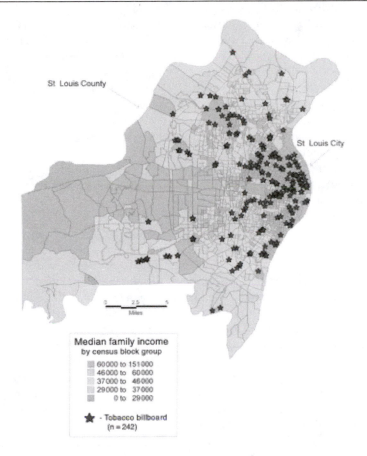

Figure 7–3 Location of tobacco billboards in St. Louis city and county. Census block groups are shaded according to median family income.

Table 7–3 Comparison of Billboard Distribution for St. Louis City and County

| | City | | County | | City:County |
Billboards	Count	Density	Count	Density	Density Ratio
Nontobacco	497	8.03	500	0.98	8.19
Tobacco	145	2.34	97	0.19	12.32

Note: $\chi^2 = 7.91$; df = 1, $p < 0.01$. Density is the number of billboards per square mile. St. Louis city is 61.9 square miles, St. Louis County is 507.7 square miles.

regression analysis, depicted in Table 7–4, shows that the proportion of tobacco billboards relative to nontobacco billboards tended to be higher in census block groups containing higher concentrations of low-income and African American populations. Investigators found a "dose-response" relationship when they included block groups with more than three billboards in their analysis.

Figure 7–4 is a map showing the distribution of tobacco billboard images in relationship to sociodemographic factors. Census block groups shading represents the percentage of African American population, whereas the figures represent images found on the billboard (African American figure[s], white figure[s], no images of people). Although billboards with white figures or no figures appear to be located throughout the city and county, billboards with African American figures seem concentrated mostly in the north side, which has the highest concentration of the African American population in the region. A statistical analysis (see Table 7–5) confirmed the map's visual impression.

The buffering feature of GIS technology allowed investigators to evaluate the relationship between locations of tobacco billboards and public schools. Figure 7–5, an overlay of billboard and school locations, shows that nearly three-fourths of tobacco billboards within St. Louis were located within 2,000 feet of public school property.

What implications do these findings have for public health practitioners? Although the results describe the location of the billboards, they do not provide reasons for their location. The absence of billboards in affluent areas could be due to many factors, including zoning regulations, political opposition, and other historical and political factors. On the other hand, figuring out the cause of the location is not always necessary for public health interventions. For example, the location of three-fourths of the tobacco billboards within sight of public schools could prompt a public health intervention without requiring a detailed analysis explaining the reason for their location. Interventions could include the passage of local ordinances requiring all billboard tobacco/alcohol advertisements to be located at least 2,000 or more feet from public schools. In addition, the study findings suggest that the tobacco industry has tailored its advertisements for specific populations, including African American populations. This information can be useful for communities interested in developing effective tobacco prevention strategies.

Although tobacco billboards are no longer with us, the tobacco industry could substitute other forms of outside advertising, such as smaller tobacco advertisements on the windows and walls of retail establishments. If so, public health officials could use similar methods to evaluate and respond to tobacco marketing. In addition, GIS technology could be effective in evaluating and developing strategies to respond to advertisements for other unhealthy products, such as alcohol. Finally, GIS technology, with its ability to incorporate multiple sources of data, could be helpful in evaluating the results of public health interventions removing advertisements. For example, in local areas, public health researchers could use the Youth Risk Behavior Survey (YRBS) or similar surveys to evaluate the effectiveness of these interventions on adolescent smoking behavior.

CANCER CLUSTERS

For several decades, in comparison to other parts of the United States, breast cancer mortality rates have been higher in the Northeast.[9,10] From 1988 to 1992, the mortality rate from breast cancer was 15.6 percent higher in 11 states in the northeastern United States and the District of Columbia than in the rest of the country.[9] Several studies have reported more localized clusters of breast cancers within this area, specifically on Long Island, New York. A disease cluster of any kind is the occurrence of a greater-than-expected number of cases of a particular disease within a group of people, a geographic area, or a period of time.

Given the public concern on Long Island over these high rates, including a concern about potential environmental causes, the U.S. Congress mandated an investigation by the National Cancer Institute (NCI). The study was to include all of Long Island and two additional counties: Tolland County, Connecticut, and Schohaire County in upstate New

Table 7–4 Relationship between Block Group Characteristics and Proportion of Tobacco Billboards

	Proportion of Tobacco Billboards			
	Block Groups with at Least 1 Billboard (n = 378)		Block Groups with > 3 Billboards (n = 125)	
Block group characteristic	r	p	r	p
Percent African American residents	0.15	0.004	0.22	0.015
Median family income	-0.13	0.012	-0.27	0.002

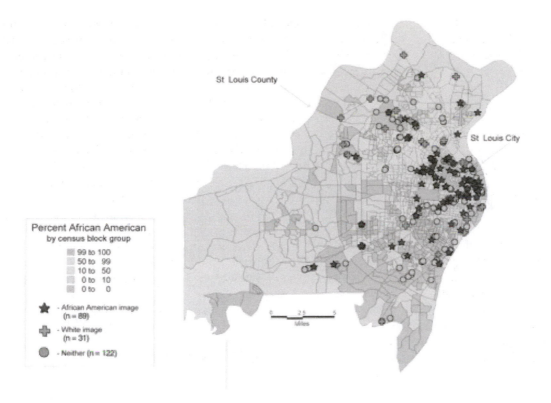

Figure 7–4 Targeted placement of tobacco billboards with African American images in St. Louis. Symbols indicate type of image found on the tobacco billboard. Census block groups are shaded according to percentage of African American residents.

Table 7–5 Relationship of Geographic Location and Type of Images Found on Tobacco Billboards, St. Louis

| | Type of Billboard Images | | |
Location	African American	White	Neither
City: north side	**53 (57%)**	5 (5%)	35 (38%)
City: south side	15 (29%)	5 (10%)	32 (61%)
County	21 (22%)	**21 (22%)**	55 (56%)

Note: $\chi^2 = 32.65$; df = 4, $p < 0.001$. Bold figures contribute most to the overall significant χ^2 (that is, standardized residuals greater than or less than 2). Percentages are row percentages.

York. Congress added these counties because they had the highest breast cancer mortality rates of all counties in the Northeast containing 30 or more cases. To avoid preselection bias, NCI investigators elected to examine a much larger area using spatial scan statistic methodology (described in Chap-

ter 3). Preselection bias typically occurs in studies of cancer (or other disease) clusters when investigators use statistical tests to see if the number of cases in the cluster is significantly higher than would be expected by chance. The cluster already has a high number of cases, so the study design introduces bias because the study ends up using the large number of cases to define as well as test the hypothesis. The spatial scan statistic (Chapter 3) eliminates this problem by scanning an area for clusters without specifying their location or size ahead of time. Additionally, while investigating areas with multiple potential clusters, the methodology avoids statistical problems associated with multiple testing (see Chapter 3).

For their study, NCI investigators selected a geographic area containing 245 counties in Maine, New Hampshire, Vermont, Massachusetts, Rhode Island, Connecticut, New York, New Jersey, Pennsylvania, Delaware, Maryland, and the District of Columbia. Attribute data included mortality data, available to the public, provided by the National Center for Health Statistics (NCHS), and demographic data, obtained from the 1994 census revision. To adjust for potential confounding variables, investigators used indirect standard-

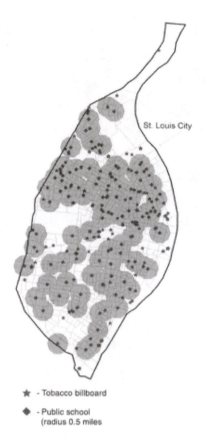

St. Louis City

★ - Tobacco billboard

◆ - Public school
(radius 0.5 miles

Figure 7–5 Locations of tobacco billboards and public schools in St. Louis city. Buffer zones have half a mile radius.

the degree of urbanization and adjacency to a metropolitan area. The USDA uses these codes in determining eligibility for several federal programs. These codes allow researchers to break county-level data down into finer residential groups than the standard metro/nonmetro. The USDA developed the codes based on the June 1993 Office of Management and Budget definition of metropolitan and nonmetropolitan counties:

Metro counties:

0: Central counties of metro areas of 1 million population or more
1: Fringe counties of metro areas of 1 million population or more
2: Counties in metro areas of 250,000 to 1 million population
3: Counties in metro areas of fewer than 250,000 population

Nonmetro counties:

4: Urban population of 20,000 or more, adjacent to a metro area
5: Urban population of 20,000 or more, not adjacent to a metro area
6: Urban population of 2,500 to 19,999, adjacent to a metro area
7: Urban population of 2,500 to 19,999, not adjacent to a metro area
8: Completely rural or fewer than 2,500 urban population, adjacent to a metro area
9: Completely rural or fewer than 2,500 urban population, not adjacent to a metro area

izared. They calculated specific mortality rates for each cross-classification of the confounding variables pooled across the entire Northeast. Next, they applied these rates to the appropriate population in each of the 245 counties to obtain expected numbers of deaths in each county adjusted for the confounders. Because the etiology of breast cancer may differ on the basis of menopausal status, they also conducted separate analyses for women older and younger than 50 years.[9]

To deal with urban/rural characteristic as a potential confounder, investigators classified each of the counties as urban or rural. Because the data set included the county of residence for each case, they could perform indirect standardization to adjust for this variable. To classify each county, they first selected counties located within U.S. census–designated metropolitan statistical areas, consolidated metropolitan statistical areas, or a New England county metropolitan area with a total population of at least 500,000. Next, using a U.S. Department of Agriculture (USDA) classification scheme, they classified central metropolitan counties as urban and fringe metropolitan counties as rural. The USDA rural-urban continuum code classifies all U.S. counties by

More information can be found at the USDA Web site, <www.ers.usda.gov/briefing/rural/Data/>. Figure 7–6 is the resulting map of urban northeastern counties.[9]

NCI investigators had a little more trouble adjusting for parity (number of births), another potentially confounding variable.[11] Because the available mortality data did not include information on parity, they had to use surrogate methods to try to adjust for parity. First, they estimated expected mortality rates as a function of parity. To do this, they used relative risks in relation to parity calculated by the Cancer and Steroid Hormone Study.[9] In determining parity-associated relative risks, the Cancer and Steroid Hormone Study adjusted for age, history of surgically confirmed benign breast disease, family history of breast cancer, menopausal status, irregular menses as a teenager, and adiposity. On the basis of that study's findings, NCI investigators assumed that each additional child lowered the risk of breast cancer mortality by the same number of percentage points. Next, NCI investigators obtained 1990 census data containing the average parity of women in each county in each of five age groups. Finally, they calculated the parity-adjusted expected

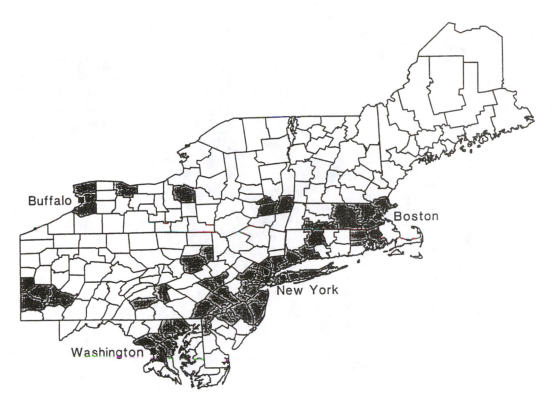

Figure 7–6 Counties classified as urban in the Northeast United States

number of deaths for each county on the basis of the estimated relative risks.

Figure 7–7 is a choropleth map showing the indirectly age-adjusted breast cancer mortality rates for each county in the Northeast. Each county's shade and pattern indicates the percentage that the county's breast cancer mortality rate was above or below the average for all counties in the Northeast. Figure 7–8 and Table 7–6 are the results of an analysis applying the age-adjusted spatial scanning statistic methodology to the same data set. This methodology found the most likely cluster in a region containing the New York City–Philadelphia metropolitan area, including Long Island, with a mortality rate 7.4 percent higher than the rest of the Northeast. This cluster had a statistically significant increase in breast cancer mortality rate at the $p = 0.0001$ level. Other secondary clusters with higher than average mortality rates from 1988 to 1992 included Buffalo, the District of Columbia, Boston and its suburbs, and eastern Maine. Unlike the finding regarding the New York City–Philadelphia metropolitan cluster, none of these findings were statistically significant.

Because of the underlying methodology, the spatial scan statistic could not define the exact border of the cluster. In addition, some counties within the cluster had rates much lower than the average for the Northeast. NCI investigators could only conclude that there was evidence for a cluster of breast cancer mortality in the northeastern United States (from 1988 to 1992) and that Long Island appeared to be part of the cluster. The next step was to examine smaller areas within the most likely cluster, or subclusters, that were strong enough themselves to be statistically significant. Four subclusters meeting this criterion were Long Island, Northeast New Jersey, Philadelphia, and central New Jersey (Figure 7–9 and Table 7–6).

Interestingly, the two counties that Congress added to the study, Schoharie and Tolland, did not emerge within either a primary or a secondary cluster because the numbers of cases discovered were less than those expected in each county. As commonly seen in small areas with small numbers, the excess number of deaths from 1983 to 1987 that led to congressional action did not recur in the following five-year period. Like all statistical and analytical procedures, GIS technology is vulnerable to biases if conclusions drawn are based on small numbers. (See Chapter 9 for a discussion of problems associated with small numbers.) If Congress had originally examined the 1988 to 1992 data instead of the 1983 to 1987 data, they might have ordered the NCI to add Essex County, New York, and Hancock County, Maine, to

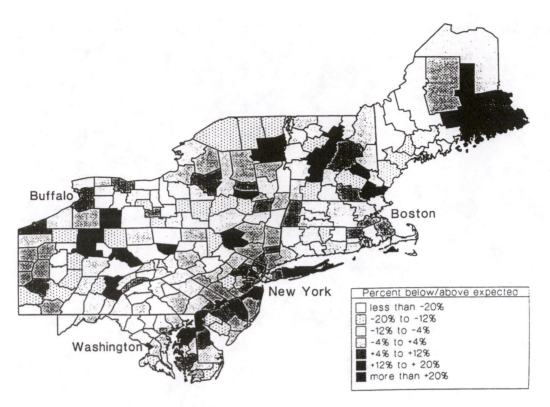

Figure 7–7 Age-adjusted breast cancer mortality rates among women in the Northeast United States, 1988–1992

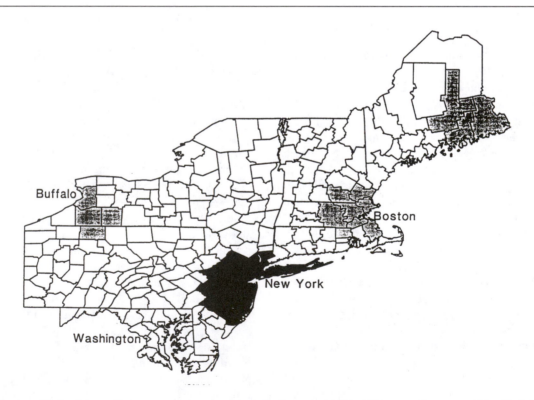

Figure 7–8 The most likely cluster of breast cancer among women for the period 1988–1992, occurring around New York, New York, and Philadelphia, Pennsylvania, as well as four secondary clusters

Table 7–6 Breast Cancer Mortality Analysis for Women in the Northeast United States, 1988–1992, Using the Spatial Scan Statistic

	Analysis			Cluster					
	Age (years)	Confounders	Type	Location	Cases	Expected	RR*	LLR*	p value
A	All	Age	M*	New York, NY-Philadelphia, PA	24,044	23,040	1.074	35.7	0.0001
			S*	Buffalo, NY	1,416	1,280	1.109	7.1	0.122
			S	Washington, DC	712	618	1.154	6.9	0.147
			S	Boston, MA	5,966	5,726	1.047	5.5	0.398
			S	Eastern Maine	267	229	1.166	3.0	0.994
			SO*	Philadelphia, PA	3,815	3,441	1.116	20.8	0.0001
			SO	Long Island, NY	2,935	2,620	1.127	19.2	0.0001
			SO	Central New Jersey	3,784	3,437	1.108	18.0	0.0001
			SO	Northeast New Jersey	2,738	2,467	1.115	15.0	0.0001
			S	Essex, NY	51	40	1.273	1.4	1
			SO	Hancock, ME	67	53	1.263	1.7	1
B	All	Age, race	M	New York, NY-Philadelphia, PA	24,044	22,973	1.079	40.7	0.0001
	All	Age, parity	M	New Jersey-Philadelphia, PA†	9,873	9,205	1.087	28.2	0.0001
			S	Long Island, NY	2,935	2,604	1.134	21.2	0.0001
	All	Age, urban	M	New Jersey-Philadelphia, PA†	9,873	9,339	1.069	17.8	0.0001
			S	Long Island, NY	2,935	2,684	1.098	11.9	0.0017
C	≥50	Age	M	New York, NY-Philadelphia, PA	20,737	19,862	1.074	31.4	0.0001
	<50	Age	M	Washington, DC	144	87	1.670	15.8	0.0002
			S	Philadelphia, PA	525	435	1.223	9.4	0.017
	<50	Age, race	M	Washington, DC	144	106	1.369	6.3	0.207
			S	Philadelphia, PA‡	753	673	1.132	5.1	0.508

* M, most likely; S, secondary; SO, secondary that overlaps with other more likely cluster; RR, relative risk within the cluster compared with the rest of the Northeast; LLR, log likelihood ratio.

† Includes Staten Island, as well as the same Pennsylvania and New Jersey counties as the larger New York City-Philadelphia cluster (Figure 7–9), with the exception of Northampton, Sussex, Passaic, Atlantic, and Gloucester.

‡ In addition to the five Philadelphia counties shown in Figure 7–9, this area also includes Ocean, Mercer, Atlantic, and Monmouth counties.

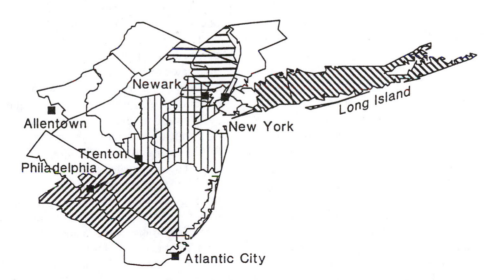

Figure 7–9 A close-up of the most likely cluster for breast cancer among women in the Northeast United States during 1988–1992, with four subclusters that are significant on their own strength. Two of the latter are overlapping, with Essex, New Jersey, as a common county.

the study because of the excess numbers of deaths in those counties. Neither of these excess numbers, however, was statistically significant.

Analysis adjusting for confounders led to slightly different results. While the analysis adjusting for race resulted in the same most likely cluster as found in the overall analysis, the most likely cluster ended up with a slightly higher likelihood value. On the other hand, adjusting for race and parity resulted in a smaller (but still significant) most likely cluster, but in the same general area, with a slightly smaller likelihood ratio, indicating that parity might explain some of the excess deaths in the region. Adjusting for urbanicity did not explain the excess number of cases in the region because the resulting most likely cluster continued to contain Philadelphia, central New Jersey, and Staten Island, with a significant secondary cluster on Long Island. In addition, simultaneous adjustment for age, race, parity, and urbanicity gave similar results. Analysis restricted to women over 50 gave similar results to the analyses including all ages. For the analysis restricted to women under 50, however, the resulting most likely cluster was the District of Columbia, which lost significance after adjustment for race.

Some Limitations of GIS in Cluster Analyses

This study illustrates some of the limitations of GIS technology in assessing potential cancer clusters. Although the methodology revealed that elevated breast cancer rates in a region of the Northeast were not due to chance, it could not pinpoint a cause for several reasons. First, even though investigators used electronic death data that included information on individuals, the data set lacked information on many potential confounders. The study could account for race and age because this information was available in the mortality data set at the individual level. Adjustment for parity and urbanicity was less satisfactory because parity could only be estimated on the basis of county averages and urbanicity was available only at the county level. In addition, the study could not account for other confounders[11] at the individual level, such as age at menarche, age at menopause, age at first birth, breastfeeding, country of birth, genetic disposition, family history, alcohol consumption, and potential environmental exposure factors. Second, the cross-sectional design could not account for the length of time between potential exposures related to geography and time of death. Third, the study could not account for access to health care, preventive (mammography) or treatment (early surgery), an important factor influencing survival from breast cancer and other preventable chronic diseases. Finally, the study lumped together all types of breast cancer, whereas different types may have different etiologies.

On the other hand, one of the benefits of using GIS technology is that negative results can be reassuring for concerned community residents. Public health officials frequently receive reports from their constituents worried about cancer and other chronic disease clusters in their communities. Often, without helpful tools, public health officials are reluctant to respond. A GIS analysis, using appropriate statistical methodology (available free from the NCI on the Web; see Chapter 3) and accompanied by easily understandable maps, can be helpful in reassuring concerned residents that they are not living within a significant cluster of cancer cases. For example, by sharing simple maps showing the location of local, countywide, and statewide pediatric cancer cases, local public health officials can frequently reassure their constituents that rumors of a local pediatric cancer cluster were unfounded.

Environmental Exposures and Cancer Clusters

Just such public concern about breast cancer led to a GIS analysis of breast cancer incidence on Cape Cod, Massachusetts, illustrating the value of the technology in addressing such concerns. In 1993, on the basis of nine years of cancer registry data, the Massachusetts Department of Public Health issued a report revealing that the age-adjusted incidence of breast cancer was significantly higher in many towns on Cape Cod than in the rest of the state.[2,12] While many cancer clusters reported to local health officials involve very small areas, such as neighborhoods, the area of concern on Cape Cod covered nine towns over a large area of 440 square miles.[2,13]

As a response to the public's concern, the state of Massachusetts funded an investigation led by Silent Spring Institute, in partnership with researchers from several academic institutions, including Harvard, Tufts, and Boston Universities.[14] As in many communities, residents concerned about high rates of cancer focus on environmental etiologies in addition to personal factors, and this was true for the communities living on Cape Cod. Consequently, researchers focused on environmental factors, including human exposure to chemical environmental contaminants.[2,13,14]

Although available demographic information before the study began indicated that people living on Cape Cod were similar to their counterparts in the rest of the state, they had lived in a unique environment.[2] Compared to others, people living on Cape Cod could have had increased risks of exposure to environmental contaminants for a couple of reasons. First, drinking water for most people on the Cape has come from groundwater lying in a shallow sand and gravel aquifer below sandy soils. Such poorly protected groundwater could have been subject to contamination from septic tanks and other land uses.[2,14] Second, the land uses on the Cape have provided a continuing source of potential chemical exposure. Cape Cod has been home to many cranberry bogs, golf courses, and trees that require eradication of gypsy moths and other pests. Such land uses have traditionally been associated with a greater use of pesticides compared to other areas. In addition, the two military installations on the Cape, including the Massachusetts Military Reservation (MMR), a Superfund site, could have exposed nearby residents to additional environmental contaminants.[2,14]

Investigators used several sources of data for the study. The Cape Cod Commission provided the geospatial data, based on parcels (residential and nonresidential lots). For calculating incidence rates, investigators used 1990 U.S. census data, with age and sex distribution down to the block group level. These data were less valid during intercensus years because different towns, parts of towns, and other areas on the Cape grew at different rates. To account for this differential growth, investigators used the parcel data as a surrogate measure for number of households (and women) to estimate populations in the intercensus years.[2,14] They were able to do this because most of the residences on Cape Cod are single-family dwellings.[14] Census data also provided housing density and housing age down to the block group level. The Massachusetts Cancer Registry provided the breast cancer data, including the addresses of 2,173 Cape Cod women diagnosed with breast cancer between 1982 and 1994.

Data for estimates on environmental exposures came from different sources. To estimate exposure to airborne contaminants, such as wind-blown pesticides, investigators used historical records and land use data to map areas of pesticide use. For example, using aerial photographs, the University of Massachusetts created land use maps for 1951, 1971, 1984, and 1990. These maps identified the location of cranberry bogs and other sites where pesticide use was likely.[13] For contaminated groundwater exposure estimates, the U.S. Geological Survey provided data on analyses of private wells conducted by the Health and Environment Department of Barnstable County. Because contamination by wastes and pesticides can increase nitrate concentrations, investigators use the nitrate concentrations of well water as an indicator of potential exposure.[2]

After geocoding the cancer registry data, the study looked at breast cancer incidence for specific geographic areas on Cape Cod. Because the incidence of breast cancer increases with age, researchers had to perform an age adjustment to account for age distribution differences between areas of Cape Cod (home to many retirees) and the rest of the state. They chose to use indirect standardization, calculating the ratio of observed cases to expected cases, the standardized incidence ratio (SIR). To calculate the SIR, investigators used several steps (Table 7–7):

1. They calculated the breast cancer incidence rate for each 10-year age group (starting with age 25) for women in Massachusetts outside Cape Cod. This is known as the age-specific rate.
2. They estimated the number of women in each 10-year age group for specific areas on the Cape, such as towns (using census and parcel data).
3. They multiplied the each age-specific rate in the non–Cape Cod region by the number of women in the corresponding age group for the area of interest on the Cape, resulting in the expected number of cases for that age group.
4. They added up the expected number of ages for each group to get the total number of expected cases. They divided the observed number of cases by the expected number of cases and multiplied by 100 to get the SIR. An SIR of 100 means that the observed (actual) number of cases was the same as the expected number, indicating that the age-adjusted rate in the area of concern was the same as the state rate. An SIR of 120 means that the observed number of cases was 20 percent higher than what would be expected; an SIR of 75 means that the observed number of cases in the area was 25 percent lower than expected.[13]

In addition, to get an idea of how the incidence changed over time, investigators calculated SIRs for overlapping three-year time periods within the study period.[13]

For the years 1982 through 1994, the incidence of breast cancer was 20 percent higher for Cape Cod compared to the rest of Massachusetts. Figure 7–10 shows that rates varied by geography within the Cape, with several census tracts having higher rates compared to others.[2]

The next step was to look at environmental factors that could be associated with higher rates of breast cancer, such as drinking-water quality and pesticide exposure. Because studies have shown a possible association between breast cancer and lifetime exposure to estrogen (as inferred from the fact that early menarche and advanced age at time of giving birth are associated with breast cancer), some investigators believe that an association between breast cancer and exposure to nonestrogen chemicals that act like estrogens is biologically plausible. These chemicals, which can be found in wastewater,[2] belong to a group of chemicals known as endocrine-disrupting compounds (EDCs)[2] or hormone-disrupting chemicals (HDCs).[13] Studies have also hypothesized that some pesticides may be endocrine disrupters.[13]

Since endocrine-disrupting chemicals can be found in wastewater, investigators decided to look at the association between drinking-water quality and breast cancer on the Cape. They believed that two factors, housing density and

Table 7–7 Calculating Expected Cases of Breast Cancer, Cape Cod, Massachusetts

Age Group	Rate, Non-Cape Area	X	No. of Women in Specific Cape Area or Town	=	Expected Cases in Town or Area
25–34		X		=	
35–44		X		=	
45–54		X		=	
55–64		X		=	
65–74		X		=	
75–84		X		=	
≥ 85		X		=	
			Expected cases (sum of all ages) →		

Note: SIR = observed cases/expected cases.

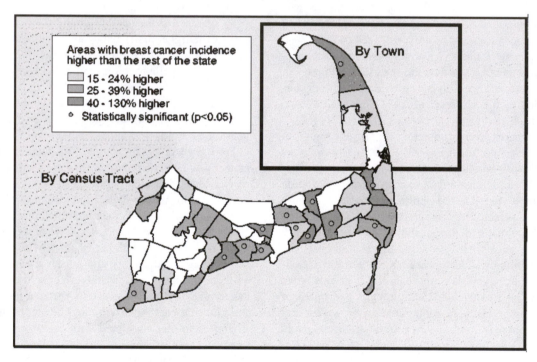

Figure 7–10 Breast cancer incidence by census tract, 1982–1994. Cape-wide breast cancer incidence was 20 percent higher than incidence for the rest of Massachusetts for this period. The circled areas are subregions of Cape Code where the excess breast cancer incidence is concentrated.

housing age, could be associated with drinking-water quality for several reasons:

- Areas with dense housing contribute more waste to the drinking-water aquifer.

- Areas with older housing may contain many homes with older disposal systems that do not meet current standards.
- The amount of waste generated is related to the length of time a septic tank has been in use.[2]

Figure 7–11 shows housing density for block groups on the lower part of Cape Cod. Figure 7–12 shows the percentage of older housing by block groups within the same area. The maps show that density and age of housing vary by block group, with town centers (particularly Wellfleet) having concentrations of dense and older housing.

To look at the association between these housing factors, their hypothesized association with drinking-water quality,

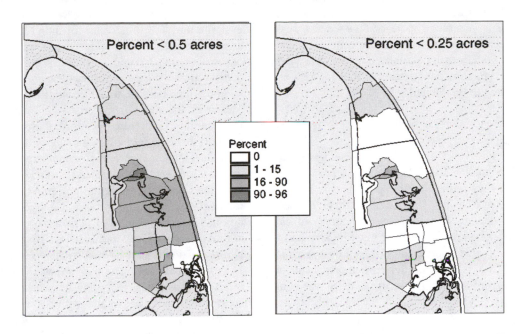

Figure 7–11 Percent high-density housing, 1971. With the Lower Cape there are differences in housing density. Areas of higher density may have more wells affected by wastewater disposed of in septic tanks.

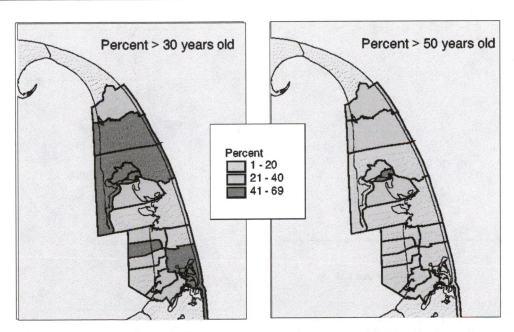

Figure 7–12 Percent old housing. The age of housing also varies within the Lower Cape. Wellfleet Center, in the middle of the figure, stands out as an area with old, dense housing.

and breast cancer, investigators calculated SIRs by census block groups for block groups dependent on private wells for drinking water. They then created a scatter plot of block group breast cancer SIRs by percentage of older housing. When they chose "more than 20 years old" as a definition of older housing, they found no association between housing age and breast cancer incidence. When they used percentage of housing older than 50 years, they found a weak association between housing age and breast cancer.[2]

To account for both housing age and housing density in their analysis, investigators next created a housing risk index (HRI) according to the formula

$$HRI = a + d$$

where a = percentage of old housing and d = percentage of residential land in smaller than half-acre lots up to a maximum value of a.[2] They limited the housing density up to a maximum value of age because they assumed that if the percentage of dense housing exceeded the percentage of old housing, then the excess dense housing must be new housing.[2] Finally, they created a scatter plot of HRI compared to SIR and found a stronger association between breast cancer incidence and housing age when housing density was considered (see Figure 7–13).[2]

Like other ecologic studies, this GIS analysis of the association between housing risk index and breast cancer proves nothing but does raise questions for further studies. Without accurate exposure data on individuals, studies like this cannot account for confounding variables. For example, breast cancer has been associated with higher socioeconomic status, which, in turn, could be associated with ownership of desirable older homes on Cape Cod.[2] Additionally, the exposure measures are subject to several sources of error. For example they fail to account for individual behaviors such as use of bottled water, which could reduce exposure, and occupation, which could increase exposure. Housing age and density are surrogate exposure measures only and may not be good indicators of actual drinking-water contamination. Moreover, the study, being cross-sectional, fails to account for duration of individual exposure. Future studies based on a cohort design could address many of these issues.

To develop a measure of potential exposure to pesticides, investigators used historical land use and parcel data obtained from the Cape Cod Commission, the State Office of Environmental Affairs, and the U.S. Geological Survey. In addition, they created digital versions of paper maps showing areas where trees had received pesticide treatments.[14] Figure 7–14 is a map of Sandwich, Massachusetts, created from these data sets. The map shows the location of areas receiving pesticides, including bogs and golf courses, and areas where trees were treated with pesticides. Next, investigators overlaid the pesticide use map with parcel data. Because some parcels were not residential, they used codes from the Department of Revenue to eliminate nonresidential parcels, such as wetlands (see Figure 7–15).[14] In addition, they

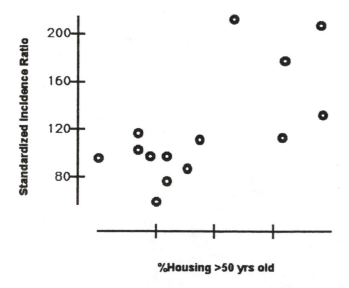

Figure 7–13 Breast cancer incidence, age of housing, and housing density in the Lower Cape. The correlation between breast cancer incidence and age of housing is stronger when the age of housing is weighted to account for housing density. Wellfleet Center was excluded from this plot.

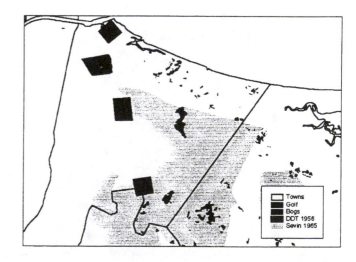

Figure 7–14 Pesticide use areas in Sandwich, Massachusetts.[4] The study was able to map large-scale pesticide use areas, including cranberry bogs, golf courses, and areas sprayed for tree pests.

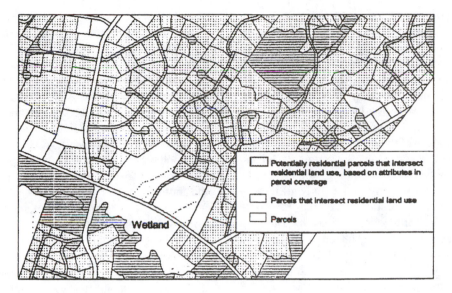

Figure 7–15 Estimating potentially exposed populations. To estimate number of households near pesticide use areas, the study first identified parcels that intersect residential land use, then used codes from the Department of Revenue to eliminate parcels that could not be residential (such as the wetland, shaded with horizontal stripes).

eliminated parcels that intersected less than one-tenth of an acre of residential land (see Figure 7–16).[14]

One problem with this methodology is that investigators used historic (1951) land use data combined with 1990 parcel data. They decided that this methodology was appropriate because (1) over the years, nearly all residential development had occurred in previously forested areas and not in already developed areas and (2) almost none of the residential land with less than half-acre lots in 1951 was broken into smaller lots.[14]

Next, using GIS software, they calculated the distance from each residential parcel to areas with pesticide use and classi-

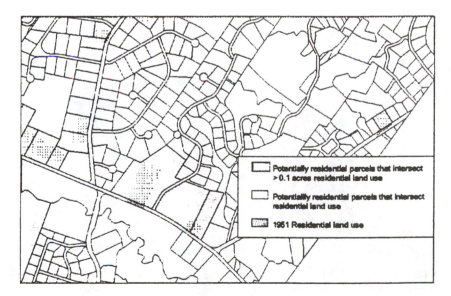

Figure 7–16 Refining estimates of exposed populations. We further refined our estimates of numbers of households by eliminating the parcels that intersected less than one-tenth of an acre of residential land, shown here shaded with vertical stripes.

fied census block groups into high- and low-exposure categories based on the distance between residential parcels in these block groups and their proximity to pesticide use areas (see Figure 7–17).[14] If they desired, they could further classify block groups by exposure to specific pesticides.[14]

Using cancer registry data, the study failed to find an association between breast cancer incidence and block groups in high-exposure categories. The limitations of this analysis are similar to the limitations of the ecologic analysis of housing age and density with breast cancer. Investigators did not have information on potential confounding variables, such as risk factors for individuals living in the study area. Census block group proximity to pesticide use areas may be a poor measure of exposure for a couple of reasons. The area of exposure to airborne pesticides may be much smaller than the block group scale,[14] and exposure may be associated with other factors, such as prevailing wind speed and direction. As in the housing study, investigators failed to account for duration of individual exposure, such as time spent in the home and years of residence in the area.[14] In addition, a more appropriate methodology, such as the spatial scan statistic, would eliminate the problem of multiple testing and give a more accurate assessment of the significance of the block group and census tract cancer clusters.

Clearly, for cancer cluster studies like this one, rather than providing answers, GIS technology may be useful for gener-ating hypotheses and identifying exposed populations for other studies. Information derived from such ecologic studies could be useful in cohort and case control studies, where it can serve as a surrogate measure of individual exposure. For example, the Cape Cod investigators are designing a case-control study involving 2,500 Cape Cod women with and without breast cancer. Through personal interviews, they plan to get information on individual risk factors, individual exposure to specific chemicals, and personal behaviors for both cases and controls. In addition, they plan to obtain measurements on environmental conditions in the homes of cases and controls, and they plan to test urine samples for the presence of estrogen-disrupting compounds.[13] Using GIS, they will also estimate other measures of environmental exposure for both cases and controls.[13]

In another example, a Nebraska study assessed the feasibility of using GIS to identify pesticide exposure in a case-control study of non-Hodgkin's lymphoma.[15] Using GIS, the Nebraska study showed how satellite imagery could help reconstruct historical crop maps and how crop type could serve as a surrogate for specific pesticide exposure. Investigators used Farm Service Agency records as a source of ground reference data to classify crop species on the basis of a 1984 satellite image identifying four major crops in a three-county area. Next, they obtained pesticide surveys, which identified the specific pesticides used most frequently

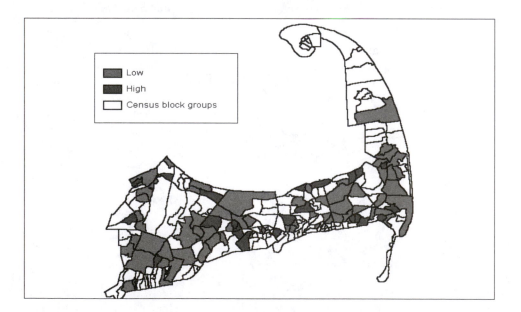

Figure 7–17 Exposure groups for cranberry bogs. The study classified the census block groups according to the number of women potentially exposed to areas of large-scale pesticide use.

on each of the four crop types. Finally, using GIS, they mapped residencies of cases and controls from the lymphoma study. Of these residencies, 22 percent were located less than 500 meters from one of the four crops, within an intermediate distance that would allow pesticides to drift via the wind after application.[15]

Exposure information like this obtained through GIS methodology is frequently preferable to historical recall of cases and controls for a couple of reasons. First, it eliminates recall bias. Second, for environmental exposures, GIS methodology can sometimes provide a more accurate measure of exposure, even if it is a surrogate measure. For example, most individuals living in agricultural areas have little knowledge of the types of pesticides historically used on fields next to their residences and could not identify a chemical when asked. If the data are available, GIS applications can incorporate databases containing historic information on these specific chemicals, eliminating the bias associated with personal recall. On the other hand, GIS technology still provides only a surrogate measure, or estimation of possible exposure, and the quality and quantity of data limit the value of surrogate measures. In the Nebraska pesticide study, a better estimation of exposure would need information on the specific pesticides used, the amount used, and climatic conditions on days that pesticides were applied (such as wind speed, wind direction, and rain). In addition, case-control studies still must rely on interviews to evaluate exposure to other risk factors, such as dietary intake and other behaviors. Later in this chapter, we will discuss the use of modeling techniques helpful in developing improved surrogate exposure measures.

The degree of resolution of the data also limits the accuracy of GIS exposure assessments. If the cancer registry did not include street address and reported residence only down to the census tract level, it would be impossible to create exposure measures (based on residence) for a chemical released over a very small area. Likewise, if the environmental data, such as pesticide use, were available only for large areas, it would be difficult to estimate exposure even if residence address were available.

PEDIATRIC CANCERS

In addition to helping assess reported cancer clusters, GIS technology can be useful in addressing public concerns about potential health risks from known hazardous sites. Pediatric cancers lend themselves to this type of analysis for several reasons. First, they tend to have briefer latent periods than adult cancers, which can develop 20 or 30 years after exposure. This is especially important in a GIS analysis because the exposure of interest occurs over a shorter time, reducing the potential number of residential exposure locations. Second, pediatric cancer registry data are usually very complete and comprehensive because of close supervision by parents and our health care system's priority for care. Third, childhood cancers, such as leukemia, have occurred in types of clusters most commonly suggesting environmental causes.[16] Finally, the short latent period and rarity of pediatric cancers are indications that a toxin may be affecting rapidly growing pediatric tissue, making pediatric cancers sentinel health events (SHEs), potential warning signals about environmental contamination.[16] Consequently, the public has been especially concerned about potential environmental causes of pediatric cancer. GIS technology is especially suited for studying the relationship between environmental hazards and cancer because of its ability to incorporate multiple sources of data in its analysis.

An exploratory study in North Carolina provides an example of the use of GIS technology in evaluating the health risks related to exposure of children to chemicals associated with hazardous waste facilities. The North Carolina Department of Public Instruction provided the spatial data, including street networks, from its Transportation Information Management System files. Attribute data came from several sources. The Agency for Toxic Substances and Disease Registry provided HazDat data (see Chapter 2) containing information on 22 National Priorities List (NPL) hazardous waste sites in the state. HazDat data included details of the location of each site, the chemicals present, and the extent of on-site and off-site chemical contamination. Because of discrepancies between the office address of the company responsible for the waste and the location of the actual waste site, investigators had to use a couple of other data sources to confirm the location of each NPL site. These included the files of the North Carolina Department of Solid Waste and cancer cluster report files at the North Carolina Central Cancer Registry (CCR). For about one-fourth of the sites, the three sources of data conflicted on ZIP code location. For those sites, investigators compared site locations on U.S. Geological Service topographic maps with GIS-produced local ZIP code maps. Figure 7–18 shows the location of the 18 counties and 22 ZIP codes containing NPL sites in North Carolina. The CCR, a population-based registry, supplied the cancer incidence data, including age, address, county, and residence ZIP code. Two different sources, the 1990 U.S. census and 1990 marketing publications, provided population data used in determining rates. At the county and state level, information was available for three age groups: 0 to 4 years old, 5 to 9 years old, and 10 to 14 years old. At the ZIP code level, population data were available only for 0- to 4-year-old and 5- to 17-year-old age groups, illustrating one of the prob-

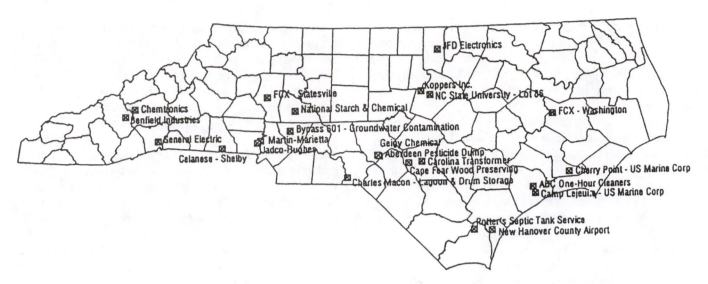

Figure 7–18 National Priority List Sites in North Carolina. The study was limited to the 18 counties and 22 ZIP codes contained in these sites

lems with analyses based at the ZIP code level, the availability of good population data.

At first, investigators calculated incidence rates at the ZIP code level because ZIP codes more closely surrounded each NPL site compared to county boundaries. This proved unsatisfactory because the ZIP codes had irregular shapes and did not have any specific geographic relationship with the waste sites. So instead, using GIS, the investigators created circular buffers, with a radius of 1.6 km (1 mile), centered at the location of each NPL site. This provided a reasonable population to study within a meaningful distance from the site. In the final phase of the study, investigators mapped pediatric cancer cases, measuring the distance from each case to the local NPL site.

For each NPL site–containing area (ZIP code or county), and for the different age groups listed above, investigators calculated standardized incidence ratios (SIRS) for all cancers. The SIRS represented the ratio of observed cases in each area divided by the number of expected cases, based on North Carolina cancer incidence. Because small numbers are associated with unstable incidence rates, investigators considered SIRS inconclusive if there were fewer than three observed cases in a given area or there were 0.5 or fewer expected cases for the area. For statistical analysis, they used a one-tailed Poisson distribution to determine the lower limit of the upper 95 percent confidence interval for each SIR.[16]

From 1990 to 1993, North Carolina experienced 238 cases of pediatric cancer. Table 7–8 shows the pediatric cancer SIRS for each of the 18 counties with an NPL site. None of the county SIRS reached statistical significance. Because of the rarity of pediatric cancer, analysis at the geographically smaller ZIP code level resulted in very small numbers of cases (see Table 7–9). Of the 22 ZIP codes studied, only two had SIRS with significantly elevated incidence. (More conservative statistical methods, accounting for multiple testing, may have had reduced this number.) One of these ZIP codes, 27889, with the highest SIR, had only three pediatric cancer cases. The other, with a greater population, had seven cases over the 1990 to 1993 period.

Figure 7–19 is an event map illustrating the results of a GIS analysis for two of the counties, Gaston and Mecklenburg. This map contains overlays of four data layers—cancer cases, county boundaries, road layers, and NPL site locations—and includes a GIS-produced buffer of 1 mile around each NPL site. This map illustrates the value of a GIS presentation in that quick inspection reveals the proximity of cases in geographic relation to the NPL sites. Table 7–10 shows the results of the GIS analysis for all 18 counties, with the number of cases found within the one-mile buffer of NPL sites. For the entire state, only three cases fell within the buffer, representing only 1.3 percent of all the pediatric cancer cases. Unfortunately, as illustrated in Table 7–9, the address-match rate was quite low in many of the counties, ranging from 0 percent in rural Moore County to 95 to 100 percent in the more urban counties of Mecklenburg and Onslow.

Table 7–8 Pediatric Cancer Case Totals and Standardized Incidence Ratios (SIRs), by County for Each County with an NPL Site

County	NPL Sites	Population	Cases	County SIR	Conf. < 90%
Beaufort	FCX, Inc. (Washington)	42,331	5	1.52	0.37
Brunswick	Potter's Septic	51,365	5	1.30	0.30
Buncombe	Chemtronics	175,173	13	1.06	0.35
Cabarrus	Bypass 601 Groundwater	99,256	5	0.66	0.16
Cleveland	Celanese Corporation	84,748	8	1.25	0.37
Cumberland	Carolina Transformer	276,791	24	0.93	0.47
	Cape Fear Wood Preserving	276,791	24	0.93	0.47
Gaston	Jadco-Hughes	175,410	19	1.39	0.56
Granville	JFD Electric	38,510	5	1.74	0.41
Haywood	Benfield Industries	46,950	4	1.34	0.23
Henderson	General Electric	69,551	11	2.46	0.70
Iredell	FCX, Inc. (Statesville)	93,193	13	1.84	0.65
Meck	Martin Marietta	514,056	41	1.01	0.47
Moore	Aberdeen Pesticides	59,228	5	1.20	0.26
	Geigy Chemical	59,228	5	1.20	0.26
New Hanover	New Hanover Co. Airport	120,691	11	1.26	0.40
Onslow	ABC 1-Hour Cleaners	150,744	6	0.53	0.14
	Camp Lejeune	150,744	6	0.53	0.14
Richmond	Charles Macon Co.	44,502	4	1.17	0.24
Rowan	National Starch and Chemical	110,886	10	1.19	0.39
Wake	Koppers Co.	426,212	48	1.49	0.68
	NCSU Lot #86	426,212	48	1.49	0.68

Note: NPL = National Priority List; Conf. < 90% = lower limit of one-tailed 95% Poisson confidence interval.

Limitations of These Studies

This study points out several lessons. First, for studies on the association between health outcomes, such as cancer, and local environmental exposures, county-level data are frequently inadequate. Locally produced environmental contaminants, even if they have human health consequences, are likely to affect only the locally exposed population. County-level analysis of health outcomes dilutes the effects of such exposures, reducing the possibility of finding associations. On the other hand, for rare diseases such as pediatric cancer, the small number of cases found at smaller geographic levels, such as ZIP codes, reduces the statistical power of the analysis. We will discuss problems with small numbers in Chapter 9. In such cases, the value of the GIS analysis is that it raises questions for further study. One possible solution is to look at the association between specific chemical exposures and pediatric cancers at NPL sites in multiple states, combining the data to achieve sufficient numbers for analysis.

An additional limitation of the study, seen in Table 7–10, is selection bias due to inaccuracies in the residential addresses of cases and failure to address-match many of the cases, especially in rural areas. One cause for address inaccuracies is the way hospitals report cases to the cancer registry. Frequently, hospitals use billing data when making the report. In many cases, especially in pediatric cases, the billing address is different from the patient's residential address. For example, the billing address may be the business address of a parent, the address of a relative responsible for the bill, or an address where the child was staying while undergoing a medical evaluation for the cancer. Any geographic study of health outcomes that relies on residential address should use a second independent source of data to validate the addresses.[16] Failure to match addresses also leads to selection bias because match failure is more common in rural areas. Reasons for this include inaccuracies in the spatial database, such as incomplete road networks, and inability to match rural route or post office box addresses. In the North Carolina study, 4 out of 11 cases address-matched in rural Iredell County, a match rate of only 31 percent (see Table 7–10). Although two of the four cases lived near the NPL site, interpretation of the data is impossible without ac-

Table 7–9 Pediatric Cancer Case Totals and Standardized Incidence Ratios (SIRs), by ZIP code for Code Areas Containing an NPL Site

Sites	ZIP code	Population	Cases	ZIP code SIR	Conf. < 90%
FCX, Inc. (Washington)	27889	865	3	24.64	7.23
Potter's Septic	28451	7,803	3	2.56	0.80
Chemtronics	28778	4,866	0	0.00	0.00
Bypass 601 Groundwater	28124	4,640	1	1.63	0.05
Celanese Corporation	28038	4,795	0	0.00	0.00
Carolina Transformer	28301	35,253	2	0.44	0.08
Cape Fear Wood Preserving	28304	33,868	3	0.58	0.18
Jadco-Hughes	28012	19,477	1	0.35	0.01
JFD Electric	27565	20,568	4	1.50	0.51
Benfield Industries	28738	1,759	0	0.00	0.00
General Electric	28726	3,770	0	0.00	0.00
FCX, Inc. (Statesville)	28677	52,895	6	0.93	0.38
Martin Marietta	28214	16,852	7	3.57	1.49
Aberdeen Pesticides	28315	7,767	0	0.00	0.00
Geigy Chemical	28315	7,767	0	0.00	0.00
New Hanover Co. Airport	28401	21,561	2	0.82	0.12
ABC 1-Hour Cleaners	28540	52,792	4	0.67	0.20
Camp Lejeune	28542	23,717	1	0.67	0.01
Charles Macon Co.	28330	24,282	1	0.30	0.01
National Starch and Chemical	28144	34,563	5	1.20	0.44
Koppers Co.	27560	3,922	0	0.00	0.00
NCSU Lot #86	27607	19,515	0	0.00	0.00

Note: NPL = National Priority List; Conf. < 90% = lower limit of one-tailed 95% Poisson confidence interval.

Gaston and Mecklenburg Counties

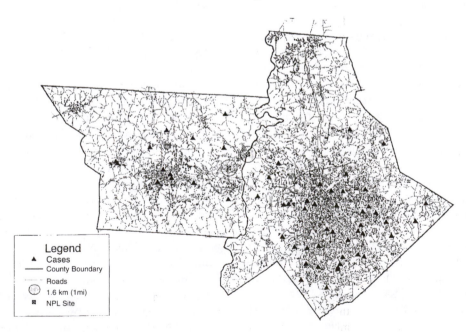

Figure 7–19 Results of GIS analysis for two counties in the study, Gaston and Mecklenburg. The map shows pediatric cancer cases, roads, and National Priority List sites with one-mile buffer.

Table 7–10 Sites, NPL Pediatric Cancer Cases, and Address-Matching Rates, by County

County	Population	No. of NPL Sites	Total Cases	Matched Cases	Address Match Rate (%)	Cases within Buffer
Beaufort	42,331	1	5	1	20	0
Brunswick	51,365	1	5	1	20	0
Buncombe	175,173	1	13	9	69	0
Cabarrus	99,256	1	5	4	80	1
Cleveland	84,748	1	9	6	67	0
Cumberland	276,791	2	24	18	75	0
Gaston	175,410	1	19	13	68	0
Granville	38,510	1	5	2	40	0
Haywood	46,950	1	4	1	25	0
Henderson	69,551	1	11	4	36	0
Iredell	93,193	1	13	4	31	2
Meck	514,056	1	41	39	95	0
Moore	59,228	2	5	0	0	0
New Hanover	120,691	1	11	10	91	0
Onslow	150,744	2	6	6	100	0
Richmond	44,502	1	4	1	25	0
Rowan	110,886	1	10	8	80	0
Wake	426,212	2	48	40	83	0
Totals		22	238	167	70	3

Note: NPL, National Priorities List.

counting for residence of the other seven cases. Other possible solutions for the rural matching problem are to match postal routes to U.S. Geological Survey 1:24,000–scale quadrangle maps by hand or to conduct field research and then enter the data on the computer. We will discuss data quality problems in depth in Chapter 9.

One additional significant limitation is the lack of accurate exposure data. Studies using only residential proximity as a surrogate measure of exposure cannot account for other potential sources of exposure. Additional sources for consideration include parents' occupation, parents' lifestyles, or even parental exposures before birth or conception. More importantly, although proximity may help predict exposure, it does not guarantee exposure. Additional information on potential exposure routes, such as wind speed, wind direction, or groundwater flow, could better predict exposure.

In spite of these limitations, the North Carolina exploratory study did suggest additional venues for research. First, to eliminate problems with small numbers, future studies could combine data from multiple sites in multiple states on the basis of type of facility, the chemical exposures, and the extent of contamination off site. To eliminate the dilution effect of analysis over large areas, the combined sites should be small enough to present a reasonable chance of residential exposure. Because GIS allows the incorporation of multiple data sets, future studies should include data on other sources of exposure and exposure routes.

MORE COMMON CANCERS: ADULT AND PEDIATRIC BRAIN CANCER

A similar study in New Jersey looked at cancers that are more common, child and adult brain cancers, in proximity to NPL sites. This study was a response to public concerns about the rates of primary brain cancer occurring near those sites, including a reported cluster of childhood brain cancer and leukemia in the Tom's River, New Jersey, area.[17] Attribute data came from the same types of sources as the North Carolina study. The Cancer Registry Program of the New Jersey Department of Health and Senior Services provided data on the street addresses of 2,556 cases of primary brain cancer, based on ICD code, diagnosed in New Jersey from 1986 through 1990. These data included residence location at the time of diagnosis, year of diagnosis, patient age, race, gender, and type of tumor. HazDat data, supplied by the ATSDR (see Chapter 2), again provided information on NPL site location, chemical content, and extent of on-site and off-site contamination. The 1990 census supplied population data used in calculating incidence rates by census tract and county.

Like the North Carolina study, the New Jersey study used SIRs to compare the incidence of brain cancer for residents living within ½-mile and 1-mile buffers of an NPL site with the cancer incidence of all New Jersey residents. They compared the observed number of brain cancer cases with the expected number of cases for each area, using the SIR and its 95 percent confidence interval. In addition, investigators looked specifically at the association between off-site contamination and the incidence of brain cancer. The Cancer Registry provided the observed number of cases within the buffer zones, while investigators calculated the expected numbers, using the average annual New Jersey age- and sex-specific incidence rates from 1986 through 1990 and applying this to the denominator population within the buffer areas.

Table 7–11 shows the observed and expected number of cases, the SIRs, and their 95 percent Poisson confidence intervals within 1 mile of an NPL site. The analysis failed to find an association between residence near a New Jersey NPL site and brain cancer diagnosis. For each age group, the observed number of cases is smaller than the expected number of cases, although none of these results is statistically significant. In addition, the specific types of brain cancer (histological tissue types) of residents living near NPL sites and the age, sex, and racial distributions of this population were not different from those of other New Jersey residents.

Lessons learned from this study were similar to those learned in the North Carolina study, and they suggest the need to improve data collection. Before they geocoded the cancer data, investigators had to remove 7 percent of the cases from the data set, either because addresses were missing or because only post office boxes were available. They had to eliminate an additional 3 percent of the cases due to lack of a street address or an unidentifiable address. One of the purposes of developing cancer registries is to provide data that could support studies of cancer etiology. Clearly, cancer registries could help this process if they improved the case ad-

dress data. Besides using the cancer registry, investigators obtained some of the data from the mortality file. Unfortunately, they also had to eliminate many of these cases (nearly 9 percent of the total) from the study because the death certificates contained an unspecified histological code, preventing them from classifying the cases as primary brain cancer. We have no way of knowing if inclusion of these cases would have made the association between residence near an NPL site and brain cancer diagnosis stronger or weaker. We do know, however, that agencies collecting data, including disease registries and vital statistics programs, will need to ensure better data quality to eliminate this problem.

In addition, because of the small numbers of observed and expected cases, investigators were unable to evaluate the SIRs within ½ mile of the NPL sites, nor could they evaluate the SIRs related to specific off-site chemical contamination. Future studies may solve this problem by combining data from at least several states, making standardization of disease registry data essential.

STUDIES USING MODELING TECHNIQUES TO DEVELOP SURROGATE MEASURES OF EXPOSURE

In Southington, Connecticut, improper disposal of chemical solvents led to chemical contamination of the air, soil, and public drinking-water supplies.[18] The problem began after 1955, when the operator of the NPL hazardous waste site, Solvents Recovery Services of New England (SRSNE), began solvent recovery operations. In 1976 and 1977, contamination with volatile organic compounds and possibly heavy metals was found in two public wells, #4 and #6, located near the facility, and in public well #5, near another disposal site for SRSNE waste. In addition, SRSNE operations contributed to air pollution by burning solvent and metal sludges without air pollution controls (until 1976) and by allow-

Table 7–11 Standardized Incidence Rates (SIRs) and 95% Confidence Intervals (CI) for Brain Cancer, One Mile from NPL Sites, New Jersey, 1986–1990

| Age Groups | Number of Cases | | SIR | 95% CI Lower–Upper |
	Observed	Expected		
0–14	19	25	0.75	0.46–1.20
15–44	41	60	0.68	0.49–0.93
45–64	50	83	0.60	0.45–0.75
65+	67	109	0.62	0.48–0.78
Total	177	277	0.64	0.55–0.74

ing evaporation from facility lagoons and storage tanks and from 25 recovery wells without air strippers. Knowledge of these practices led to public concerns that people living in neighborhoods near the SRSNE Superfund site had higher rates of cancer than the general population, which in turn prompted an ATSDR-funded Connecticut Department of Public Health study.

Study investigators used an enhanced TIGER file, Dynamap/2000, as the spatial database. The Connecticut Department of Health (DPH) provided the attribute data from their tumor registry. The registry contained information on patient age and gender, date of diagnosis, residential address at the time of diagnosis, and primary site of diagnosis. Two of the 424 cases could not be geocoded because the registry data did not include an address. The 1980 U.S. census, chosen because 1980 was the midpoint of the study period, provided population estimates for calculating incidence rates.

Because individual exposure data were unavailable, investigators used modeling (see Chapter 3) to develop surrogate measures of human exposure to contaminated water and air. The ATSDR and the Georgia Institute of Technology analyzed the public water supply to determine geographic areas with the highest likelihood of trichloroethylene (TCE) contamination of drinking water. In developing their model, they used several sources of data. The Southington Water Company (SWC) provided information on the water supply, including pipe location, diameter, elevation, and junctures. Next, the University of Connecticut Department of Geography converted these data into a digitized map. In addition, the SWC provided data on the elevation and location of reservoirs, location of wells, and the proportion and quantity of water that these sources delivered during the relevant years of the study. The DPH and the SWC also provided data on water contaminants measured through sampling.

On the basis of these data, the model assigned a relative contaminated-water exposure ranking for each census block. To develop the ranking, investigators used a U.S. Environmental Protection Agency (EPA) software program, EPANET, which tracks the flow of water within each pipe segment, the pressure at each pipe junction, the height of water in each reservoir, and the concentration of each contaminant throughout the distribution system. Criteria for the model's exposure rankings included whether the census block received public water, whether it was on a noncontaminated well, and whether high hydraulic pressure within the drinking-water system was likely to send contaminated water preferentially to a specific census block. For the analysis, investigators grouped census blocks subject to a similar degree of exposure on the basis of the model.

Table 7–12 and a map (Figure 7–20) show the estimated daily exposure, grouped into four categories, based on the

model. According to the model, two-thirds of the Southington population was not subject to water contaminated with TCE. The model assigned populations living in areas northeast of the contaminated wells the highest estimated level of exposure. Model variables of water usage, competing source of water, and hydraulic pressures in the distribution system influenced the size and shape of the polygons, aggregations of census blocks with similar estimated levels of exposure.

Because human exposure was not limited to drinking water, investigators developed a second model as a surrogate measure of airborne exposure. The SciTech Corporation, Wethersfield, Connecticut, developed this model, based on the EPA Industrial Source Complex Long-Term (ISCLT2) model. The Connecticut Departments of Environmental Protection (DEP) and Public Health (DPH) and the EPA provided data on source emissions based on SRSNE record reviews. A nearby National Weather Service station supplied climatological data used to complete the model.

The EPA provided data and equations that allowed investigators to estimate emissions from several sources. Investigators estimated emissions from the solvent reclamation process and the receiving/storage and blend tanks using standard emission factors. Using mass balance equations based on groundwater flow rates and groundwater and effluent concentrations, they estimated air stripper emissions. Finally, using engineering equations, they estimated air emissions from the lagoons and pit incineration. The completed model estimated the air exposure to TCE by summing the individual contributions of each source during the 24-year study period and then calculating an average level over that time. This relatively simple model only used one pollutant, TCE, even though the SRSNE facility had released many other potential carcinogens. In addition, the model used average levels, even though TCE air emissions had probably fluctuated over time.

Unfortunately, in studies like this, investigators can only create models based on available data. Consequently, even the best models have limitations in how well they predict exposure. As we will discuss in Chapter 9, models are only as accurate as the data used to create them, they consider only some of the conditions related to exposure, and they become less accurate as the distance increases from the source of exposure. In addition, models can be unstable when the number of potential variables is equal to or greater than the number of cases of disease.

The final model contains four categories of air exposure shown in Table 7–13. Figure 7–21 is a map showing the geographic distribution of the exposure categories. On the basis of estimations from the model, most of the town suffered no impact from TCE-containing air emissions from the SRSNE facility. Seventy-one percent of Southington was in

Table 7–12 Population and Contaminant Levels of Water Exposure Categories, Southington, Connecticut

Water Exposure Category	Estimated TCE Level per Category (µg/l)	Population*	No. of Census Blocks
Southington		36,723	295
Level 1	No exposure	24,374	236
Level 2	1 to < 10	7,186	39
Level 3	10 to < 50	5,163	18
Level 4	50 or greater	0	2

*1980 census figures.

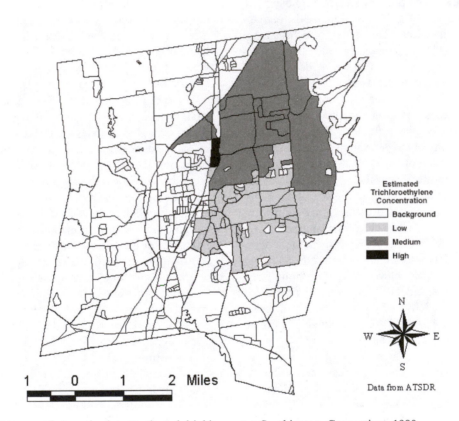

Figure 7–20 Geographic areas that received contaminated drinking water, Southington, Connecticut, 1980

Table 7–13 Population and Contaminant Levels of Air Exposure Categories, Southington, Connecticut

Air Exposure Category	Estimated TCE Level per Category (µg/m³)	Population*	No. of Census Blocks
Southington		36,723	295
Level 1	less than 0.01	25,895	200
Level 2	0.01 to < 0.015	5,585	46
Level 3	0.015 to < 0.10	5,243	46
Level 4	0.10 or greater	0	3

*1980 census figures.

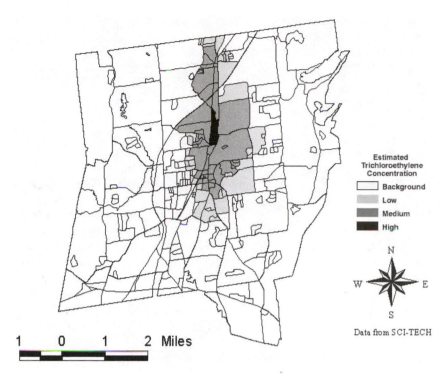

Estimated Trichloroethylene Concentration

☐ Background
▨ Low
▨ Medium
■ High

Data from SCI-TECH

1 0 1 2 **Miles**

Figure 7–21 Geographic areas exposed to air emissions from solvents recovery systems of New England, Southington, Connecticut, 1980

category one, the lowest exposure category, and no area of town was in the highest exposure category. Topography and prevailing winds, accounted for in the climatologically influenced model, influenced the size and shape of the affected areas.

The completed models estimating air and water exposures allowed investigators to compare cancer incidence based on exposure, using the indirect method of age standardization. For each primary tumor site and for all tumor sites combined, they divided the observed number of cases for each drinking-water and air exposure ranking by the expected number, based on the Connecticut state incidence rates. This gave them SIRs and associated confidence intervals for each exposure area, for each type of tumor. To adjust for multiple comparisons, they used a Bonferroni correction.

Study results failed to find any significant increase in the incidence of cancer of the bladder, kidney, liver, or testis, leukemia, non-Hodgkin's lymphoma (NHL), or Hodgkin's disease for any of the exposure categories compared to the state of Connecticut. Table 7–14 shows the results for all air exposure categories for all tumor types combined. Although the results failed to achieve statistical significance, the SIR was higher for NHL for women in the highest–air exposure areas. Additionally, the proportion of a specific tissue type (nodular) was higher compared to the rest of the state, suggesting a need for further study (see Table 7–15).

Like the other GIS studies of cancer incidence, this study highlights the value of GIS analyses in raising hypotheses for further study. In addition, it suggests improvements and additions to our data system. For example, tumor registries may want to consider adding data on potential confounding individual risk factors, such as smoking, alcohol use, family history, and occupation. These exploratory studies also suggest that collaboration between two or more states might be helpful. With collaboration among researchers from multiple states using the same modeling techniques, future studies could combine similarly exposed populations to achieve greater statistical power.

A case-control study of breast cancer on Long Island, New York, also used modeling techniques to establish exposure measures for cases and controls.[19] Chemicals suspected but not proven to contribute to breast cancer are those that can affect estrogen production and metabolism. These chemicals, produced by industry and automobiles, include chlorinated organic compounds such as dichlorodiphenyltrichloroethane (DDT) and polychlorinated biphenyls (PCBs), among others. For this study, investigators developed models of residential exposure to these chemicals from industry and automobile traffic.

An earlier case-control study, with history based on interviews, provided cases and controls for this study. Personal risk factor data were available and included family history,

Table 7–14 Cancer Incidence by Gender for Air Exposure Categories, Southington, Connecticut, 1968–1991

Cancer Type	Cancer Incidence in Total Population				Cancer Incidence in Females				Cancer Incidence in Males			
	OBS	EXP	SIR	95% CI	OBS	EXP	SIR	95% CI	OBS	EXP	SIR	95% CI
Southington	424	453.11	0.94	0.78, 1.09	126	160.58	0.78	0.54, 1.03	298	296.39	1.01	0.80, 1.21
Air level 1	265	298.41	0.89	0.70, 1.08	73	105.13	0.69	0.41, 0.98	192	196.21	0.98	0.73, 1.22
Air level 2	84	84.53	0.99	0.62, 1.37	27	30.28	0.89	0.29, 1.49	57	54.90	1.04	0.56, 1.52
Air level 3	73	70.17	1.04	0.62, 1.47	26	25.17	1.03	0.33, 1.74	47	45.27	1.04	0.51, 1.57
Air level 2+3 (any air exposure)	157	154.70	1.01	0.73, 1.30	53	55.45	0.96	0.50, 1.41	104	100.18	1.04	0.68, 1.39

Note: OBS = Number of observed cancer cases; EXP = Number of expected cancer cases; SIR = standardized incidence ratios; CI = confidence interval.

Table 7–15 Incidence of Non-Hodgkin's Lymphoma (NHL) by Gender for Air Exposure Categories, Southington, Connecticut, 1968–1991

	NHL Incidence in Total Population				NHL Incidence in Females				NHL Incidence in Males			
	OBS	EXP	SIR	95% CI	OBS	EXP	SIR	95% CI	OBS	EXP	SIR	95% CI
Southington	80	92.75	0.86	0.53, 1.20	39	44.37	0.88	0.39, 1.37	41	48.62	0.84	0.38, 1.30
Air level 1	44	61.08	0.72	0.34, 1.10	17	28.79	0.59	0.09, 1.09	27	32.45	0.83	0.27, 1.39
Air level 2	13	17.34	0.75	0.02, 1.48	5	8.54	0.59	0.00, 1.50	8	8.85	0.90	0.00, 2.02
Air level 3	22	14.33	1.54	0.39, 2.68	17	7.03	2.42	0.37, 4.46	5	7.32	0.68	0.00, 1.75
Air level 2+3 (any air exposure)	35	31.67	1.11	0.45, 1.76	22	15.57	1.41	0.39, 2.46	13	16.17	0.80	0.03, 1.58

Note: OBS = Number of observed cancer cases; EXP = Number of expected cancer cases; SIR = standardized incidence ratios; CI = confidence interval.

history of benign breast disease, and age at first live birth. Menopausal status was also available. In addition, the data set contained information on each woman's residential history from birth. Investigators excluded cases and controls from the study if they had not lived on Long Island continuously for 20 years or if address information was inaccurate.

To develop exposure models, study investigators used a couple of sources of data. The New York State Industrial Directory for 1965 and 1975 provided historical data on addresses, standard industrial-classification (SIC) codes, and the number of workers at each facility employing 20 or more workers. Investigators were able to create two subsets of industrial facilities, chemical and other manufacturing, based on the likelihood that they would have emitted toxic chemicals of concern. The New York State Department of Transportation supplied computerized traffic data, including vehicle counts on selected highways from 1990 through 1992. The data set aggregated the traffic data into 25 km² grid cells. Using these data, investigators developed an estimate of traffic density within each cell based on the vehicle miles of travel divided by the cumulative number of miles of highway. This measure accounted for only about 60 percent of the traffic because the data set did not count vehicles on nonprincipal roads.

Using GIS software, investigators divided Long Island into nearly 6,000 1 km² grid cells and placed each industrial facility within the appropriate cell. They assigned summary chemical exposure values to each cell for both 1965 and 1975 on the basis of the number of facilities of each subset present within the cell that year. Figures 7–22 and 7–23 show the distribution of these facilities in 1965 and 1975 respectively. Investigators also gave each grid cell an exposure value, the sum of the industries of each subset within the 8 adjacent grid cells. In addition, they assigned each 1 km² grid cell the traffic value associated with the much larger 25 km² grid within which it was located.

Next, using GIS software, they assigned case and control participant residences to the appropriate 1 km² grid cell. Investigators calculated exposure values for each study participant on the basis of both the chemical values and the traf-

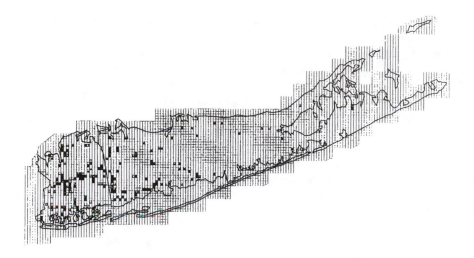

Note: Chemical and other manufacturing facilities include Standard Industrial Classification (SIC) Major Groups: 28, Chemicals and allied products; 29, petroleum refining and related industries; 30, rubber and miscellaneous plastics products; 33, primary metal industries; 34, fabricated metal products; 35, machinery, except electrical; 36, electrical machinery, equipment and supplies; 37, transportation equipment; 38, professional, scientific and controlling instruments, photographic and optical goods.

1 km Grid Cells

■ 4 to 30 Facilities
▨ 1 to 3 Facilities

Figure 7–22 Chemical and other manufacturing facilities with 20 or more workers: Nassau and Suffolk counties, Long Island, New York (1965)

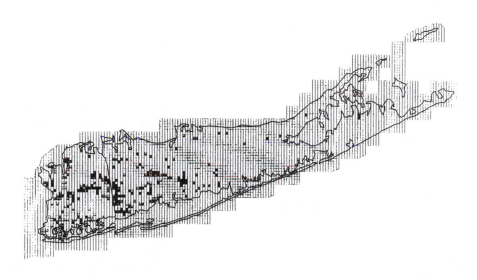

Note: Chemical and other manufacturing facilities include Standard Industrial Classification (SIC) Major Groups: 28, Chemicals and allied products; 29, petroleum refining and related industries; 30, rubber and miscellaneous plastics products; 33, primary metal industries; 34, fabricated metal products; 35, machinery, except electrical; 36, electrical machinery, equipment and supplies; 37, transportation equipment; 38, professional, scientific and controlling instruments, photographic and optical goods.

1 km Grid Cells

■ 4 to 33 Facilities
▨ 1 to 3 Facilities

Figure 7–23 Chemical and other manufacturing facilities with 20 or more workers: Nassau and Suffolk counties, Long Island, New York (1975)

fic values within the cell where each participant lived. Because many of the women did not live at a specific site for the full 20 years studied, investigators used the duration of residence within each grid cell to calculate weighted exposure values over the 20 years for each participant. They used 1965 industry data to assign exposure values for the first 10 years and 1975 data for the second 10 years.

On the basis of the exposure values, investigators next classified case and control exposures as "ever" or "never." The cutoff value for "ever exposure to traffic" was a density of 100,000 vehicles per mile of highway. This represented the 95th percentile rank of traffic density for all participants. The cutoff point for industrial exposure was one or more facilities within the grid cell or residence. Because some of the grid cells without facilities were adjacent to cells with facilities, investigators used the exposure value based on adjacent cell facilities in a second analysis looking at dose-response relationships. (A positive dose-response relationship, or the association between cancer outcome and exposure to increasing doses of a suspected carcinogen, provides evidence, but does not prove, that the chemical causes the cancer.)

Tables 7–16 and 7–17 show the results of the case-control study, using model-determined exposures for pre- and postmenopausal women. Residence in 1 km^2 grids containing any industrial facility, chemical or other, was not associated with breast cancer in either group of women. For postmenopausal Nassau County women only, residence in a grid cell with a chemical facility was statistically associated with breast cancer. Previously recognized risk factors, such as family history and reproductive history, were also associated with breast cancer for Nassau County participants. The association between breast cancer (in postmenopausal women) and residence in a grid cell with chemical facilities in Nassau County remained after controlling for these other risk factors, as shown in Table 7–18. Exposure to high-density traffic was not associated statistically with breast cancer for pre- or postmenopausal women in either county.

Interestingly, for Nassau County postmenopausal participants, the association between chemical facility exposure and breast cancer was stronger for those exposed for at least one year during the first 10 years of the study period, suggesting that this could be due to the long latency period from exposure to clinical disease. Accounting for exposure from chemical facilities in adjacent grid cells did not alter the study findings, suggesting that risk diminishes with increasing distance. In addition, the results in Table 7–15 suggest a dose-response relationship for postmenopausal women in Nassau County. As expressed by the odds ratio, higher levels of exposure (based on residence in grid cells averaging more than one chemical facility) had a stronger association with breast cancer compared to lower exposure levels.

This study further illustrates the use and limitations of GIS technology in developing exposure models for case-control studies, mostly related to data quality and availability. The traffic data were aggregated into geographic grids (25 km^2) that were probably too large to be meaningful for human exposure. In addition, the data included information on traffic only for principal roads, eliminating 40 percent of traffic mileage from the study. In developing its exposure model, the study failed to account for many potential exposures besides physical proximity to industrial facilities, such as diesel truck and train traffic. Proximity alone may be a poor measure for exposure. Climatic data, such as wind speed, wind direction, and precipitation, data on actual air and water emissions involving specific chemicals, and data on drinking-water contamination are relevant for human exposure, and investigators should consider including such data in improved models. In addition, future studies should account for other relevant factors, such as occupational exposure measures and the amount of time that participants spent at their residence, either outdoors or indoors.

Like other case-control studies, this study was also subject to confounding and selection bias. For example, residential proximity to industrial facilities could be associated with socioeconomic status and other demographic factors, which could also be associated with breast cancer incidence. In addition, while 88 percent of the eligible study cases agreed to be interviewed, only 67 percent of controls agreed. If women living in close proximity were more likely to respond, such selection bias could inflate the measured association between residential proximity to industrial facilities and breast cancer. Once again, this GIS study raised questions for future studies to address. All issues of bias, reliability, and validity that apply to other forms of data analysis also apply to the use of GIS technology. Researchers are responsible for clearly identifying the limitations of the results that they present.

HEART DISEASE

Cancer is not the only chronic disease amenable to geographic analysis. Mapping heart disease mortality is useful in guiding public health activities and may also be helpful in addressing racial and ethnic health disparities. Recognizing this potential benefit of GIS technology, the CDC collaborated with West Virginia University to publish "Women and Heart Disease: An Atlas of Racial and Ethnic Disparities in Mortality."[20] The atlas includes maps showing the geographic pattern of heart disease in women at the national, state, and county levels. To develop the atlas, the staff at the Office of Social Environment and Health Research at West Virginia (OSEHR) abstracted death certificate data for 1991

Table 7–16 Distribution of Breast Cancer Risk Factors among Cases and Controls, Unadjusted Exposure Odds Ratios, and 95% Confidence Intervals: Premenopausal Women (Nassau and Suffolk Counties)

	Cases		Controls			
	Number (n = 93)	Percentage of Cases	Number (n = 85)	Percentage of Controls	Unadjusted Exposure OR	95% CI
Nassau (n = 178)						
Family history of breast cancer	13	14.0	6	7.1	2.14	.78–5.91
History of benign breast disease	53	57.0	26	30.6	3.01 ‡	1.62–5.58
Over age 30 at first live birth or no live births	18	19.4	8	9.4	2.31	.95–5.63
One or more facilities in grid cell of residence						
Chemical or other*	33	35.5	28	32.9	1.12	.60–2.08
Chemical	11	11.8	12	14.2	.82	.34–1.96
High-density traffic†	8	8.6	6	7.1	1.24	.41–3.73
Suffolk (n = 143)§						
Family history of breast cancer	7	9.6	2	2.9	3.61	.72–18.0
History of benign breast disease	35	48.0	16	22.9	3.11 ‡	1.51–6.40
Over age 30 at first live birth or no live births	8	11.0	12	17.1	.60	.23–1.56
One or more facilities in grid cell of residence						
Chemical or other*	15	20.6	15	21.4	.95	.42–2.12
Chemical	3	4.1	5	7.1	.56	.13–2.43
High-density traffic†	2	2.7	2	2.9	.96	.13–7.00

*Chemical facilities subset included Standard Industrial Classification (SIC) major groups: 28, chemicals and allied products; 29, petroleum refining and related industries; 30, rubber and miscellaneous plastics products. Other facilities subset included Standard Industrial Classification (SIC) major groups: 33, primary metal industries; 34, fabricated metal products; 35, machinery, except electrical; 36, electrical machinery, equipment and supplies; 37, transportation equipment; 38, professional, scientific and controlling instruments, and photographic and optical goods.

†High-density traffic was defined as more than 100,000 vehicle miles of travel (in 1990) per cumulative linear miles of highway included in traffic counts.

‡Significant at α = .05 level.

§Number of cases and controls in Suffolk County were 73 and 70, respectively.

---

through 1995 from the National Vital Statistics System at the National Center for Health Statistics (NCHS; see Chapter 2). They defined heart disease deaths on the basis of the underlying cause of death on the death certificate according to ICD-9 codes 390–398, 402, and 404–429. The NCHS defines these codes as "diseases of the heart." Death certificate data included information on age, race, ethnicity, gender, and county of residence at the time of death. The Bureau of the Census provided denominator data for each county (population estimates for the years 1991–1995), including gender, race, ethnicity, and age.

Using these data, the OSEHR was able to develop choropleth maps of heart disease mortality rates for women in counties across the United States. One of the problems

they faced in creating these maps was due to the small populations of many of the counties. As we will discuss in Chapter 9, small numbers of numerators and denominators can lead to unstable rates in that small changes in the number of deaths, merely related to chance, could result in large changes in rates over time. This is especially problematic when analyzing rates by race and ethnicity because racial and ethnic minority populations may be quite small in certain geographic areas, particularly many rural areas. Mapping these unstable rates could misrepresent the geographic pattern of disease mortality.

To reduce the problem of rate instability, OSEHR staff used two approaches, temporal aggregation and spatial smoothing. For temporal aggregation, they summed all heart

Table 7–17 Distribution of Breast Cancer Risk Factors among Cases and Controls, Unadjusted Exposure Odds Ratios, and 95% Confidence Intervals: Postmenopausal Women (Nassau and Suffolk Counties)

	Cases		Controls			
	Number (n = 401)	Percentage of Cases	Number (n = 507)	Percentage of Controls	Unadjusted Exposure OR	95% CI
Nassau (n = 908)						
Family history of breast cancer	68	17.0	56	11.1	1.65 [†]	1.12–2.41
History of benign breast disease	153	38.2	156	30.8	1.39 [†]	1.05–1.83
Over age 30 at first live birth or no live births	110	27.4	95	18.7	1.64 [†]	1.20–2.24
One or more facilities in grid cell of residence						
Chemical or other*	127	31.7	149	29.4	1.11	.84–1.48
Chemical	58	14.5	48	9.5	1.62 [†]	1.08–2.43
High-density traffic [‡]	33	8.2	32	6.3	1.33	.80–2.21
Suffolk (n = 530)[§]						
Family history of breast cancer	38	16.8	38	12.5	1.42	.87–2.30
History of benign breast disease	74	32.7	82	27.0	1.32	.91–1.92
Over age 30 at first live birth or no live births	56	24.8	76	25.0	.99	.66–1.47
One or more facilities in grid cell of residence						
Chemical or other*	44	19.5	54	17.8	1.12	.72–1.74
Chemical	14	6.2	12	4.0	1.61	.73–3.54
High-density traffic [‡]	11	4.9	16	5.3	.92	.42–2.03

*Chemical facilities subset included Standard Industrial Classification (SIC) major groups: 28, chemicals and allied products; 29, petroleum refining and related industries; 30, rubber and miscellaneous plastics products. Other facilities subset included Standard Industrial Classification (SIC) major groups: 33, primary metal industries; 34, fabricated metal products; 35, machinery, except electrical; 36, electrical machinery, equipment and supplies; 37, transportation equipment; 38, professional, scientific and controlling instruments, and photographic and optical goods.

[†]Significant at α = .05 level.

[‡]High-density traffic was defined as more than 100,000 vehicle miles of travel (in 1990) per cumulative linear miles of highway included in traffic counts.

[§]Number of cases and controls in Suffolk County were 226 and 304, respectively.

---

disease deaths and population counts over a five-year period, from 1991 to 1995. This resulted in larger numbers of numerators and denominators but also in a loss of data for specific years within the five-year period. Next, they created smoothed rates using a spatial moving average. To produce the average rate, they added the numerators and denominators of each county to the numerators and denominators of contiguous counties and then divided by the number of contiguous counties plus one to produce the average rate. The resulting smoothed county death rates represent the average death rates for each specific county and its neighboring counties.

OSEHR calculated smoothed age-specific heart disease death rates for each county and then directly adjusted these rates to the 1970 U.S. population standard. They performed the same procedure to calculate smoothed rates for ethnic and racial groups. To avoid problems with rate instability, they did not calculate rates for small numerators (deaths) or denominators (population). Specifically, they did not calculate rates for counties where the number of heart disease deaths (numerators) for the county and its neighbors was below 20 for the five-year period. In addition, they did not calculate rates for ethnic or racial populations (denominators) whose numbers were below five in a given county, even if neighboring counties had significant populations.

Figures 7–24 through 7–27 are the resulting choropleth maps showing the pattern of heart disease mortality for

Table 7–18 Association of Industry or Traffic in Grid Cell of Residence and Postmenopausal Breast Cancer Risk, Controlling for Other Risk Factors (Nassau and Suffolk Counties)

County	Potential Exposure in Grid Cell of Residence	Parameter Estimate	Adjusted* OR	95% CI
Nassau (*n* = 908)	Chemical or other[†]	.11	1.11	.83–1.48
	Chemical	.48	1.61 [§]	1.06–2.43
	Other	.08	1.08	.80–1.46
	High-density traffic[‡]	.25	1.29	.77–2.15
Suffolk (*n* = 530)	Chemical or other[†]	.11	1.12	.72–1.74
	Chemical	.46	1.58	.71–3.51
	Other	-.01	.99	.62–1.56
	High-density traffic [‡]	-.11	.89	.40–1.99

*Each parameter was estimated in a separate model. Each model also included family history of breast cancer; history of benign breast disease; age at first live birth (if no live birth: current age if under 50, age 50 if over 50); years of education; and years of age.

[†]Chemical facilities subset included Standard Industrial Classification (SIC) major groups: 28, chemicals and allied products; 29, petroleum refining and related industries; 30, rubber and miscellaneous plastics products. Other facilities subset included Standard Industrial Classification (SIC) major groups: 33, primary metal industries; 34, fabricated metal products; 35, machinery, except electrical; 36, electrical machinery, equipment and supplies; 37, transportation equipment; 38, professional, scientific and controlling instruments, and photographic and optical goods.

[‡]High-density traffic was defined as more than 100,000 vehicle miles of travel (in 1990) per cumulative linear miles of highway included in traffic counts.

[§]Significant at α = .05 level.

women in the United States.[15] Cartographers used quintiles of heart mortality rates to determine county shades, so there are an equal number of counties in each shaded group. Counties with the darkest shade had smoothed heart disease mortality rates lying in the top quintile (top 20 percent) of all U.S. counties, while counties with the lightest shade were in the lowest quintile of heart disease mortality. Figure 7–24, the map of heart disease mortality for all women, shows that counties in the eastern United States tended to have the highest cardiovascular mortality rates for women, while counties in western states tended to have lower rates. Figures 7–25 through 7–29 show cardiovascular mortality rates for women in U.S. counties by ethnicity. Counties listed as having insufficient data are not shaded because numerators (fewer than 20 heart disease deaths) were small or denominators (fewer than five women of a particular ethnicity living within the county) were small. As with other ecologic studies, these maps do not explain why the rates vary, or even whether the differences are significant, but they do suggest the need for further evaluation. Further studies could focus on individual risk factors within the higher-rate counties. Depending on the results, public health officials might consider health promotion efforts aimed at addressing identified risk factors.

In developing these health promotion programs, public health officials might also be interested in looking within

their states to determine where to target their efforts. The next six figures are maps depicting smoothed county heart disease mortality rates by quintile within Oregon. Figure 7–30 depicts rates for all women, while Figures 7–31 through 7–35 show the rates for white women, black women, American Indian and Alaska Native women, Asian and Pacific Islander women, and Hispanic women respectively. Table 7–19 displays an Oregon state profile for heart disease in women.

The overall age-adjusted mortality rate for women over 35 years in Oregon was 307 per 100,000 between 1991 and 1995. During those years, counties in the southeastern and southwestern parts of the state had the highest rates of heart disease mortality. One county in the highest quintile in the north central part of the state was not contiguous with the other high-rate counties. The map for white women looks almost identical to that for all women because 95.5 percent of women over age 35 in Oregon were white in 1995. The statewide age-adjusted heart disease mortality rate for white women was 307 per 100,000. Compared to white women, black women had a higher statewide age-adjusted heart disease mortality rate of 463 per 100,000. Because of the rate differences, the quintile ranges depicted in the map legends are different for white and black women, with rates for black women higher in each quintile. For the top three quintiles, the lowest rate for black women was higher than the highest

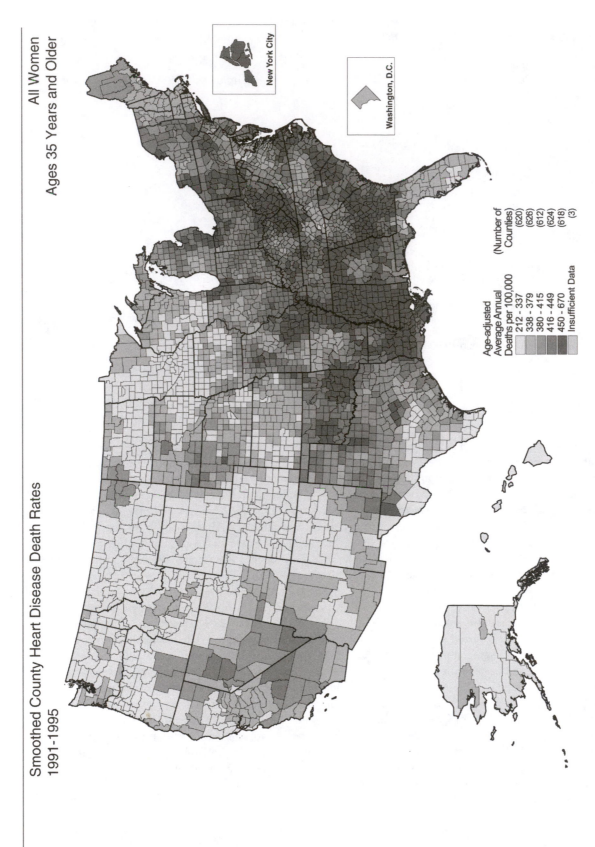

Figure 7–24 Smoothed county heart disease death rates for all U.S. women aged 35 years and older, 1991–1995

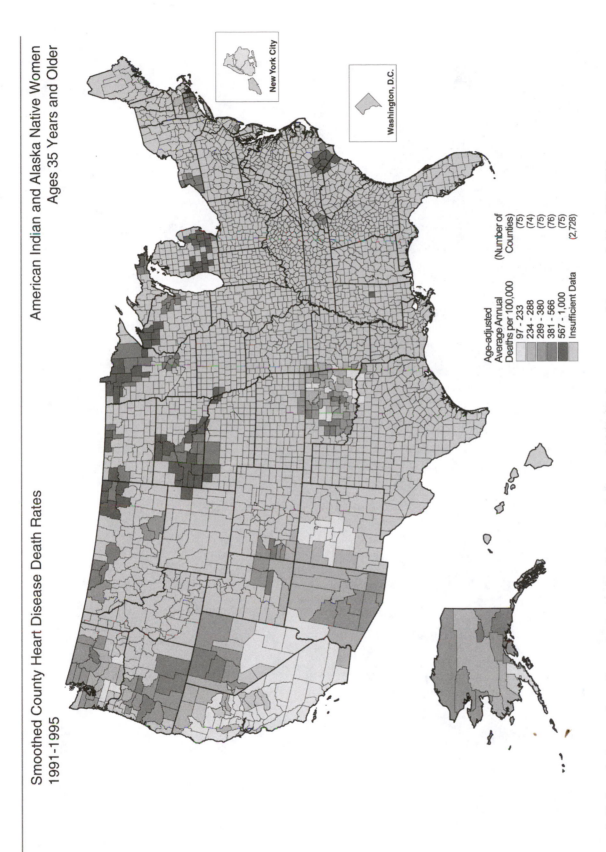

Smoothed County Heart Disease Death Rates
1991-1995

American Indian and Alaska Native Women
Ages 35 Years and Older

Age-adjusted
Average Annual
Deaths per 100,000   (Number of Counties)

97 - 233	(75)
234 - 288	(74)
289 - 380	(75)
381 - 566	(76)
567 - 1,000	(75)
Insufficient Data	(2,728)

Figure 7–25 Smoothed county heart disease death rates for all American Indian and Alaska Native women ages 35 years and older, 1991–1995

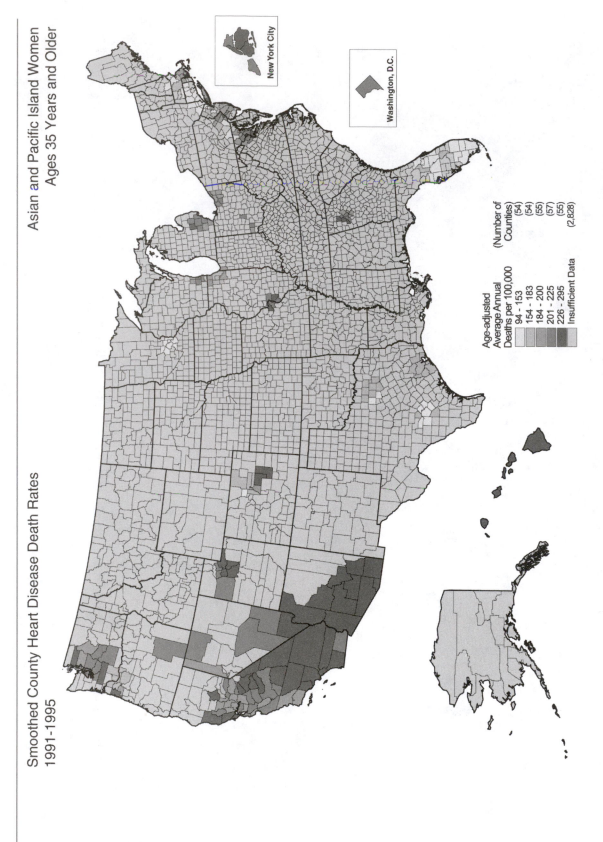

Figure 7–26 Smoothed county heart disease death rates for U.S. Asian and Pacific Island women, ages 35 years and older, 1991–1995

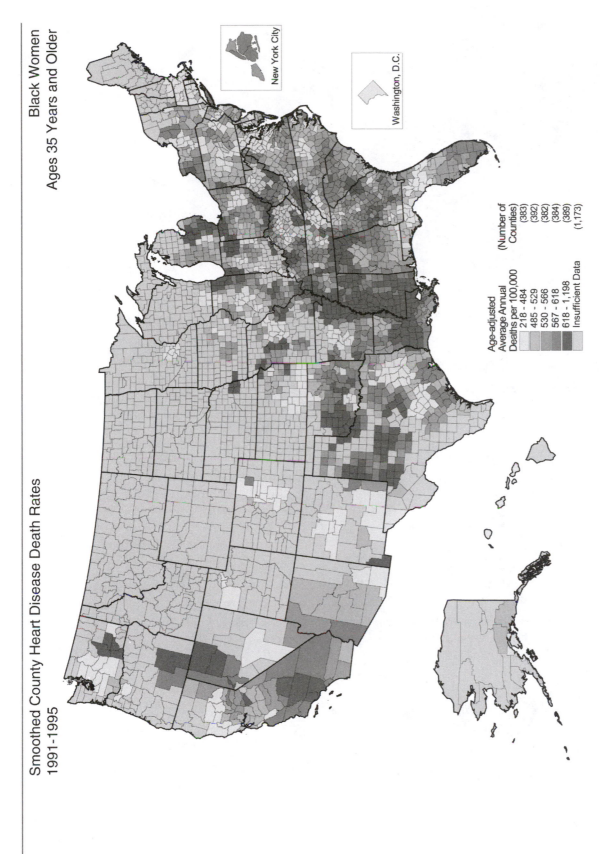

Smoothed County Heart Disease Death Rates
1991-1995

Black Women
Ages 35 Years and Older

Age-adjusted
Average Annual
Deaths per 100,000

		(Number of Counties)
	218 - 484	(383)
	485 - 529	(392)
	530 - 566	(382)
	567 - 618	(384)
	618 - 1,198	(389)
	Insufficient Data	(1,173)

New York City

Washington, D.C.

Figure 7–27 Smoothed county heart disease death rates for U.S. black women ages 35 years and older, 1991–1995

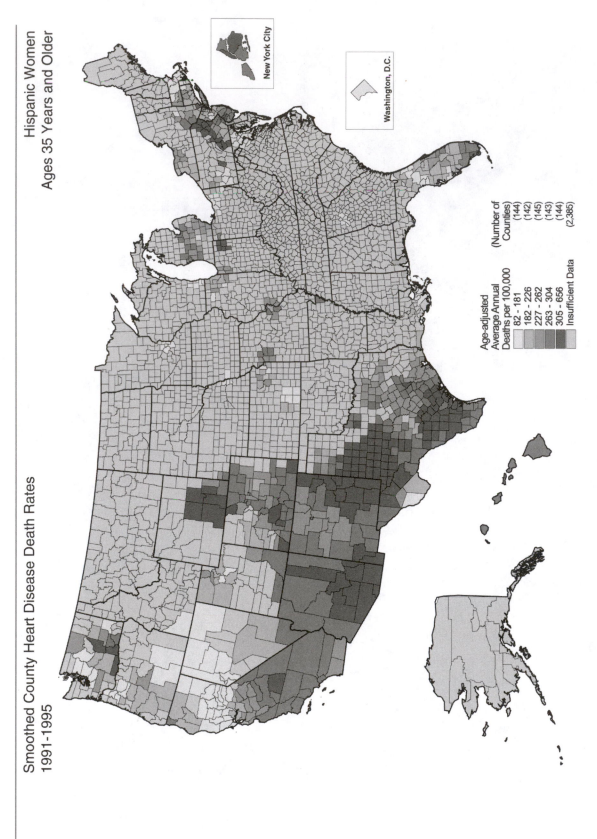

Figure 7–28 Smoothed county heart disease death rates for U.S. Hispanic women ages 35 years and older, 1991–1995

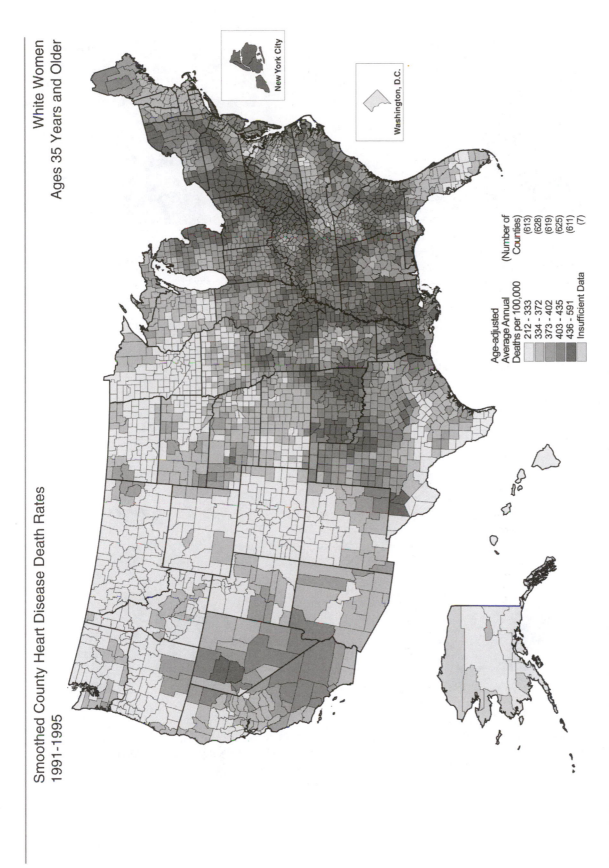

Smoothed County Heart Disease Death Rates
1991-1995

White Women
Ages 35 Years and Older

New York City

Washington, D.C.

Age-adjusted Average Annual Deaths per 100,000	(Number of Counties)
212 - 333	(613)
334 - 372	(628)
373 - 402	(619)
403 - 435	(625)
436 - 591	(611)
Insufficient Data	(7)

Figure 7–29 Smoothed county heart disease death rates for U.S. white women ages 35 years and older, 1991–1995

All Women

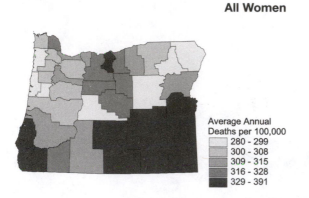

Figure 7–30 Smoothed county heart disease death rates for all women in Oregon, 1991–1995

White Women

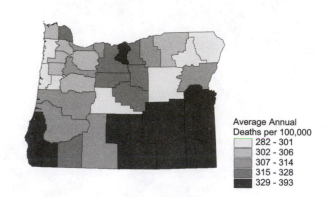

Figure 7–31 Smoothed county heart disease death rates for white women in Oregon, 1991–1995

Black Women

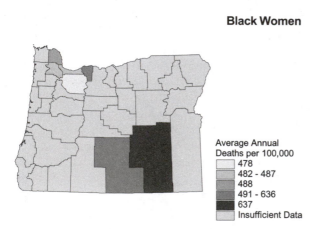

Figure 7–32 Smoothed county heart disease death rates for black women in Oregon, 1991–1995

American Indian and Alaska Native Women

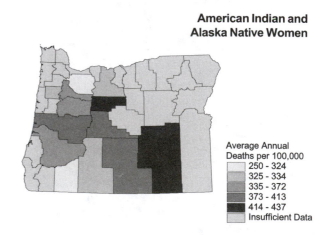

Figure 7–33 Smoothed county heart disease death rates for American Indian and Alaska Native women in Oregon, 1991–1995

Asian and Pacific Islander Women

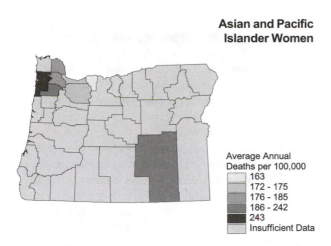

Hispanic Women

Average Annual
Deaths per 100,000
- 163
- 172 - 175
- 176 - 185
- 186 - 242
- 243
- Insufficient Data

Average Annual
Deaths per 100,000
- 91 - 123
- 124 - 165
- 166 - 194
- 195 - 207
- 208 - 250
- Insufficient Data

Figure 7–34 Smoothed county heart disease death rates for Asian and Pacific Islander women in Oregon, 1991–1995

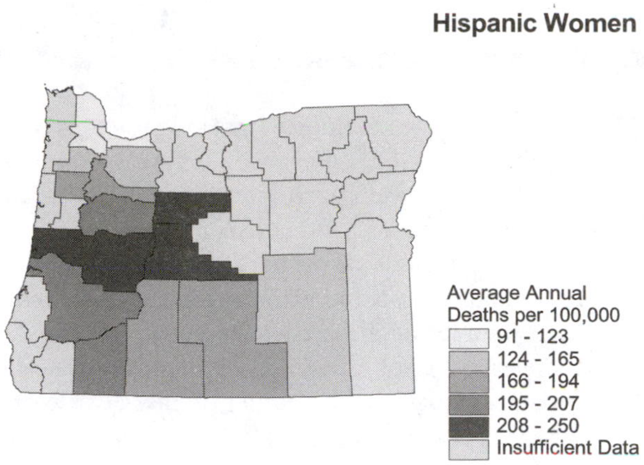

Figure 7–35 Smoothed county heart disease death rates for Hispanic women in Oregon, 1991–1995

Table 7–19 State Profile—Oregon

Race or Ethnicity	State Population 1995	State Heart Disease Death Rate, 1991–1995*
All Women	848,184	307
American Indian and Alaska Native Women	8,954	277
Asian and Pacific Islander Women	19,208	187
Black Women	10,036	463
Hispanic Women	21,680	142
White Women	809,986	307

*Average annual age-adjusted rate (deaths per 100,000) for women ages 35 years and older. Data for Hispanics are also included within each of the four categories of race.

rate for white women. The geographic distribution of heart disease mortality rates for black women was also different, with the highest rates located in nearly contiguous counties in the northwestern part of the state, around the Portland, Oregon, metropolitan area. In many of the counties, the small population of black women prevented calculation of stable mortality rates.

What are the advantages of such a geographic representation of heart disease mortality? Although the maps do not address the reasons for the geographic distribution of heart disease mortality, they identify populations for further study. Future public health efforts could evaluate specific risk factors within counties with higher rates, leading to interventions that are more effective. In addition, maps like these could identify different geographic patterns of chronic disease mortality for different racial and ethnic populations, which could further help public health officials target appropriate interventions aimed at reducing ethnic and racial health disparities. One other advantage of GIS technology is that it can link multiple data sources. Future studies could compare chronic disease mortality with other factors, such as socioeconomic status and availability of health care resources. In this particular study, investigators used GIS technology to map county rates. As we will describe in the next chapter, the same technology is capable of analyzing communities within counties, allowing health officials to evaluate health status at the neighborhood level.

CHAPTER REVIEW

1. Chronic diseases—illnesses that are prolonged, do not resolve spontaneously, and are rarely completely cured—affect over 90 million Americans and account for 70 percent of all deaths in the United States. Chronic illnesses disproportionately affect women and minority populations. Cancer and heart disease are examples of chronic diseases.

2. A disease cluster of any kind is the occurrence of a greater-than-expected number of cases of a particular disease within a group of people, a geographic area, or a period of time.

3. Studies based on cancer registry data have revealed that incidence rates for specific cancers frequently vary by region. People living in areas with high incidence rates, or clusters, are beginning to ask public health officials why and are requesting formal assessments and interventions. Many communities are concerned that local environmental hazards may be causing cancer, yet differences in rates of chronic disease, including cancer, have many additional determinants, such as the behavioral, genetic, and socioeconomic characteristics of underlying populations.

4. Public health officials can respond to the challenge of chronic disease in their communities by using GIS technology to help
   - Target communities with relevant health education and health promotion messages.
   - Evaluate many potential risk factors simultaneously. Health officials can use GIS technology to investigate possible associations between socioeconomic, behavioral, environmental, and other factors and local chronic disease incidence.
   - Show quickly, clearly, and convincingly the results of a complex analysis to concerned constituents.

5. Studies using GIS technology to analyze cancer clusters, while helpful, suffer from several limitations that prevent them from pinpointing causes:
   - Incorporated data usually lack information on many potential confounders, such as personal behaviors and other risk factors.
   - Data do not contain adequate measures of exposure to environmental hazards.
   - Typical cross-sectional study designs cannot account for the length of time between potential exposures related to geography and time of death.
   - Studies frequently cannot account for access to health care, preventive services (such as mammography), or treatment (early surgery), important factors influencing survival from cancer and other chronic diseases.
   - Studies often lump together all cell types of a particular cancer (such as breast or lung cancer), whereas different types may have different etiologies.

6. On the other hand, one of the benefits of using GIS technology is that negative results can be reassuring for concerned community residents. For example, by sharing simple maps showing the location of local, countywide, and statewide pediatric cancer cases, local public health officials can frequently reassure their constituents that rumors of a local pediatric cancer cluster were unfounded.

7. Rather than providing answers for the cause of chronic disease clusters, GIS technology may be useful for generating hypotheses and identifying exposed populations for other studies. Information derived from such ecologic studies could be useful in cohort and case-control studies, where it can serve as a surrogate measure of individual exposure.

8. GIS analyses of pediatric cancers are helpful in improving our understanding of the relationship between environmental hazards and cancer for several reasons:
   - Pediatric cancers tend to have briefer latent periods than adult cancers, which can develop 20 or 30 years after exposure. This is especially important in a GIS analysis because the exposure of interest occurs over a shorter time, reducing the potential number of residential exposure locations.
   - Pediatric cancer registry data are usually very complete and comprehensive because of close supervision by parents and our health care system's priority for care.
   - Childhood cancers, such as leukemia, have occurred in types of clusters most commonly suggesting environmental causes.
   - The short latent period and rarity of pediatric cancers are indications that a toxin may be affecting rapidly growing pediatric tissue, making pediatric cancers sentinel health events (SHEs), potential warning signals about environmental contamination.

9. GIS technology is especially suited for studying the relationship between environmental hazards and can-

cer because of its ability to incorporate multiple sources of data in its analysis.

10. Although helpful, GIS studies of pediatric cancer have several limitations:
    - County-level data for studies on associations between pediatric cancer and environmental exposures are frequently inadequate. Locally produced environmental contaminants, even if they have human health consequences, are likely to affect only the exposed population in very small areas. County-level analysis of health outcomes dilutes the effects of such exposures, reducing the possibility of finding associations.
    - If investigators try to compensate by studying pediatric cancer in smaller geographic areas, the small number of cases found at these levels, such as ZIP codes, reduces the statistical power of the analysis. One possible solution is to look at the association between specific chemical exposures and pediatric cancers at National Priorities List hazardous sites in multiple states, combining the data to achieve sufficient numbers for analysis.
    - Selection bias occurs due to inaccuracies in the residential addresses of cases and failure to address-

match many of the cases, especially in rural areas. One cause for address inaccuracies is the way hospitals report cases to the cancer registry. Frequently, hospitals use billing data when making the report. In many cases, especially in pediatric cases, the billing address is different from the patient's residential address.
    - Accurate exposure data are lacking.

11. Modeling techniques are useful in developing surrogate measures of human exposure in GIS studies of the association between environmental contaminants and chronic disease. However, models are only as accurate as the data used to create them, they consider only some of the conditions related to exposure, and they become less accurate as the distance increases from the source of exposure. In addition, models can be unstable when the number of potential variables is equal to or greater than the number of cases of disease.

12. Cancer is not the only chronic disease amenable to geographic analysis. Mapping heart disease mortality is useful in guiding public health activities and may also be helpful in addressing racial and ethnic health disparities.

REFERENCES

1. Centers for Disease Control and Prevention, National Center for Chronic Disease Prevention and Health Promotion. "Chronic Disease Prevention: About Chronic Disease." <www.cdc.gov/nccdphp/about.htm>.

2. S.J. Melly et al. "Exploratory Data Analysis in a Study of Breast Cancer and the Environment," in *Geographic Information Systems in Public Health: Proceedings from the Third National Conference*, eds. R.C. Williams et al.: U.S. Department of Health and Human Services, Agency for Toxic Substances and Disease Registry, 1998; San Diego, CA: 461–467.

3. Centers for Disease Control and Prevention, National Center for Chronic Disease Prevention and Health Promotion. "Cancer Prevention and Control: About the Program." <www.cdc.gov/cancer/npcr/register.htm>.

4. Centers for Disease Control and Prevention. "State Cancer Registries: Status of Authorizing Legislation and Enabling Regulations—United States, October, 1993." *Morbidity and Mortality Weekly Report* 43, no. 4 (1994): 71–75.

5. A.L. Melnick and D.W. Fleming. "Modern Geographic Information Systems: Promise and Pitfalls." *Journal of Public Health Management and Practice* 5, no. 2 (1999): viii–x.

6. M.Y. Rogers. "Using Marketing Information To Focus Smoking Cessation Programs in Specific Census Block Groups along the Buford Highway Corridor, DeKalb County, Georgia, 1996." *Public Health Management and Practice* 5, no. 2 (1999): 55–56.

7. Claritas PRIZM Lifestyle Cluster data sets were licensed through Claritas, Inc., by the Georgia Department of Human Resources, Division of Public Health, for local public health planning.

8. D. Luke et al. "Smoke Signs: Patterns of Tobacco Billboard Advertising in a Metropolitan Region." *Tobacco Control* 9 (2000): 16–23.

9. M. Kulldorff et al. "Breast Cancer Clusters in the Northeast United States: A Geographic Analysis." *American Journal of Epidemiology* 146, no. 2 (1997): 161–170.

10. B.A. Miller et al, eds. "SEER Cancer Statistics Review, 1973–1990." Pub. No. 93–2789. Bethesda, MD: National Institutes of Health, 1993.

11. P.M. Layde et al. "The Independent Associations of Parity, Age at First Full Time Pregnancy, and Duration of Breastfeeding with the Risk of Breast Cancer." *Journal of Clinical Epidemiology* 42 (1989): 963–973.

12. L. Lang. "Finding the Link." Chapter 3 of *GIS for Health Organizations*. Redlands, CA: Environmental Systems Research Institute, Inc., 2000.

13. Silent Spring Institute Inc. "Breast Cancer on Cape Cod." <www.silentspring.org/Projects/Capestudy/Capebrca.html>. 1997.

14. S.J. Melly et al. "Characterizing the Environmental Features of a Region for a Community-Level Health Study of Breast Cancer," in *Geographic Information Systems in Public Health: Proceedings from the Third National Conference*, eds. R.C. Williams et al.: U.S. Department of Health and Human Services, Agency for Toxic Substances and Disease Registry, 1998; San Diego, CA: 461–467.

15. M.H. Ward et al. "Identifying Populations Potentially Exposed to Agricultural Pesticides Using Remote Sensing and a Geographic Information System." *Environmental Health Perspectives* 108, no. 1 (2000): 5–12.

16. E. White and T. Aldrich. "Geographic Studies of Pediatric Cancer Near Hazardous Waste Sites." *Archives of Environmental Health* 54 (1999): 390–397.

17. O.I. Muravov et al. "GIS Analysis of Brain Cancer Incidence Near National Priorities List Sites in New Jersey," in *Geographic Information Systems in Public Health: Proceedings from the Third National Conference,* eds. R.C. Williams et al.: U.S. Department of Health and Human Services, Agency for Toxic Substances and Disease Registry, 1998; San Diego, CA: 323–329.

18. D.D. Aye et al. "Cancer Incidence in Southington, Connecticut, 1968–1991, in Relation to Emissions from Solvents Recovery Services of New England," in *Geographic Information Systems in Public Health: Proceedings from the Third National Conference*, eds. R.C. Williams et al.: U.S. Department of Health and Human Services, Agency for Toxic Substances and Disease Registry, 1998; San Diego, CA: 365–376.

19. E.L. Lewis-Michi et al. "Breast Cancer Risk and Residence Near Industry or Traffic in Nassau and Suffolk Counties, Long Island, New York." *Archives of Environmental Health* 51, no. 4 (1996): 255–265.

20. M.L. Casper et al. "Women and Heart Disease: An Atlas of Racial and Ethnic Disparities in Mortality." Office for Social Environment and Health Research, West Virginia University, Morgantown, West Virginia, and Centers for Disease Control and Prevention, National Center for Chronic Disease Prevention and Health Promotion. December 1999. <www.cdc.gov/nccdphp/cvd/womensatlas/>.

CHAPTER 8

Public Health GIS Applications: Community Health Assessment and Planning

For many public health practitioners, the most exciting aspect of GIS technology is its potential to revolutionize the process of community health improvement by improving access to health-related data. Every community or neighborhood has assets and capacities in addition to needs.[1] GIS technology can help public health practitioners and their community partners assess many of these factors, strengths and weaknesses, related to community well-being and allow them to evaluate actions that they take to improve their health status.[2] This potential is a consequence of several features inherent in GIS.

The relational and overlay features of GIS described in previous chapters encourage the rapid incorporation of multiple attribute data sets, including data sets not traditionally viewed as related to public health. One vision for community health assessment suggests adding data such as high school dropout rates, commuting time, and domestic abuse.[2] Communities can add data on neighborhood assets, such as local business, religious, and cultural organizations.[1] Software "Data Wizards" make it easy for partners to incorporate additional data sets into the system, further encouraging multiple agencies to share data.[2]

The feature of unlimited scale of analysis is particularly helpful when performing community health assessments and program evaluations in densely populated counties. Large counties often contain many diverse and sizable communities whose borders do not necessarily coincide with county boundaries. Summaries based on these boundaries may not accurately capture community characteristics. For example, a large county may have low teen birth rates compared to the state, while several communities within the county may have markedly elevated rates. In this instance, county-level data are not useful in targeting teen pregnancy prevention efforts to neighborhoods with the high rates. Using GIS, public

health practitioners and their community partners can analyze and display the data at local, subcounty community levels. They can compare their teen birth rate measures statistically with state data, national data, and benchmarks. They can display available resources for teen pregnancy prevention by overlaying physical features such as health and social work facilities, roads, public transit routes, and travel time.[2,3] Over time, they can use the analytical features of GIS to evaluate the outcomes of pregnancy prevention or other public health efforts within their communities.[2]

The flexibility to define community geographically is invaluable in community health planning. GIS software can aggregate census block groups into a variety of community definitions, such as high school attendance areas or legislative districts. Likewise, the GIS software can aggregate attribute data, such as vital statistics data, into the same areas for analysis. For example, a GIS prototype application that we will fully describe in this chapter analyzed teen birth rates, teen male arrest rates, and adequacy of prenatal care by high school attendance area and compared these rates with overall county and state rates and benchmarks.[2] Overlays allow users to look at two variables simultaneously so that they can visualize spatial patterns and relationships. For example, GIS could depict teen birth rates with Youth Risk Behavior Survey (YRBS) results for high school attendance areas. Alternatively, those interested in improving prenatal care could evaluate percentage of first trimester care and income level by legislative district.

Depending on the state and locality, many data sets are easily obtainable, such as vital statistics data (perinatal and mortality), health care expenditures, access to primary care, hospital discharge data, and behavioral risk factor data.[4,5] Table 8–1 lists a few examples of data sets commonly available (also see Chapter 2).

Table 8–1 Types and Potential Sources of Attribute Data

Category (Examples)	Source (Varies by State)	Level of Analysis (Varies by State and Locality)
Demographic data (e.g., age, sex, race and ethnic distribution)	U.S. Bureau of the Census	Census block group, county, state
Perinatal indicators by age and population subgroups (e.g., births, repeat births, prenatal care, low birth weight)	State vital statistics	Census block group (if address included on birth certificate), county, state
Pregnancies, abortions	State vital statistics	County (abortion data do not contain street address), state
Mortality (by age and population subgroups), including years of potential life lost	State vital statistics	Census block group if address included on death certificate; otherwise county and state
Hospitalization (causes by age and population subgroup)	Depends on state—may be Medicaid agency	Varies (census block group, ZIP code, county, state, depending on how residence is reported)
Ambulatory encounter data (by diagnosis, age, and population subgroup) for Medicaid population	State Medicaid agency	Census block group, county, state
Reportable disease (communicable disease, including sexually transmitted disease, lead poisoning, pesticide exposure)	Local health department, state epidemiologist	Census block group, county, state
Immunization of two-year-olds	Depends on state—may be state health department	Varies
Cancer incidence (by age and population subgroup)	State cancer registry	Census block group, county, state
Behavioral risk factors	Centers for Disease Control and Prevention (CDC)	ZIP code, state
Youth risk behaviors (Youth Risk Behavior Survey)	CDC, state health department	High school, state
Synar reports (reports of tobacco outlet inspections)	Depends on state—agency responsible for alcohol and drug treatment planning	Census block group, county, state
Arrests by residence (causes by age and population subgroup)	County law enforcement (e.g., sheriff's office), state justice department	Census block group, county, state

Perhaps the greatest strength of GIS technology in community health assessment is that its product is a picture.[6] Epidemiologists often present analyses in formats comprehensible only to other epidemiologists. Program managers, policy makers, and others who must act on results need these results in a way they can digest and therefore believe. GIS translates complex data into easily understandable information in a visual format. A GIS visual presentation allows viewers to see "at a glance" complex interactions between two or more variables. This feature promises to enhance collaboration between all partners involved in community health improvement.

In this chapter, we will describe several GIS applications in community health assessment and planning, including health services management and planning. We will begin by discussing how GIS can help public health agencies evaluate and ensure health care access in their communities. Then we will illustrate the use of GIS technology in the comprehensive assessment of community health needs. In addition to needs assessments, we will show how public health agencies and their partners can map community assets or community capacity. We will give examples of the use of needs-based maps, assets-based maps, and both in community health assessment and planning.

PLANNING SERVICE DELIVERY: PRIMARY CARE AND OTHER HUMAN SERVICES

Health Care Access

Public health agencies have historically been responsible for ensuring access to health care. The Division of Public Health Systems within the Public Health Practice Program Office (PHPPO) of the Centers for Disease Control and Prevention (CDC) has developed performance standards for public health agencies based on 10 essential public health services, of which two address health care access. Essential service #7 sets an expectation for public health agencies to "link people to needed personal health services (e.g., services that increase access to health care)," and essential service #9 sets an expectation for public health agencies to "evaluate effectiveness, accessibility, and quality of personal and population-based health services (e.g., continuous evaluation of public health programs)."[7]

GIS applications are quite useful in assessing an important aspect of accessibility to health care services, the geographic relationship between the location of potential clients and service utilization. For example, GIS technology can measure the distance from clients to clinics by actual distance (as the crow flies) or by the shortest path distance by roads. If travel time data are available, GIS software can assess the time it takes to travel from home to clinic, even at different times of day with different traffic densities.

GIS technology can help local health departments and other health care providers determine the market area for their services. After entering client encounter data, which must include client home address, agencies can use GIS to map the location of their clients. Agencies having more than one clinic site can identify persons served by their different facilities by using different symbols and by drawing lines from clients' home location to the clinics that they use. Depending on the extent of overlap of symbols and signs, agencies can quickly identify whether their facilities are efficiently serving different geographic areas.[8]

Similarly, public health departments and other health care providers can use GIS to determine the proportion of the eligible population, or market share, that is receiving services from their agency.[8] Two sources of attribute data contribute to measuring market share. Census data supply population denominators broken down by age, gender, and other demographic variables at the block group level, and client encounter data serve as the numerator. For public health agencies interested in ensuring access, this information is helpful because it can quickly identify underserved neighborhoods with large proportions of eligible persons failing to receive services. On the basis of this information, public health departments can target services, including new clinic locations, to improve services for these neighborhoods. Repeat analysis can reveal whether utilization in these areas increases following service improvements.

Public health departments can use GIS technology to evaluate the relationship between client geographic access, health care utilization, and health outcomes.[8] For example, GIS analysis can examine whether the proportion of eligible clients receiving services declines as the distance to the nearest health care facility increases. A simple way to do this is to create buffers of different sizes around clinic sites and measure the proportion of eligible clients receiving services at each buffered distance. Other utilization measures amenable to GIS analysis are the relationships between patient distance from the clinic and the frequency of clinic visits, the proportion of clinic appointments kept, and, for prenatal patients, the time that trimester care began. An example of a health outcome amenable to GIS analysis is the relationship between low birth weight (and other pregnancy outcomes) and patient distance from the nearest clinic site.

Like other GIS analyses we have discussed in this book, these studies cannot give reasons for associations found between distance to health care facilities and health care utilization and health outcomes for a couple reasons. First, even if the studies use individual exposures (with distance being the exposure) and individual outcomes, many of the data sets do not include potential confounders of any association. Second, ecological designs involving aggregate data and cross-sectional study designs preclude drawing any causation conclusions. On the other hand, these studies raise additional questions about access and health outcomes, and they are useful for program planning. For example, local health departments can use the results of GIS analyses to decide where to site new clinics or which clinics to remove when overlapping services exist.[7] Using GIS software in combination with spreadsheets, public health practitioners can locate clinics on the basis of minimizing the average distance or maximum distance of clients to the closest clinic.[8] In addition, using previous analyses of the relationship between proportion of eligible patients served and distance to facilities, health departments can predict the number of eligible clients in a specific neighborhood who would use a new clinic sited at a given distance from the neighborhood.[7] Then, after making program changes such as adding or removing facilities, adding services such as translation or transportation, or changing the hours of operation, local health departments can use the results of such studies to evaluate whether health care utilization for specific population subgroups in underserved areas increased, decreased, or remained the same.

Figure 8–1 is a map illustrating the use of GIS analyses in planning health service delivery. In the four years prior to production of this map, patient visits had decreased by 60 percent at five community-based pediatric clinics operated by the Akron, Ohio, Health Department.[9] Although the health department had no data indicating why utilization had decreased, health officials thought that privatization of Medicaid had contributed to the decline. In response to the drop in utilization, the health department was considering whether consolidating four part-time pediatric clinics into two full-time staffed sites would increase efficiencies. Because a potential outcome of the consolidation would be diminished access, the health department created four maps illustrating residence of children seen at each site to determine whether accessibility would suffer after clinic consolidation. Figure 8–1, one of the four maps, shows the location of the North Hill Clinic in relation to the residence of children seen there. Six bus routes stopping within one-half block serve the clinic, located on a major north-south street running

through Akron. This map, illustrating that clinic patients came from all over the city, was similar to the maps for the three other clinics. Once they saw these maps, city council members easily understood that each "community-based" facility had patients coming from all over the city. This information was very helpful to the health department and the city in countering political concerns that low-income children would suffer from diminished access if the health department were to consolidate clinics. Clearly, the GIS application helped the Akron Health Department make decisions about how to efficiently allocate available resources.[8,9]

GIS technology can also aid health departments in deciding what services to offer at specific clinic sites. Figure 8–2 is a map from Austin/Travis County, Texas, showing the patient demographics at low-income clinics within the county.[10] Brackenridge Hospital, in partnership with the local health department, produced this map as part of its annual report on the use of Medicaid Disproportionate Share funds. The partners created the map because they were concerned that low-income persons without access to a regular source of health care were using the hospital emergency room for nonemergent diagnoses. They felt that the clinic sites, by providing a clinical home, could more appropriately deliver

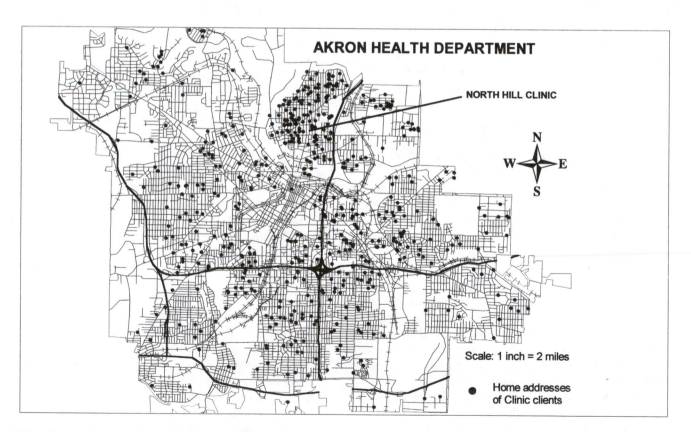

Figure 8–1 Active patients attending the North Hill Child Health Clinic, Akron, Ohio, 1997

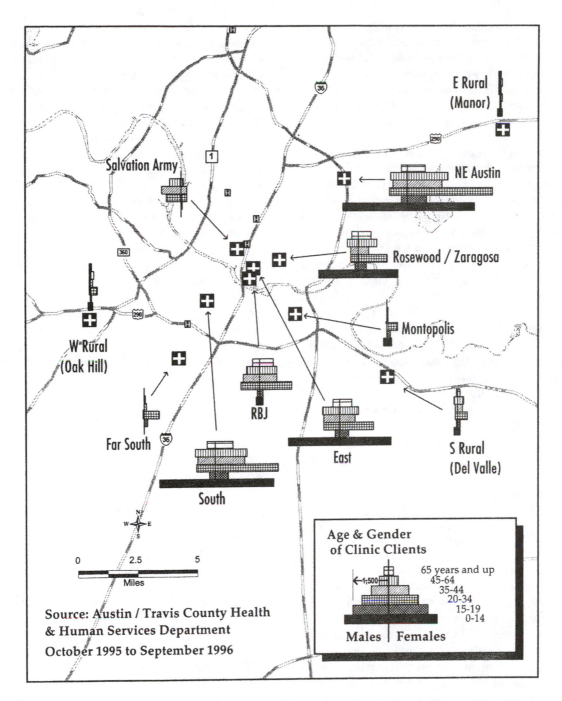

Figure 8–2 Client demographics (age and gender) at low-income clinics in Austin/Travis County, Texas, 1995–1996

comprehensive primary care services. The map shows that clinics in different locations in the county encounter very different patient populations. For example, the Salvation Army clinic in downtown Austin sees mostly middle-aged homeless men, while the North East Austin Clinic mainly serves young adult women and their children. This map helped the local health department improve primary care services (and hopefully utilization) by making it easier for them to decide what services and providers to have available at each clinic site.

Insurance coverage, another important factor affecting access to health care, can vary by geography. Figure 3–15, a map showing the percentage of adults without health insurance in Ingham County, Michigan, illustrates the use of GIS in estimating the geographic distribution of health care insurance coverage.[11] To create this map, cartographers used "synthetic methods" based on results from local behavioral risk factor survey.[11] The 1994 survey of 923 county residents, with a response rate of 63 percent, asked respondents if they had health care insurance, including Medicare and Medicaid. Fourteen percent of the respondents reported that they were uninsured.

Next, the cartographers developed their estimates on those most likely to be uninsured by cross-tabulating insurance status by demographic variables such as age, household income, household type, and "an interaction term" that included poverty status by gender. They then applied these results to the population in a circle one mile with a one-mile diameter around grid points on an Ingham County map. The cartographers used a hypothetical example to describe their methodology. Suppose that the survey results and the cross-tabulations showed that 18 percent of the males were uninsured compared with 10 percent of the females. Next, suppose that one drew a one-mile diameter circle around each grid point on the map. Using GIS (with census denominator data), one determined that 100 persons, 50 male and 50 female, lived within that circle. Then, if one assumed that the behavioral survey results applied to the entire county (one reason that this is an estimate), the circle would contain nine uninsured males (18 percent of 50) and five uninsured females. Using the following formula, the final estimate of percentage of uninsured at that particular grid point would be 14 percent:

$$\% \text{ Uninsured} = \frac{(\text{Uninsured Males} + \text{Uninsured Females})}{(\text{No. of Males} + \text{No. of Females})} = \frac{(9 + 5)}{(50 + 50)} = 14\%$$

Using a similar process, one could then develop estimates for each demographic variable cross-tabulated with insurance status. The final step would be to create a "surface map" with the height at each grid point based on the average of all the estimates at that point.[11] This surface map is similar to the topographic maps used by hikers and mountain climbers. In this case, the height at each grid point represents the estimated percentage of uninsured respondents rather than the altitude. Of course, any form of averaging loses part of the information and may not represent the full range of values behind a given average.

In Figure 3–15, a map based on this methodology, the height of the surface at each point where grid lines intersect represents the estimated percentage of adults without health insurance within a one-mile diameter circle around the point. The map suggests that uninsured adults are concentrated in Lansing, the capital of Michigan and the largest city in the county. The highs and the lows on the map are probably underestimations because they are a result of county-level survey data projected down to much smaller areas and thus miss potential small area variations.[11]

Although the map represents estimates of uninsured persons, it has been useful for the community in improving health care access.[11] After seeing the map, community leaders in Ingham County understood that significant numbers of county residents lacked health insurance. They became aware that low-income people in Lansing and young adults living in low-income housing near Michigan State were the populations most likely to be without coverage. In addition, service providers have used the map in grant proposals that were successful in obtaining additional health care resources. Students and practitioners interested in more information about the methodology used in producing the map can visit the project Web site at <http://pages.prodigy.com/BRLP95A/index.htm>.

Another important aspect of health care access (and a community asset) is the local supply of health care providers with adequate skills and knowledge. To increase the number of providers, particularly in underserved rural communities, many training institutions are turning to telemedicine technology. Telemedicine is a means of using dial-up phone lines that allow audio and audiovisual connections with university faculty for medical and other students working in remote locations such as rural hospitals, practitioners' offices, schools, community health clinics, and patient homes. An East Carolina University (ECU) study illustrates the use of GIS in planning where to locate telemedicine sites in eastern North Carolina, a medically underserved area.[12] Figure 8–3 is a map of eastern North Carolina counties showing where ECU telemedicine sites are in relation to federally designated primary care health professional shortage areas (HPSAs) and shortage population groups, specific underserved populations within a non-HPSA. The Health Resources Services Administration (HRSA) designates these shortage areas on the basis of the local supply of health care providers. More information on HPSA designations is available at the HRSA Web site at <www.hrsa.gov>.

To create this map, ECU obtained the HPSA designations from the *Federal Register* 62(104), May 30, 1997.[13] The ECU Center for Health Sciences Communication supplied the data on telemedicine sites, and the ECU Center for Health Services Research and Development supplied the spatial data. This map served two purposes. First, telemedicine administrators, public health practitioners, medical consultants, and educators have used the portrayed information of the local demographic milieu and provider supply to tailor their educational programs in specific areas. Second, the map has helped ECU plan where to locate additional telemedicine sites.

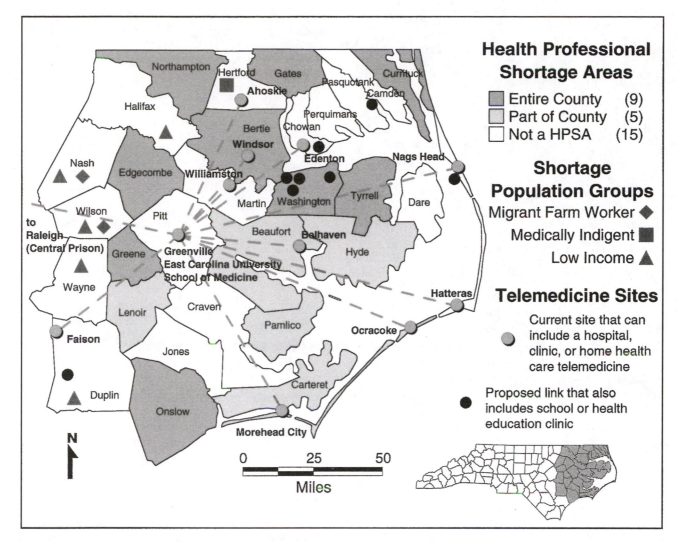

Figure 8–3 Location of East Carolina University School of Medicine telemedicine sites in relation to primary care health professional shortage areas for North Carolina's Health Service Area VI, 1997

USING GIS IN PERFORMING COMMUNITY HEALTH ASSESSMENTS

Historically, in many communities, state agencies and their partners frequently delivered health and human services in a nonintegrated, haphazard manner. The pattern of service delivery was independent of local needs (which were frequently unidentified) and was broken into separate categories (silos) of programs, so that recipients often had to interact with several different agencies to receive services, a barrier to access. To improve access to service and make the level and type of services responsive to local needs, many states are now beginning to develop service integration ini-

tiatives. These initiatives are requiring state agencies and their partners to collaborate in offering services in convenient, accessible locations, based on comprehensive assessments of community health status.

In 1997, directed by the Governor's Family Services Cabinet Council, the state of Delaware embarked on such a service integration project. The council asked the state Health Statistics Center to prioritize needs across the state. Using the integrative capacity of GIS technology, the center assessed health needs by census tract throughout Delaware and ranked them by priority.[14] To do this, center staff first identified 10 factors related to community health needs for which data on two measures for the factor were available down to the census tract level (see Table 8–2). The first measure for each factor was an absolute number: the number of people affected or the number of events, such as births. Absolute numbers were helpful for planning because they indicated the potential number of clients needing services for each factor in each census tract. The second measure for each of the same factors was a proportion: the percentage of people affected or the incidence rate of events. Proportions and rates were helpful because they indicated the relative impact of each factor for each census tract. The center staff then calculated both measures for all 10 factors for each census tract in Delaware and ranked each census tract for each measurement. For the third step, they developed a summary rank for every census tract based on an average of rankings for all the measures, which they termed a "mean priority score." To do this, they added the ranking for each measure and then divided the total score by 20, the total number of measures. On the basis of the mean priority scores, Table 8–3 sorts all 168 census tracts into quintiles. Figure 8–4 displays the same information on a choropleth map of New Castle County,

Table 8–3 Census Tracts Divided into Quintiles (Five Priority Groups) Based on Their Mean Priority Scores

Priority Group	Number of Census Tracts	Priority Level	Population
1	34	Highest	170,725
2	34	↑	163,455
3	34	↑	116,407
4	33	↑	127,171
5	33	Lowest	88,410

Delaware, with census tract polygon shades and patterns representing the priority ranking by quintile.

Following a presentation by the Health Statistics Center, the Family Services Council officially endorsed the priority maps and targeted the highest-priority census tracts for Delaware's new service integration project. In comparison to the old categorical approach, the service integration project

Table 8–2 Selected Factors Where Census Tract–Level Data Were Available for the Entire State

Factor	Specific Measure	Source
Teen mothers	Number of births to teen mothers (< 20 years old)	1991–1995 vital statistics data
	Estimated teen birth rate (15–19 years of age)	1991–1995 vital statistics data 1990 Census data, and Delaware Population Consortium Estimates
Prenatal care	Number of births with less than adequate care (Kessner Index)	1991–1995 vital statistics data
	Percent of births with less than adequate care (Kessner Index)	1991–1995 vital statistics data
Poverty	Number of persons below 200 percent of poverty	1990 Census data
	Percent of persons below 200 percent of poverty	1990 Census data
Employment	Number of unemployed persons	1990 Census data
	Percent of unemployed persons	1990 Census data
Public assistance	Number of persons receiving public assistance	1990 Census data
	Percent of persons receiving public assistance	1990 Census data
Transportation	Number of households with no vehicle available	1990 Census data
	Percent of households with no vehicle available	1990 Census data
Home ownership	Number of renter-occupied housing units	1990 Census data
	Percent of renter-occupied housing units	1990 Census data
Education	Number of persons 25 and older with less than a high school diploma	1990 Census data
	Percent of persons 25 and older with less than a high school diploma	1990 Census data
Language	Number of persons who do not speak English well or at all	1990 Census data
	Percent of persons who do not speak English well or at all	1990 Census data
Children in single-parent households	Number of children < 18 years of age living in female-headed households (no husband present)	1990 Census data
	Percent of children < 18 years of age living in female-headed households (no husband present)	1990 Census data

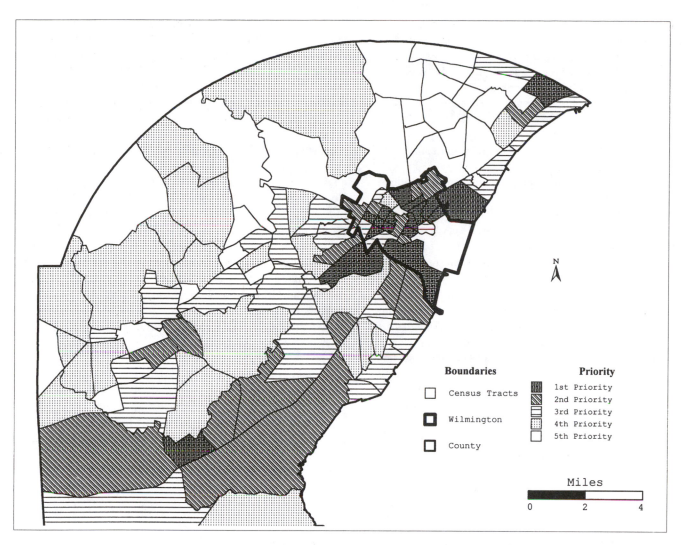

Figure 8–4 Ranking priorities for a state family service integration initiative by census tract in northern New Castle County, Delaware, 1997

promises to involve a community-based partnership model. Using information from the maps, several state agencies, school districts, and nonprofit organizations are beginning to collaborate to provide multiple services with a client-centered focus. The Health Statistics Center is planning to survey residents of the highest-priority census tracts to gather additional information about access to specific services and service utilization. On the basis of this information, they will develop a "menu" of services available for those communities within the priority census tracts. The communities could then select services from the menu that best meet their needs. Future versions of the GIS application will map the location of community assets, such as schools, nonprofit agencies, shelters, and food banks.[14] We will discuss community asset mapping in more detail later in this chapter.

BRINGING COMMUNITY HEALTH ASSESSMENT TO THE COMMUNITY

GIS technology promises to bring the process of community health assessment to communities by making health data more accessible, localized, and community based.[15] The term *accessible data* means that community members and interested agencies are able to obtain relevant information about the health status of their communities at a variety of sites, including local libraries and home computers. *Localized* means that community-level health data are available for analysis at the neighborhood/community level. *Community based* means that local communities should be able to determine for themselves what information about their community is relevant; it also means that local and state governments should be a resource for these communities in providing for their data needs. We will discuss a couple of GIS applications that bring community health assessment tools to the local level. The first application, in Seattle, Washington, allows local health department staff without sophisticated computer skills or programming expertise to analyze a variety of data sets related to community health status. The second application, in Clackamas County, Oregon, shows how local public health agencies can make the technology available to community partners.

The Seattle-King County Health Department developed its application, VISTA/PH, to make it easy for local health departments to analyze data at the local level.[16] VISTA/PH has several features that allow this. First, it serves as sort of a data warehouse by incorporating different data sets in one location. Second, it makes these data available for analysis in a flexible, easy-to-use format. Third, it standardizes the analysis methods, ensuring that the same methodology is used across jurisdictions. Finally, the output is in a simple database (*.dbf) format. This allows local health department staff to import the results into spreadsheets, tables, graphics, or GIS mapping software, allowing multiple presentation formats.

Table 8–4 shows the type of health data, the years available, and the level of possible geographic analysis in VISTA/PH. Besides rates, VISTA/PH can produce counts of each event listed under the assessment topics in the table. Users can simply click on appropriate buttons to specify analysis for subpopulations (such as age, race, and gender), geo-graphic areas, and time periods. The application allows users to combine census tracts or ZIP codes into larger areas of their choice and to combine more than one year of data for analysis. For mortality analyses, users can choose to calculate crude, age-specific, and age-adjusted rates, and they can analyze the data by one or more causes of death. Because VISTA/PH contains a statistical package, SPSS, it performs several statistical tests, such as 95 percent confidence intervals for rates. Its flexibility allows users to specify other confidence intervals. In addition, users can perform statistical analyses for trends in rates over time, a capacity that is particularly helpful in program evaluation.

Another benefit for VISTA/PH users without formal computer or epidemiologic skills is the help button feature. By simply clicking on the appropriate button, users can get help on definitions of measures such as fertility rates and cause of death groupings by ICD-9 code. Other help buttons lead the user to explanations of the various statistical tests, such as time-trend analyses. Still other help features allow users to save groupings of geographic areas of interest so that they do not have to redefine them later.

Figure 3–7 in Chapter 3, a map of childhood asthma hospitalization rates by ZIP code of residence in King County, illustrates how VISTA/PH can help local health officials target local interventions to improve community health. The local health department produced this map because childhood asthma hospitalizations in the county had increased by 22 percent over the previous 10 years. To produce this map, they used VISTA/PH to analyze age-specific asthma hospi-

Table 8–4 Assessment Topics, Years, and Geographic Units of Analysis Available in VISTA/PH

Assessment Topic*	Years Available	Geographic Units†
Fertility rates	1980–1996	Census tract, county, state
Birth risk factors	1980–1996	Census tract, county, state
Abortion/pregnancy rates	1981–1996	Seattle, county, state
Infant death rates and causes	1980–1996	Census tract, county, state
Birth risk factors for infant death	1980–1996	Census tract, county, state
Death rates	1980–1996	Census tract, county, state
Hospitalization rates	1987–1996	ZIP code, county, state
Life expectancy tables	1980–1996	Census tract, county, state
Tuberculosis rates	1980–1996	ZIP code, county, state
STD rates	1987–1996	Census tract, county, state
Other communicable disease rates	1988–1996	Census tract, ZIP code, county, state
Population tables	1988–2002	Census tract, ZIP code, county, state
Census measures	1990	Census tract, ZIP code, county, state
Case file input‡	Data dependent	Data dependent

*Data are available for Washington State only. The data sources for VISTA/PH include Washington State Department of Health, Washington State Department of Social and Health Services, and the 1990 U.S. Census.

†Units can be grouped into larger areas by the user.

‡The case file input option allows analysis of any user-defined data set that meets simple format criteria.

talization data by ZIP code and then imported the results into GIS software, MapInfo Professional 4.5. They were able to do this because the VISTA/PH-produced results, in spreadsheet format, contained the same ZIP code variable as the spatial data stored in MapInfo. ZIP code served as the local geographic area for analysis because ZIP code was the only geographic variable in the hospitalization data. The health department defined asthma hospitalizations as hospital discharges with a principal ICD-9 diagnosis code of 493 and counted each hospitalization for individuals with multiple hospitalizations as a separate event. The census population tables served as denominators for rate calculations by ZIP code. Because individual year rates (due to small numbers) were unstable, the researchers aggregated the data into a seven-year period (1990–1996) in calculating rates.

Figure 3–7 groups the ZIP code polygons into four quartiles of hospitalization rates over the seven-year period for childhood asthma. The background map includes all of King County, while the main map provides a close-up view of Seattle and its inner suburbs. Local health officials, working with community partners, used the results of this analysis to target a research and evaluation project, Seattle Healthy Homes, to reduce exposure to indoor asthma triggers in central/south Seattle area. This area contains the ZIP code aggregations bordered by the dark, thick line. They were able to obtain funding for the project from the National Institute of Environmental Health Sciences. In deciding where to implement Seattle Healthy Homes, the partnership used VISTA/PH to look at several other ZIP code characteristics, including percentage living below the federal poverty level, percentage without a high school education, and ethnicity.

In addition to facilitating the development of the Healthy Homes project, local health officials have used VISTA/PH to produce at least a dozen reports on many community health issues and to answer hundreds of data requests from other agencies, researchers, and the public. Local public health officials are also using VISTA/PH to produce state-mandated community assessment reports. Future versions of VISTA/PH may include Internet access, allowing community members to perform their own analyses and produce their own reports.

The VISTA/PH example points out the benefits and limitations of geographic analysis of community health status. Certainly, health officials can use the results of analyses such as this one to target and evaluate health promotion programs. On the other hand, as we discussed in Chapter 2, health officials have to be careful in drawing conclusions from such ecologic data. The VISTA/PH analyses looked at hospitalization rates, not asthma illness. Many other factors besides illness (and beside indoor air quality) could lead to hospital admissions. For example, a higher hospital bed supply, proximity and accessibility of hospitals, and physician practice, including whether local physicians prescribe the most effec-

tive asthma medications, could be better predictors of asthma hospitalization.[17] The maps in Figure 8–4 clearly raise some interesting questions begging further analyses.

The Clackamas County, Oregon, Department of Human Services has designed a prototype of another GIS application, the Community Health Mapping Engine (CHiME), to improve access to data by local health consumers and planners and allow local government to engage diverse communities in partnerships to improve community health.[2] The design of CHiME facilitates the rapid on-line incorporation of multiple geographically referenced attribute data sets, allowing analyses at the local, subcounty level. Through the Healthy Communities partnership process, many local agencies, both private and governmental, could share data, allowing their incorporation into the CHiME application. Planners foresee CHiME serving as an enterprise model and as a tool to facilitate community health planning. As an enterprise GIS, CHiME could provide a centralized assessment tool for use by many county agencies (in addition to the human services department) and partners. The Web-based CHiME, with its help features, could be publicly available to community-based groups and consumers interested in performing community health assessments.

When fully developed, CHiME could provide communities within Clackamas County with a tool to help themselves in at least two ways: (1) by enabling them to assess a variety of factors related to community well-being and (2) by allowing them to evaluate any actions they take directed at improving their health status. The developers have already involved community residents in a variety of ways, such as through the Local Public Safety Coordinating Council, the Reduce Adolescent Pregnancy Project, the Healthy Communities Council, and the Robert Wood Johnson–funded Turning Point Partnership. The vision for the Clackamas County CHiME includes several useful features:

- A user-friendly interactive system accessible through the Internet
- An initial screen containing text describing the project, listing data and data sources (metadata), and providing instructions on how to use the system
- Help icons and screens available at all times
- Features designed for community members without formal epidemiological skills as well as advanced epidemiological investigators. Such features will include
  - An epidemiology tutorial, with instructions on how to use the system
  - Explanations of concepts such as incidence rates, prevalence, confidence intervals, and the need for age adjustment when evaluating mortality rates
  - Pop-up help screens containing messages discussing the concept of ecologic fallacy and the need for caution about drawing conclusions when cause-and-ef-

fect relationships have not been established previously[18]

- Data analysis at the community level, the county level, and the state level, with findings presented in table, chart, and polygon/map format
- Census data (and estimated intercensus data) with information about demographic characteristics and population counts. For the prototype application, CHiME developers purchased intercensus data from a private provider, Equifax National Decision Systems (ENDS). ENDS provides current year estimates of demographic and population data in several formats, including ArcView GIS, and has a history of providing such data for commercial use.
- Capacity to
  - Compare community level measures with countywide data, statewide data, state benchmarks, and national data
  - Compare measures for each geographical area over time
  - Calculate confidence intervals automatically
  - Aggregate data over time periods when rates for a single year are unstable due to small numbers
  - Display data in chart or table form by clicking on a state, county, or community
  - Zoom in or out among geographic levels
- Information displayed for each geographic level that includes absolute numbers, rates, means, and confidence intervals (with the capability to make a Bonferroni adjustment for multiple comparisons)
- Capacity to evaluate two variables simultaneously to visualize spatial patterns and relationships (for example, to evaluate relationships between teen birth rates and risk factors such as poverty)
- Community areas defined by aggregation of census block groups:
  - For compatibility with population data sources (used for the denominators), CHiME developers defined communities as census block groups aggregated to approximate high school attendance areas. They chose not to use ZIP codes or the larger census tracts because these cross community and city boundaries. In addition, it is difficult to obtain denominator data for ZIP codes.
  - CHiME developers conducted several focus groups, including those with the elderly, teens, and minority populations, who concurred with the initial decision to use high school attendance areas as geographic community definitions. Following community input, the Data Wizard could aggregate census block group data to create maps for alternative target areas such as legislative districts, elementary school attendance areas, or other user-defined small areas.

- A "Data Wizard" feature that allows project administrators to incorporate additional data sets into the system easily and rapidly. The Wizard facilitates the process of geocoding and adding new data to CHiME and supports several data formats.
- Assurance of confidentiality:
  - The CHiME developers could make copies of the Data Wizard available for their data-sharing partners. Then agencies sharing data could use the Data Wizard to geocode individual records and aggregate the records into the defined geographic communities. After aggregation into the appropriate geographic area, they could use the Wizard to remove all individual identifiers before sharing the data with the county's Web-based CHiME. Not only does the Wizard help ensure confidentiality, but its geocoding and aggregating properties have already encouraged formerly reluctant agencies such as hospitals to share their data with the county public health officials.
  - Developers can further ensure confidentiality by designing CHiME to automatically restrict analysis, reporting, and depiction of very small numbers, especially when users perform multiple stratification.
- Inclusion in each incorporated data set of an address field for geocoding. Table 8–5 lists the type of data initially included in the CHiME GIS application. Currently, several of these data sets allow geographic analysis only at the county level or above. Developers plan to add data sets allowing analysis at the subcounty level once complete address fields are available. Their vision for CHiME is that all health-related data eventually will include an accurate address field to enable analysis at the community level. Examples of data of special local interest are
  - Mortality, including years of potential life lost (YPLL), age-adjusted mortality rates, and standardized mortality rates
  - Immunization rates for children at age two
  - Cancer registry data
  - High school dropout rates
  - Commuting time
  - Domestic abuse (including elder, child, and spousal abuse)
  - Hospital discharge diagnoses (obtained through working partnerships with health care systems and health care providers)
  - Links to appropriate county health officials, allowing community users to ask questions and obtain consultation. Links to other on-line information sources could also be available.

In the sample map of Figure 8–5, the CHiME shows teen male arrest rates by high school attendance areas in

Table 8–5 Data Sets, Geographic Level of Analysis, and Years Available

Variables	County Level of Analysis	Community Level of Analysis	Years	Data Source
Age, gender, and race	X	X	Single years: 1990 to 1996	Equifax
Personal income	X	X	Single years: 1990 to 1996	Equifax
Births (including repeat births)	X	X	Single years: 1990 to 1996 Aggregate: 1991 to 1995	Oregon Health Division, Vital Statistics
Abortions	X		Single years: 1990 to 1996 Aggregate: 1991 to 1995	Oregon Health Division, Vital Statistics
Pregnancies	X		Single years: 1990 to 1996 Aggregate: 1991 to 1995	Oregon Health Division, Vital Statistics
Deaths	X		Single years: 1990 to 1996 Aggregate: 1991 to 1995	Oregon Health Division, Vital Statistics
Suicides	X	X	Single years: 1990 to 1996 Aggregate: 1991 to 1995	Oregon Health Division, Vital Statistics
Arrests	X	X	Single years: 1990 to 1996 Aggregate: 1991 to 1995	Clackamas County Sheriff's Department
Reported crimes	X	X	Single years: 1990 to 1996 Aggregate: 1991 to 1995	Clackamas County Sheriff's Department

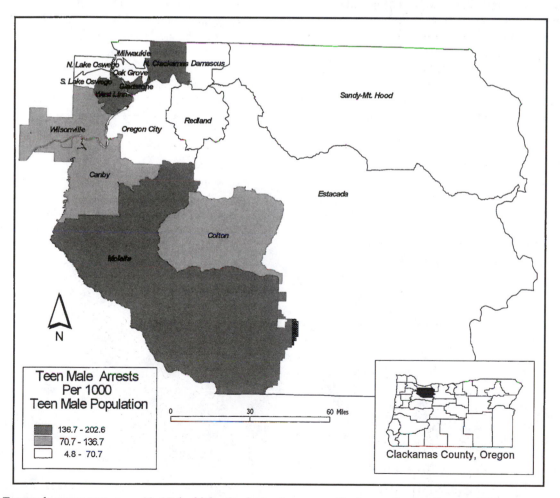

Figure 8–5 Teen male arrest rates, ages 10–17, by high school attendance area, Clackamas County, Oregon, 1995

Clackamas County. Juvenile (teen) arrests are one of Oregon's benchmarks, measurable indicators for which data are reliably, regularly, and economically available. The Oregon Progress Board, an independent state planning and oversight agency, develops the benchmarks through a public process.[19] Oregon currently has 92 benchmarks. Created by the state legislature in 1989, the Oregon Progress Board is responsible for implementing the state's 20-year strategic plan, Oregon Shines. The newest version of the strategic plan, Oregon Shines II, has three major goals: (1) quality jobs for all Oregonians; (2) safe, caring, and engaged communities; and (3) healthy, sustainable surroundings.[20]

Ten of the current Oregon benchmarks focus on traditional public health indicators such as teen pregnancy, access to prenatal care, infant mortality, and percentage of adequately immunized two-year-olds. Figures 8–6 and 8–7 show how CHiME can display some traditional indicators, teen birth rates and the proportion of pregnant women beginning prenatal care in the first trimester, at the subcounty level: high school attendance area in Clackamas County. CHiME developers had to use teen birth rates rather than teen pregnancy rates because abortion data did not include address information below the county level (pregnancies are calculated by adding births plus abortions).

However, many of the other benchmarks also have public health implications. The Oregon Progress Board realizes that connections exist between all three goals and most benchmarks. Using a public process involving thousands of Oregon residents, the Progress Board established the juvenile arrest rate as one of the benchmarks for the goal of safe, caring, and engaged communities. The Clackamas County Public Department of Human Services and its Public Health Division have viewed the juvenile arrest rate as a benchmark with public health implications for which CHiME potentially could play an important role in community partnerships.

Before the development of CHiME, Clackamas County law enforcement agencies used the location of crime and arrest events (rather than rates) in determining where to deploy resources. Following input from its Department of Human Services member, and in consideration of the established juvenile arrest rate benchmark, the Juvenile Crime Subcommittee of the Clackamas County Local Public Safety Coordinating Council became interested in looking at juvenile arrest rates as a measure of community health and safety. Their interest increased when they found that the CHiME could allow them to map and analyze juvenile arrest rates, and potential associated risk factors, at the subcounty, community level.

In Figure 8–5, the case definition for a teen male arrest is age 10–17 years, male gender, and an arrest report by a law enforcement agency. CHiME calculated rates based on the residence of the arrested teen (see Table 8–6). The analysis could just as easily calculate rates based on location of the reported crime. As mentioned earlier, CHiME developers decided on high school attendance areas as a community definition for analysis. An additional benefit of using this definition for juvenile arrest rates is its potential to design

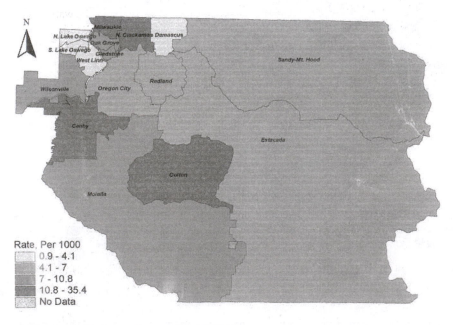

Figure 8–6 1996 community-level teen birth rates by quartile (CHiME)

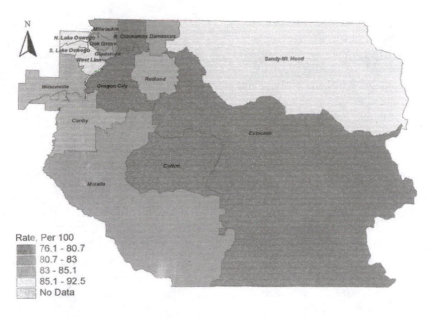

Figure 8–7 1996 community-level percentage of first-trimester care by quartile (CHiME)

Table 8–6 Teen Male Arrest Rates, Ages 10 to 17, per 1,000 Teen Male Population, by High School Attendance Area, Clackamas County, Oregon, 1995

High School Attendance Area	Number of Teen Male Arrests	Teen Male Population	Rate per 1,000
Canby	171	1,325	129.1
N. Clackamas	207	1,091	189.7
Damascus	7	843	8.3
Estacada	47	1,835	25.6
Gladstone	140	691	202.6
Milwaukie	82	1,904	43.1
Molalla	196	1,218	160.9
N. Lake Oswego	39	1,137	34.3
Oak Grove	79	1,858	42.5
Oregon City	118	2,566	46.0
Redland	20	447	44.7
S. Lake Oswego	6	1,249	4.8
Sandy–Mt. Hood	110	1,823	60.3
West Linn	212	1,486	142.7
Wilsonville	77	707	108.9
Colton	34	430	79.1

interventions and educational messages targeted at high school teachers, students, and parents.

Because the Clackamas County Sheriff provided the reported crime data in raw format, CHiME can help the Juvenile Crime Subcommittee visualize patterns of juvenile arrests in relation to demographic factors, specific crimes committed, and community health indicators such as the poverty rate. In addition, by obtaining other data sets, such as the Youth Risk Behavior Survey data, Clackamas County health officials can use CHiME to help the community look at relationships between juvenile arrest rates and behavioral risk factors. When calculating arrest rates, CHiME enables communities to calculate confidence intervals to determine whether their arrest rates are significantly above or below benchmark rates. In addition, the capability to make Bonferroni adjustments avoids the statistical problems associated with multiple simultaneous comparisons. By adding a time-trend analysis feature, future versions of CHiME could enable the Public Safety Coordinating Council, the Human Services Department, and other community partners to evaluate the effectiveness of neighborhood juvenile crime prevention initiatives.

USING GIS TO MAP COMMUNITY ASSETS FOR PUBLIC HEALTH AND HEALTH SERVICES PLANNING

Traditional public health approaches to planning have used a disease, or problem-based, approach. The first step in this approach entails evaluating the health needs of populations. Typically, such needs concern problems like teen pregnancy, neighborhood illiteracy, and neighborhood crime and drug abuse. On the basis of the results of these needs assessments, health and human service organizations develop programs to address the identified needs. One potential result for communities subjected to this approach, especially low-income communities, is that they begin to see themselves as service environments in which individual well-being depends on being a client.[1] As a result, residents gradually become consumers, rather than producers, of services in their communities, resulting in the loss of valuable human resources that could be otherwise helpful in improving community health.[1]

The development of GIS technology has facilitated an alternative approach based on evaluating community assets in addition to community needs by providing public health officials and their community partners a tool to easily map community resources. In effect, the technology assists communities in taking a new role in community development. Unlike a "top-down" approach, in which health and human service organizations target programs to communities with problems and deficiencies, GIS mapping of community assets can help communities identify and develop their own resources. Compared to traditional programs, which are frequently dependent on public or foundation financing, such community-developed resources are more likely to remain after funding sources disappear.[1]

What are some examples of community resources amenable to GIS mapping? One way to describe them is to categorize them by how accessible they are for community residents and whether their control rests within the community. The most accessible resources, "primary building blocks," are community resources located within neighborhoods and largely under neighborhood control. The next category includes assets located within the community but controlled from the outside. The third category contains the least accessible resources, those located and controlled from outside the neighborhood.[1]

Primary building blocks (see Table 8–7) include individual and organizational capacities within communities. Among individual capacities are individual skills, knowledge, abilities, personal income, individual local businesses, and home-based enterprises. Surveys useful in identifying these resources are available, and if individuals are willing to share

their addresses, survey data are available for mapping. With this information, communities can pool individual talents. Even marginalized individuals, traditional recipients of human services, carrying "labels" such as developmentally disabled or chronically mentally ill, frequently have talents and skills to contribute to their communities. Outcomes of identifying and mapping such individual talents have included the development of local business, associations of neighborhood home health care providers, and corporations of residents capable of managing local public housing developments.[1] Likewise, the location of individual business, easily obtainable from telephone books and surveys, can help communities identify and map the location of entrepreneurs potentially willing to share their skills with others.[1]

Organizations in the primary building block category include citizens' organizations, business associations, financial institutions, cultural organizations, communications organizations, and religious organizations. Examples of citizens' organizations are fraternities, women's organizations, artistic groups, and athletic clubs. Surveys to identify and map these organizations are available.[1] Frequently, especially in older neighborhoods, local business people do not belong to business associations, or if they do they may not be aware of the effectiveness of partnerships in developing their community. By mapping and sharing their locations, GIS technology can be a useful tool to help connect local businesses with each other. Mapping the location of cultural and religious organizations is also essential because these organizations contribute to neighborhood cohesion, have members who are potential volunteers, and can frequently call on external organizations for additional support and financial resources.[1]

Secondary building blocks, assets located within the community but controlled from the outside, fall into three subcategories, private and not-for-profit organizations, public institutions and services, and other physical resources (see Table 8–8).[1] Data containing locations of all of these assets are available with location for mapping purposes. Libraries are particularly important because they usually contain personal computers providing access to the Internet. Public health officials can take advantage of this resource by making their GIS applications Web based,[2] allowing community-based groups and consumers to perform their own geographic analysis of community health status in the comfort of their neighborhood libraries.

Potential building blocks, assets originating outside the community and controlled by outsiders, include welfare expenditures, public capital improvement expenditures, and public information.[1] With some creative thinking, enhanced by GIS-produced maps, planners can discover ways for welfare and capital improvement expenditures to contribute to community development activities. Welfare expenditures consist of cash and services, with the cost of the services

Table 8–7 Primary Building Blocks (Assets and Capacities Located inside the Neighborhood, Largely under Neighborhood Control)

Individual Assets	Organizational Assets
Skills, talents, and experience of residents	Associations of business
Individual businesses	Citizens' associations
Home-based enterprises	Cultural organizations
Personal income	Communications organizations
Gifts of labeled people	Religious organizations

Table 8–8 Secondary Building Blocks (Assets and Capacities Located within the Community but Controlled Largely by Outsiders)

Private and Nonprofit Organizations	Public Institutions and Services	Physical Resources
Higher education institutions	Public schools	Vacant land, commercial and industrial structures, housing
Hospitals	Police	Energy and waste (recycling) resources
Social service agencies, including community health clinics	Libraries	
	Fire departments Parks	

sometimes exceeding the cash assistance.[1] On the basis of the data available through welfare agencies, GIS users could create maps displaying information on these expenditures, such as the amount spent for cash and services within specific neighborhoods. This information could be useful for community groups interested in exploring the potential of reinvesting these expenditures into enterprises supporting individual and community independence. Likewise, similar maps displaying localized public capital investments could be useful for community groups investigating the possibility of redirecting capital improvement resources into community development activities.

Public information, the third potential building block, lies at the heart of GIS technology. Many of the data sets discussed in the previous chapters contain address information, making them amenable to analysis at the community or neighborhood level. The key is to make these data, and the software to analyze them, accessible. GIS programs can be Internet compatible, making them easily accessible. Most communities have access to Internet-capable libraries, where they can create customized maps to meet their needs.[2]

In addition, public health agencies can design GIS Internet packages for users without formal epidemiologic skills, and they can add tutorials. For example, tutorials can provide explanations of concepts such as incidence rates, prevalence, confidence intervals, and the need for age adjustment when evaluating mortality rates.[2]

In addition to the traditional public health data sets discussed in previous chapters, future community-based GIS applications could contain data of importance to specific communities. For example, community-added data could contain information on the vacancy ratios in neighborhood buildings, the amount of city money slated for capital improvements, and the amount of neighborhood property off the tax rolls.[1] In addition, communities could map issues like the skills of local teachers useful for development corporations and the time of day most frequent for neighborhood crimes.

One advantage of the assets-based approach is that it identifies locally controlled assets and their representatives, facilitating their involvement in the community health planning process. We will discuss the use of needs-based and assets-based maps throughout the rest of this chapter. Both are useful in community health planning.

ACCESS TO OTHER HUMAN SERVICES

Socioeconomic independence, a major determinant of health and well being, is dependent on many factors, including the availability of child care, transportation, and training. A study in South Carolina illustrates how GIS technology can map these community assets in relationship to potential recipients of services to facilitate community health planning.[21] Figure 8–8 is a map of Columbia, South Carolina, depicting the location of several community assets such as child care facilities, job centers, training facilities, primary care clinics, and bus routes. The map also shows the residence of clients enrolled in an Aid to Families with Dependent Children (AFDC) welfare reform program. This map is a result of a collaborative effort between two state agencies, the Health and Demographics Section of the Carolina State Budget and Control Board and the South Carolina Department of Social Services (DSS). In South Carolina, DSS administers the federally funded AFDC program, which provides cash assistance and training for job entry. Mapping the location of these services and potential recipients facilitates the efficient targeting of resources essential to improving independence, a necessary ingredient of welfare reform.

GIS technology can help identify day care centers requiring increased food reimbursements based on providing care for low-income children. As a response to federal welfare reform legislation, a study in North Carolina used GIS technology to locate family day care homes in relation to areas with high levels of child poverty.[22] The specific legislation, the Personal Responsibility and Work Opportunity Recon-

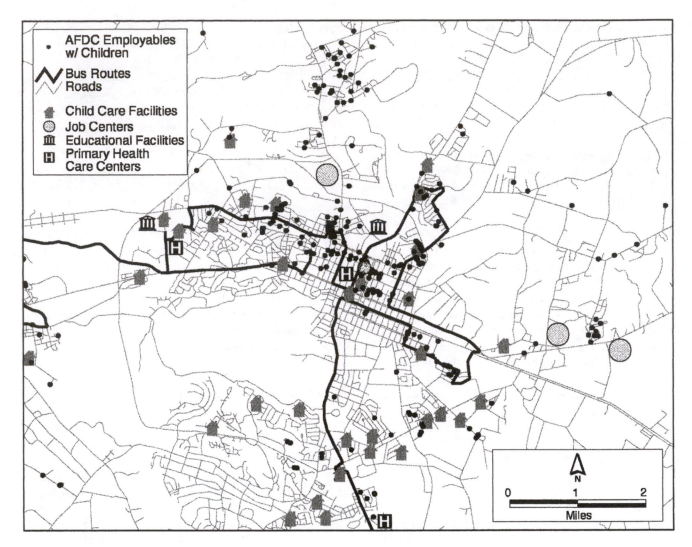

Figure 8–8 Improving delivery of health and community services to welfare recipients, Columbia, South Carolina, 1997

ciliation Act of 1996 (P.L. 104–193), changed the U.S. Department of Agriculture (USDA)–administered Child and Adult Food Program to target public funds more efficiently to people with greater needs. The food program provides food reimbursements to family day care homes (FDCHs) that provide home care to up to five children while their parents are working. The level of community need determines the level of reimbursement. FDCHs in areas with high levels of child poverty receive higher reimbursements, while those in other areas must either receive reduced reimbursements or demonstrate that they individually meet income eligibility requirements.

To perform the study, GIS staff at the North Carolina Center for Geographic Information and Analysis (NCCGIA) worked with their public health partners at the Nutrition Services Section of the Division of Women's and Children's Health. They converted attribute data containing the address information in Microsoft Excel format into a database (*.dBase) format, and then imported the data into GIS software, ArcView GIS. The NCCGIA supplied the spatial database for the study. The software matched 81 percent of more than 3,600 FDCHs located throughout the state; GIS staff manually mapped the others on the basis of locational information supplied by the Nutrition Services Section.

They then decided to define areas with high levels of child poverty on the basis of two criteria. The first criterion defined high–child poverty areas as those with school base areas where 50 percent or more of the children were eligible for free or reduced-price meals. Unfortunately, the NCCGIA was unable to use this criterion as a measure for a couple of reasons. First, the State Department of Public Instruction did not have a geographic map of school base areas. Instead, the

100 individual counties in North Carolina had their own databases with this information, at variable levels of accuracy. Second, some of the urban counties within the state operated magnet programs attracting children to inner-city schools from out of the area. As a result, the proportion of children eligible for reduced-price lunch in those schools did not reflect the proportion of such children living in the school base area.

The second criterion, census block groups where more than 50 percent of children aged 0 through 12 were at or below 185 percent of the federal poverty threshold, proved more useful. To use this measure, the USDA had to provide a special run of census data because the file supplied by the U.S. Bureau of the Census did not break these data down by age groups. NCCGIA staff linked these data with TIGER files to identify census block groups with high levels of child poverty. They then used overlays to create the final map, as illustrated in Figure 8–9, a map of one North Carolina county. In this "point-in-polygon" analysis, points representing individual family day care homes overlie census block group polygons, shaded on the basis of the second child poverty criterion. This map enables the state to determine quickly which family day care homes automatically qualify for food reimbursement at the higher level.[22]

Another GIS application, addressing community needs and assets, shows how federal agencies can support community development by making GIS technology available to communities. To fully understand, it is helpful to have some background information on the federal agency that created it. The goal of the U.S. Department of Housing and Urban Development (HUD) is to ensure a decent, safe, and sanitary home and suitable living environment for every American. To reach this goal, HUD's mission is to help the nation's communities meet their development needs, spur economic growth in distressed neighborhoods, provide housing assistance for the poor, help rehabilitate and develop moderate- and low-cost housing, and enforce the nation's fair housing laws. Specific strategies include

- Fighting for fair housing
- Increasing affordable housing and home ownership
- Reducing homelessness

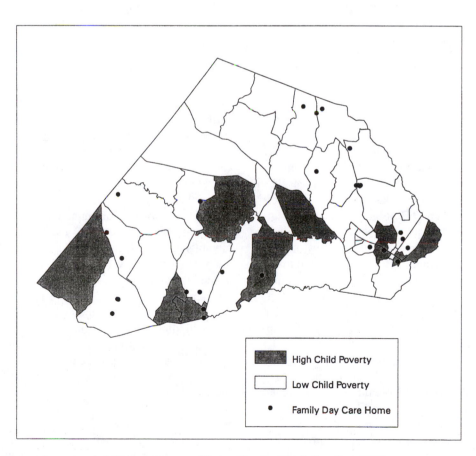

Figure 8–9 Family day care homes and child poverty areas, Harnett County, North Carolina, 1997

- Promoting jobs and economic opportunity
- Empowering people and communities
- Restoring the public trust

Certainly, many of these goals and strategies are consistent with community and public health improvement. Some examples of HUD programs directed at community empowerment and development are the urban Empowerment Zones, designed to stimulate development of jobs and the economy in inner cities, programs to redevelop environmentally contaminated industrial or commercial sites, and the Community Development Block Grant program (CDBG). The CDBG program, created in 1974 and under the Assistant Secretary for Community Planning and Development, combined a variety of old, narrow, categorical programs into block grants to aid states and communities. CDBG program funds are available for a wide range of activities, directed at three national goals: (1) aid low- and moderate-income persons; (2) prevent or eliminate slum or blight conditions; or (3) meet an urgent need that threatens health or safety. Grantees must use at least 70 percent of the funds for activities that benefit low- and moderate-income persons. As part of local empowerment, state and local jurisdictions determine the actual uses of the funds through a comprehensive strategic planning process, and they are accountable to HUD for how funds are spent. Communities have used CDBG funds to renovate housing; construct or improve public facilities, such as water, sewer, streets, and neighborhood centers; purchase real property; and assist private businesses in economic development activities.[23]

During the past decade, in an effort to further improve the way it works with local communities, HUD developed the Community 2020 Management Reform Plan.[23,24] One of the main goals of the plan is to have community priorities, rather than federal categories, drive federal funding allocations. The plan has several strategies aimed at supporting communities. For example, "Community Builders" are staff who understand local communities, provide consultation to help communities solve problems and build partnerships, and use HUD funds effectively in planning efforts. HUD "Storefront" offices and "Next Door" electronic kiosks in local communities provide residents 24-hour, 7-day-a-week access to information on issues such as affordable rental housing, home ownership, how to file a housing discrimination complaint, and local CDBG programs. In keeping with this agenda, HUD developed its GIS software, Community 2020, to improve community health and community development in three ways: (1) improved consolidated planning, (2) improved communication, and (3) improved decision making.

The integrative features of GIS technology that we have already discussed make it an ideal tool for comprehensive, consolidated health planning. By mapping community assets and making these maps freely available, GIS can help residents and their elected officials easily see where federal agencies such as HUD allocate funds locally. In addition, officials and their constituents can visualize local characteristics such as demographic factors (age, income, education), the housing market, and the locations of other assets such as schools, parks, and public facilities. At the same time, the technology can map needs, such as homelessness and unemployment, and health status (e.g., morbidity and mortality). By mapping needs and assets together, the technology facilitates the development of comprehensive strategies to link the needs with appropriate interventions. By visualizing the location of potential partners, the maps can also help community agencies develop the partnerships essential to improving the coordination of services to community residents. The capability of GIS technology to change the scale of analysis by zooming in or out allows neighborhood residents to see and understand their neighborhood in the context of their city and region, further facilitating community development and health improvement.

Community 2020 also improves communication between HUD and communities because it provides current information to program managers and the public about programs and activities through regular HUD updates. The software is capable of mapping and describing local projects and their budgets for all HUD programs within the United States. Improved consolidated planning and improved communication support the third aspect of Community 2020, improved decision making. By giving communities and their partners maps of community assets and needs, by encouraging the formation of community participation and partnerships, and by providing a means for communities to obtain information on available funding for new projects, Community 2020 can improve the capability for community residents to participate in strategic decisions to improve the health of their community.

HUD developed Community 2020 GIS software for a couple of reasons. First, HUD and its grantees generate large amounts of spatially referenced data amenable to geographic analysis. Second, development of the GIS software fits with a couple of underlying themes of the Community 2020 Management Reform Plan. These are (1) to use new developments in information technology to ensure that information about funding for local projects can help achieve multiple goals and (2) to empower communities by encouraging citizen participation through access to good information on community needs and assets. Key features of Community 2020 include data, forms, queries, a HUD map library, markers, data analysis and display, travel routes, bands, and user support. We will describe each in detail.

Spatial data included in the package are a U.S. Streets File plus geographic boundaries for states, counties, congressional districts, ZIP codes, Empowerment Zones/Enterprise Communities (HUD terms), census tracts, and census block groups. Attribute data come from several sources. First, the 1990 census data down to the block group level are included, with demographic data containing over 640 variables. The package also contains demographic estimates for 1997 and projections for 2002 and 2007 for a subset of 180 variables. Second, Community 2020 contains data that housing and community development agencies and nonprofit organizations report to HUD. Examples include data on community planning entitlement projects and competitive projects, Empowerment Zones/Enterprise Communities activities, public housing developments, and Federal Housing Administration (FHA) single-family and multifamily housing. Community 2020 provides individual program data for one or more years from 1992 to 1998. The HUD home page provides monthly updates of program data for downloading at <www.hud.gov/index.html>.

If an individual wishes to add attribute data for his or her own interest, Community 2020 will accept data in about 20 different formats. The software creates a live link between the user's data and a map layer so that maps will automatically reflect any changes that users make to the data. Users can analyze their local data in relation to the data supplied in Community 2020 for any geographic area down to buffers around specific points. In addition, Community 2020 can import maps and data created with other GIS software, such as MapInfo, ARC/INFO, and ArcView (see Chapter 10 for a description of these software applications).

Figure 8–10 shows how Community 2020 makes it easier to ask and answer questions about HUD programs. The software has forms organizing the fields in a single record. Users can explore, view, and print information on each record within the data files. Users cannot edit or change the data on these forms, but by using a Users Projects form they can create and edit their own user project data.[22] By simply pointing and clicking with a mouse, users can create queries on HUD's activities within a neighborhood by program, activity, and year. They can display information on specific projects, housing, and activities within a neighborhood or other area, including details about funding for specific neighborhood organizations, contact numbers, and progress toward program benchmarks.

The map library feature in Community 2020 allows users without sophisticated computer skills to create over 100 maps for any location within the United States. The maps can contain overlays for issues like housing, jobs, ethnicity, income, and education. Users can add their own map categories containing their own imported data. Another feature, the marker feature, allows users to return quickly to a location of interest by saving the map center and scale as a marker for that location. To make this task easier, the software prompts users to establish markers at locations they are interested in after setting up default markers for that location at different scales, ranging from the neighborhood scale all the way up to the state scale. With markers, users can create "cutouts," placing the data into smaller files that allow them to access the data more rapidly and thereby increasing the speed of the application.[24]

Community 2020 allows users to develop community profiles on a variety of factors, such as demographic characteristics. Public health officials can use the software to compare HUD investments and projects in their jurisdiction with others. Other public health applications could include evaluating location of assets such as child care facilities and hospitals, monitoring risk factors (such as older housing) for childhood lead exposure, and planning for emergency response. As a tool to improve access, Community 2020 can determine best travel routes for services such as Meals on Wheels or home nurse visits. The software evaluates several factors in defining best travel routes, such as minimum distance or minimum time, and can calculate mileage and print driving directions. Because it is a full-featured GIS application, Community 2020 allows users to create buffers around points and lines. This feature is particularly helpful in evaluating communities at risk from environmental hazards, as discussed in previous chapters.

HUD collaborated with a private corporation, the Caliper Corporation, in developing Community 2020 GIS software. Community 2020 is a special edition of version 3.0 Caliper's Maptitude GIS software (for more information on Maptitude software, go to their Web site at <www.caliper.com>). HUD released the most current version of Community 2020, Version 2.0, in 1998. In addition to the capabilities of Maptitude 3.0, Community 2020 adds data sets, programming wizards to make the software easier to use, and a map library.

Community 2020, a full-featured GIS package, requires the dedication and time investment needed to learn how to use GIS software.[25] However, for community users without sophisticated computer skills, the Community 2020 package includes a Community 2020 User's Guide, a Maptitude User's Guide, and a Maptitude tutorial. The tutorial helps novice users master several tasks, including installation, map making, and data access. In addition, the package provides a guide, "Mapping Your Community," that contains a framework and approach for using geographic data, as well as case study examples for community practitioners new to the use of GIS. Those still needing assistance can call a Community 2020 help desk. The HUD Community 2020 home page provides a discussion forum and the location of training sessions, and in partnership with Project SCOPE Inc., a nonprofit organization, HUD promotes an e-mail listserv providing news and support for local GIS users.

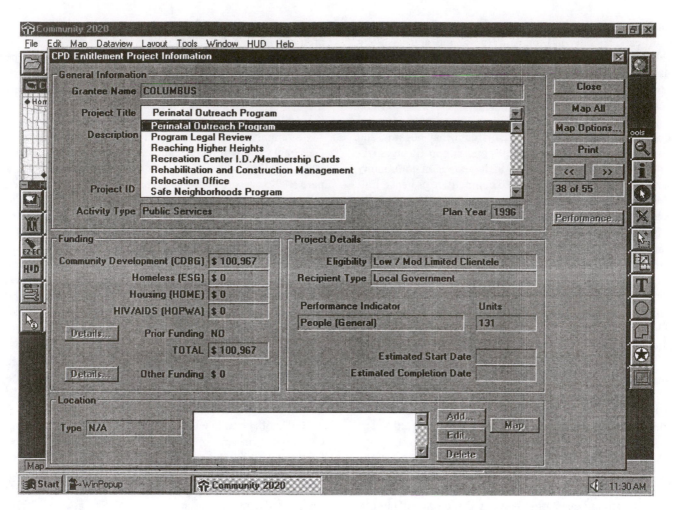

Figure 8–10 How forms are used in *Community 2020:* computer screen showing a form for community planning and development (CPD) entitlement project information for perinatal outreach programs in Columbus, Ohio, in 1996

A few local examples provide a picture of how Community 2020 can facilitate community health improvement.[23] The first case scenario involved developing programs to improve the health status of the homeless population. A consortium of 23 local and regional agencies, public and private, used Community 2020 to count homeless persons and evaluate why they became and remained homeless. Volunteers, including homeless and formerly homeless people, helped design and implement a survey used to collect the necessary data. Besides improving the health of the homeless, the project increased their involvement in improving their own community. Specific project results included the following changes:

- The local planning process now considers substance abuse treatment and other service providers as crucial components of a comprehensive community health improvement process.
- The city used the data to successfully apply for over $1 million for its project to improve the well-being of the homeless population.
- The community used the results to apply CDBG funds more efficiently to the specific needs of homeless individuals.
- The planning team developed a standardized process to survey homeless individuals, allowing them to document trends over time and evaluate the effectiveness of their programs.

- Agencies can now ensure access to services for a sub-population of chemically dependent homeless males. These services include outreach and referral, job training, and case management.
- The community created physical improvements, including permanent supportive housing for homeless adults.
- By building a GIS database that identified the location of properties with code violations, the city was better able to target housing rehabilitation funds to low-income neighborhoods with high concentrations of older or substandard housing.

Another city used Community 2020 as a tool to decide where to locate community development projects.[24] For example:

- City staff used the software to develop and use digital flood insurance maps. To create the maps, they obtained attribute data from the Federal Emergency Management Agency (FEMA). They overlaid FEMA Flood Data on the Community 2020 street address files. The resulting maps allowed them to determine automatically whether specific community development projects were within flood risk zones.
- Using the buffer function, the city mapped noise zones around railroads and the airport to help evaluate rehabilitation projects.
- With cooperation from the state, they used the software to identify thermal and blast hazards near proposed projects.
- They developed digital files with the location of community assets such as fire departments, police, and libraries.

Nonprofit organizations involved in housing issues are particularly interested in some of the maps because they identify the relationship between potential housing developments and community assets and hazards, such as environmental contamination sites. Because of this interest, the city has placed many of these maps on its Web site.

Another positive result of this city's use of Community 2020 is its increased ability to raise taxes and identify properties for low- and moderate-income housing development. With cooperation from the county and a local university, the city converted county parcel maps into GIS-based parcel maps for more than 6,000 inner-city properties. One of the variables included in the GIS data set was the location of properties adjudicated for nonpayment of taxes. The city can now regularly map and view the location of such properties, estimated to be worth over $63 million. This in turn has facilitated the efficient collection of back taxes and has enabled the city to identify properties available for low- and moderate-income housing development.[24]

The third example illustrates how Community 2020 can facilitate the entry of novice health departments and community partners into the regular use of GIS technology. As we will describe below, Community 2020 is inexpensive and easy to use, allowing health departments to avoid the investment of large amounts of money or staff time. Using HUD's fellowship program and federal work-study program, this third community was able to acquire the assistance of student interns from local universities to help them use Community 2020. To convert parcel data into digital maps, the community was able to hire students from a local university GIS laboratory. Finally, as with the other community, using GIS enabled this community to generate additional revenue by identifying properties for collection of unpaid taxes.[24]

In spite of its successes, Community 2020 has some significant limitations.[23] First, it uses an older version of Maptitude (Version 3.0) rather than the more recent version (Version 4.0), which contains several enhancements. HUD has no plan to base Community 2020 on any future Maptitude upgrades. In addition, although Community 2020 templates display HUD program data easily and efficiently, public health practitioners will find that Community 2020 does not include templates they could efficiently use to display state and local public health program data. If a local health department and its partners are interested in using HUD data, purchasing Community 2020 makes sense. If not the product probably has little value.[25]

Those interested in purchasing Community 2020 have several options. A regional edition, on a single CD-ROM disc, contains neighborhood-level geographic, demographic, and HUD program data for one region of the United States (eastern, southern, central, or western). It retails for $240. The Deluxe Edition, containing four CD-ROM discs covering the entire United States, retails for $299. The software can be ordered by calling (800) 998–9999. Currently, HUD supplies the software to (1) local and state jurisdictions involved in HUD consolidated planning; (2) HUD Empowerment Zones; and (3) HUD Community Builders (already trained to use the software). Of course, HUD field and headquarters staff also use the software. HUD has placed abbreviated versions of Community 2020 in kiosks at HUD neighborhood storefronts and on a Web site, <www.hud.gov/cio/c2020/> allowing anyone to locate funded projects and identify any HUD activities in their own neighborhoods.

CHAPTER   REVIEW

1. GIS technology has the potential to revolutionize the process of community health improvement by improving access to health-related data. GIS technology can help public health practitioners and their community partners assess many factors, strengths and weaknesses, related to community well-being and allow them to evaluate actions they take to improve their health status. This potential is a consequence of several features inherent in GIS:

   - The relational and overlay features of GIS encourage the rapid incorporation of multiple attribute data sets, including data sets not traditionally viewed as related to public health.
   - The feature of unlimited scale of analysis is particularly helpful when performing community health assessments and program evaluations in densely populated counties. Using GIS, public health practitioners and their community partners can analyze and display the data at local, subcounty, community levels. Over time, they can use the analytical features of GIS to evaluate the outcomes of public health efforts within their communities.
   - The flexibility to define community geographically is invaluable in community health planning. GIS software can aggregate census block groups into a variety of community definitions, such as high school attendance areas or legislative districts. Likewise, the GIS software can aggregate attribute data, such as vital statistics data, into the same areas for analysis.
   - Depending on the state and locality, many data sets are easily obtainable, such as vital statistics data (perinatal and mortality), health care expenditures, access to primary care, hospital discharge data, and behavioral risk factor data.
   - GIS takes complex data and translates it into easily understandable information in a visual format.

2. Public health agencies have historically been responsible for ensuring access to health care. Health officials can use GIS technology to evaluate and improve health care access by

   - Assessing the geographic relationship between the location of potential clients and available services
   - Determining the market area for their services by mapping the location of their clients
   - Determining the proportion of the eligible population that is receiving services from their agency

   - Evaluating the relationship between client geographic access, health care utilization, and health outcomes
   - Deciding what services to offer at specific clinic sites, based on neighborhood demographics
   - Estimating the proportion and the location of people without health insurance
   - Assessing the local supply of health care providers with adequate skills and knowledge

3. Studies using GIS technology to improve health care access, while helpful, suffer from several limitations that prevent them from pinpointing reasons for associations found between distance to health care facilities and health care utilization and health outcomes for a couple reasons:

   - Even if the studies use individual exposures (with distance being the exposure) and individual outcomes, many of the data sets do not include potential confounders of any association.
   - Ecological designs involving aggregate data and cross-sectional study designs preclude drawing any causation conclusions.

   On the other hand, these studies raise additional questions about access and health outcomes, and they are useful for program planning.

4. GIS technology is helpful for state and local health agencies and their partners interested in changing service delivery models from a categorical approach to an approach based on local needs. Different agencies can combine their data into GIS applications that help them locate multiple, integrated services in convenient, accessible locations on the basis of comprehensive assessments of community health status.

5. GIS technology promises to bring the process of community health assessment to communities by making health data more accessible, localized, and community based. The term *accessible data* means that community members and interested agencies are able to obtain relevant information about the health status of their communities at a variety of sites, including local libraries and home computers. *Localized* means that community-level health data are available for analysis at the neighborhood/community level. *Community based* means that local communities should be able to determine for themselves what information about their community is relevant, and it means that local and state governments should be a

resource for these communities in providing for their data needs.

6. GIS community health assessment applications under development have several common features:

- They serve as sort of a data warehouse by incorporating different data sets in one location. In addition, the applications have features such as Data Wizards that simplify the process of adding additional data sets.

- The applications make data available for analysis in a flexible, easy-to-use format. They have help buttons, allowing users without formal computer or epidemiologic skills to obtain assistance from health officials.

- The applications standardize the analysis methods, ensuring that the same methodology is used across jurisdictions.

- Their output is in a simple format, allowing health department staff and other users to produce tables and maps.

- The applications can display events and can calculate proportions and rates. In addition, they have the capacity to specify analyses for subpopulations (such as age, race, and gender), specific geographic areas, and specific time periods.

- The applications can perform simple statistical tests, such as 95 percent confidence intervals for rates, allowing users to make comparisons and analyze trends over time.

7. Although these new community health applications are helpful in raising questions about community health status and evaluating programs, health officials must ensure that users avoid drawing conclusions from ecologic data.

8. Traditional public health approaches to planning have used a disease-, or problem-based, approach, based on two steps:

- Evaluating the health needs of populations, including problems like teen pregnancy, neighborhood illiteracy, and neighborhood crime and drug abuse

- On the basis of the results of these needs assessments, developing programs to address the identified needs

9. GIS technology has facilitated an alternative approach based on evaluating community assets in addition to community. Examples of community resources amenable to GIS mapping are

- Primary building blocks: community resources located within neighborhoods and largely under neighborhood control

- Secondary building blocks: assets located within the community but controlled from the outside

- Potential building blocks: resources located and controlled from outside the neighborhood

GIS technology can assist communities in taking a new role in community development. Unlike a "top-down" approach, in which health and human service organizations target programs to communities with problems and deficiencies, GIS mapping of community assets can help communities identify and develop their own resources.

10. Community 2020 GIS software, developed by the Federal Department of Housing and Urban Development (HUD), makes GIS technology available to support community development. By allowing communities to map needs and assets simultaneously, the easy-to-use software tool can

- Facilitate the development of comprehensive strategies to link needs with appropriate interventions

- Help community agencies develop the partnerships essential to improving the coordination of services to community residents

- Allow neighborhood residents to see and understand their neighborhood in the context of their city and region, further facilitating community development and health improvement

- Improve community residents' ability to participate in strategic decisions to improve the health of their community

REFERENCES

1. J.L. McKnight and J.P. Kretzman. "Mapping Community Capacity: The Asset-Based Community Development Institute." Evanston, IL: Northwestern University, Institute for Policy Research, 1990. Revised 1996; http://www.nwu.edu/IPR/abcd.html; http://www.northwestern.edu/IPR/publications/papers/mcc.pdf.

2. A. Melnick et al. "Clackamas County Department of Human Services Community Health Mapping Engine (CHiME) Geographic Information Systems Project." *Journal of Public Health Management and Practice* 5, no. 2 (1999): 64–69.

3. A. Gordon and J. Womersley. "The Use of Mapping in Public Health and Planning Health Services." *Journal of Public Health Medicine* 19, no. 2 (1997): 139–147.

4. C.V. Lee and J.L. Irving. "Sources of Data for Community Health Planning." *Journal of Public Health Management and Practice* 5, no. 4 (1999):7–22.

5. A. Melnick. "Geographic Information Systems for Public Health," in *Public Health Administration. Principles for Population-Based*

Management, eds. L.F. Novick and G.P. Mays. Gaithersburg, MD: Aspen Publishers, Inc., 2001: 248–265.

6. A.L. Melnick and D.W. Fleming. "Modern Geographic Information Systems: Promise and Pitfalls." *Journal of Public Health Management and Practice* 5, no. 2 (1999): viii–x.

7. Centers for Disease Control and Prevention. Public Health Program Planning Office. National Public Health Performance Standards Program. "The Essential Services of Public Health." <www.phppo.cdc.gov//nphpsp/phdpp/10es.htm>.

8. G. Rushton. "Methods To Evaluate Geographic Access to Health Services." *Journal of Public Health Management and Practice* 5, no. 2 (1999): 93–100.

9. N.M. Casey et al. "Active Patients Attending the North Hill Child Health Clinic, Akron, Ohio, 1997." *Journal of Public Health Management and Practice* 5, no. 2 (1999): 51–52.

10. G.F. White and K.C. Cerny. "Client Demographics (Age and Gender) at Low-Income Clinics in Austin/Travis County, Texas, 1995–1996." *Journal of Public Health Management and Practice* 5, no. 2 (1999): 47–48.

11. M. Cheatham. "Percent of Adults without Health Insurance in Ingham County, Michigan, 1994." *Journal of Public Health Management and Practice* 5, no. 2 (1999): 53–54.

12. J.L. Wilson and A. Branigan. "Location of East Carolina University School of Medicine Telemedicine Sites in Relation to Primary Care Health Professional Shortage Areas for North Carolina's Health Service Area VI, 1997." *Journal of Public Health Management and Practice* 5, no. 2 (1999): 45–46.

13. Federal Register. "Lists of Designated Primary Medical Care, Mental Health, and Dental Health Professional Shortage Areas; Notice." *Federal Register* 62(104), May 30, 1997.

14. D. Berry and T.W. Jarrell. "Ranking Priorities for a State Family Service Integration Initiative by Census Tract in Northern New Castle County, Delaware, 1997." *Journal of Public Health Management and Practice* 5, no. 2 (1999): 57–59.

15. A. Melnick et al. "GIS in Community Health Assessment and Improvement," in *Geographic Information Systems in Public Health: Proceedings from the Third National Conference,* eds. R.C. Williams et al.: U.S. Department of Health and Human Services, Agency for Toxic Substances and Disease Registry. San Diego, CA, 1998: 593–606.

16. D. Solet et al. "VISTA/PH Software for Community Health Assessment." *Journal of Public Health Management and Practice* 5, no. 2 (1999): 60–63.

17. D.C. Goodman and J.E. Wennberg. "Maps and Health: The Challenges of Interpretation." *Journal of Public Health Management and Practice* 5, no. 4 (1999): xiii–xvii.

18. H. Morgenstern. "Ecologic Studes," in *Modern Epidemiology,* 2nd ed., eds. K.J. Rothman and S. Greenland. Philadelphia: Lippincott-Raven, 1998.

19. Oregon Progress Board. "Achieving the Oregon Shines Vision: The 2001 Benchmark Performance Report." March 2001. <http://www.econ.state.or.us/opb/2001report/2001new.html>.

20. Oregon Progress Board. "Oregon Shines II. Updating Oregon's Strategic Plan. Highlights. A Report to the People of Oregon from the Oregon Progress Board and the Governor's Oregon Shines Task Force." Salem, Oregon, 1997. <http://www.econ.state.or.us/opb/orsh2.htm>.

21. D. Morrison et al. "Improving Delivery of Health and Community Services to Welfare Recipients, Columbia, South Carolina, 1997." *Journal of Public Health Management and Practice* 5, no. 2 (1999): 49–50.

22. C.L. Hanchette. "GIS and Decision Making for Public Health Agencies: Childhood Lead Poisoning and Welfare Reform." *Journal of Public Health Management and Practice* 5, no. 4 (1999): 41–47.

23. U.S. Department of Housing and Urban Development. "Celebrating 25 Years of the CDBG Program May 27, 1999." <www.hud.gov/cpd/cdbg/anniv25.html>.

24. L. Dean. "Revitalizing Communities with Geographic Information Systems (GIS): HUD's Community 2020 Software." *Journal of Public Health Management and Practice* 5, no. 4 (1999): 47–53.

25. S.E. Thrall. "Geographic Information System (GIS) Hardware and Software." *Journal of Public Health Management and Practice* 5, no. 2 (1999): 82–90.

CHAPTER 9

Limitations of GIS:
Lessons Learned and Challenges

Like any other new promising technology, GIS come with limitations and potential for problems. Limitations include data availability, data quality, trained workforce, and costs. Potential problems include community definitions, confidentiality, and misinterpretation of results.

DATA QUALITY AND AVAILABILITY

As with any analysis, useful GIS output is dependent on useful input. Many important data sets are not available, and when they are, users must be careful to evaluate their completeness and quality.[1,2] For example, commonly used attribute databases, such as mortality data or hospital discharge data, frequently lack an address field. Numerator address data may be missing, wrong, or (particularly in rural areas) impossible to match.[1,2] Inaccuracies in vital record data, including birth and mortality data, are well documented.[3] Birth and death records contain information on whether the newborn's mother or the decedent's residences are within or outside specific city limits. This information can be inaccurate for two reasons. First, the person filling out the birth or death record may not ask sufficiently detailed questions of the respondent (the birth mother or the next of kin of the decedent) to determine the municipal location of the residence. Second, even if asked, the respondent may not know whether the residence was within or outside the city limits.[3]

Inaccuracies may exist in denominator data and in the spatial data file, especially if they are outdated. The match rate between geospatial and attribute databases is directly dependent on the quality of both. Misspellings, empty address fields, and geographic files that are not up to date with the latest road maps lead to low match rates. For example, new housing developments often create new roads that may not be present on an old file.[4] In rural areas, a trailer park address, acceptable to the post office for mail delivery, may not be included in available spatial databases. Low match rates, in turn, lead to selection bias in subsequent analyses. Public health professionals need to ensure that GIS users carefully assess and account for these limitations in their analyses. Depending on the quality of the data, unmatched records often need to be evaluated one at a time, a potentially cumbersome process. In DeKalb County, Georgia, geocoding 6,545 motor vehicle crashes took an entire month of staff time. The process was particularly cumbersome in high growth and rural areas of the county.[4]

Public health and other users of data should not use data sets without details on their source, quality, currency, and reliability. Clearly, data producers and users will need to develop and adhere to standards for currency, quality, and completeness of data incorporated into GIS. Public health professionals will have to encourage their data-sharing partners to include address fields to make their data useful for community health planning. Low-cost or free spatial databases, like the Census Bureau TIGER/line files, need continuous updating as an alternative to expensive commercial products. Many public health departments obtain spatial data from other local government agencies, such as county and city planning offices. Public health departments will need to develop partnerships with these agencies to allow timely sharing of spatial data, also at low cost.[4]

At this time, national standards are not available for spatial data that could be useful in public health applications. In addition, many commercial spatial data products do not contain adequate metadata (data about the data), such as the methods used in determining population estimates. Although standards are not available, the Department of the Interior's Federal Geographic Data Committee (FGDC) has developed guidelines for metadata that could help. If governmental and commercial data suppliers were to follow these guidelines, public health and spatial data users could better evaluate data quality because they could more easily share and compare data. The FGDC has more information on these guidelines, including fact sheets and tutorials, on their Web site at <www.fgdc.gov>.[4]

Encouraging data producers such as state vital statistics programs to geocode the data before release could further facilitate the incorporation of the data into effective GIS applications. However, even if states geocode vital records data, inaccuracies can occur because many city and county codes can change during the geocoding process. For example, during geocoding of the New York State birth file (excluding New York City), more than 9 percent of the Federal Information Processing Standards (FIPS) place codes changed.[3] Better information on the geocoding practices of different data suppliers could help reduce such inaccuracies. In an attempt to gather such information, the National Center for Health Statistics (NCHS) and the National Association for Public Health Statistics and Information Systems (NAPHSIS) surveyed 54 state vital statistics project directors. The purpose of the 1997 survey was to determine how states' vital statistics programs were handling their data, including their geocoding practices, and their interest in automating geocoding the address data. In addition to the 50 states, the vital statistics directors represented New York City, Washington, D.C., Puerto Rico, and the U.S. Virgin Islands.

Results available from 49 of the vital statistics programs revealed that 21 out of 49 were participating to some extent in automated geocoding. They used different software products, several of which we will explore in Chapter 10. Five states subcontracted out the geocoding operations to private vendors or universities. Some were limiting automated geocoding to a selected region of the state, while some were limiting geocoding to selected data files, such as birth records. Ninety-three percent (13/14) of vital statistics directors who represented states that performed some automated geocoding and who had an opinion felt that the process improved data quality. In addition, 95 percent (18/19) felt that geocoded data were useful for research, policy analysis, planning, or administration.[3] Of 27 directors whose states did not geocode and who provided an opinion, 93 percent (25/27) were interested in developing automated geocoding capability for their vital records.[3] Several state vital statistics directors commented that the process was too slow to allow the corrected geocoded data to be included in data shipments to NCHS or even standard state vital statistics data files.

Clearly, these early efforts reveal the promise and the limitations of automated geocoding practice. Future developments need to address the timeliness of the process. At the same time, public health data users should support additional efforts to create a local, state, and national spatial database infrastructure, including GIS clearinghouses at all levels, because these efforts could help build local and state geographic data libraries.[4]

In addition to spatial data, quantitative information regarding the measured attributes, such as environmental hazard exposure, must be present and accurate. Unfortunately, even if the residential address data are accurately geocoded, studies of health outcomes related to environmental exposures may be inaccurate for a couple of reasons. First, the relevant site of exposure may be somewhere other than residence.[1] In some cases, exposure through occupation may be more important than residential exposure (or possibly additive to residential exposure). Second, even if the residence is the site of potential exposure, the distance from the residence to the source of environmental contamination may not accurately reflect the degree of exposure. For airborne contaminants, wind speed and direction can significantly affect exposure levels, with people living downwind from a source experiencing higher exposures than those living closer but upwind from the source. Similarly, groundwater flow direction is relevant for exposure to groundwater contaminants.

Considering these problems, GIS researchers can improve the accuracy of their environmental exposure studies in a couple of ways. First, they can account for the time subjects spend in different locations with varying levels of exposure, such as occupation and residence.[1] Second, they can use GIS technology to develop better estimates of exposure. One way to do this is to measure exposures directly at different locations, such as air-monitoring stations, and then estimate the exposure levels between the points.[1] Another way is to use the modeling techniques discussed in Chapter 3.[1] Of course, even these models have limitations in how well they predict exposure. They are only as accurate as the data used to create them, they consider only some of the conditions related to exposure, and they become less accurate as the distance increases from the source of exposure.[1]

TRAINED WORKFORCE AND COSTS

Many local public health departments will have to invest in hardware, software, and trained staff to apply GIS successfully. National Association of County and City Health Officials (NACCHO) case studies have shown that successful GIS applications require six components: hardware, software, trained staff, data, methods, and partnerships. One NACCHO study revealed that the cost of hardware and software needed to do relatively small projects was $5,000 to $10,000, beyond the reach of small, rural health departments.[5]

There are over 3,000 local health departments within the United States, most of them small or rural, with limited resources. Equipping all of these local health departments with the necessary hardware and software would cost $15 to $30 million.[5] While these costs are substantial, they are potentially within reach and may become smaller as the technology improves.[5]

As the NACCHO studies demonstrated, hardware and software are only two of the six components of successful GIS applications. Local health departments and other agencies can fully develop GIS applications only by making significant commitments to training staff and building data libraries. Without such a commitment, the hardware and software are likely to sit on a shelf unused. Staff time is required to acquire data sets, geocode the data, check the quality of the data, perform the analyses, and answer questions about the data. Given the diversity of local public health agencies, ranging in size from one to thousands of employees, support for GIS technology will vary. Large or midsized agencies may have sufficient resources to train and dedicate one or more staff members to develop the GIS application and perform relatively sophisticated analyses. Smaller and rural local health departments with fewer resources may consider several other alternatives, such as

- *Vertical partnerships*: States with many small health departments might consider developing and maintaining an enterprise GIS on their Web site, available for use by local health agencies and others.
- *Horizontal partnerships*: Small health departments might consider partnerships with other local government and private agencies to combine resources to develop a local GIS application. These efforts have the additional benefit of encouraging collaborations on other projects beside GIS.
- *"Off-the-shelf" applications*: Federal and state agencies could consider designing low-cost, user-friendly GIS software tools for small health agencies with limited staff and resources.

DEFINING COMMUNITY

When using GIS for community health improvement, public health officials and their partners will need to be both careful and flexible in defining community. How to portray a community will be constrained by the quality of the data and the perceptions of those within the depicted community. Although GIS projects can define communities in many geographic ways—ZIP codes, census tracts, census block groups, high school attendance areas, legislative districts, cities, and counties—in any given situation, all are not equally appro-

priate.[2] For example, ZIP codes, intended primarily by the U.S. Postal Service for mail delivery, cross community and city boundaries and frequently do not correspond to socioeconomic/demographic characteristics of populations.[6] On a case-by-case basis, public health officials can share their community maps with community partners to obtain comments. Then, using GIS, they can easily redraw the community boundaries, selecting the most appropriate mapping strategy.[2]

The Clackamas County, Oregon, GIS application CHiME, described in Chapter 8, illustrates how public health officials can work with their constituents to characterize communities.[6,7] In developing CHiME, county public health officials considered high school attendance areas as a community definition because for two of the measures (teen arrests and teen birth), using high school attendance areas facilitated targeting interventions and educational messages at high school teachers, students, and their parents. They then conducted several focus groups of county residents, including the elderly, teens, and minorities, who concurred with the initial decision to use high school areas as community definitions. Clackamas County health officials learned that successful GIS applications must involve the public early in the process of defining community and in determining what issues community health assessments address. In the case of CHiME, high school attendance areas proved useful as units for analysis because they were meaningful as a community definition for the public. Flexible GIS applications encouraging ongoing public input could lead to maps based on alternative useful community definitions, such as legislative districts, elementary school attendance areas, or other user-defined small areas.

CONFIDENTIALITY

The balance between the public's right to health-related information and the individual's right to privacy poses a significant limitation for public health officials intending to share health-related data with community partners or place data on the Internet.[8] Improvements in GIS technology and attendant improvements in the accessibility of health-related data increase the risk of violating confidentiality. Data containing personal addresses can be as identifying as data with names. Without appropriate, clear laws, guidelines, and standards regarding confidentiality and data release, health agencies and consumers may be unwilling to provide needed information.[9] Those responsible for maintaining the data files should ensure appropriate precautions to prevent unauthorized access. Great care and thought must precede the depiction of address data linked to confidential information.

There are three ways that data release can identify individuals: direct release of individual information, indirect identification of individuals, and group disclosure.

1. *Direct release of individual information.* This occurs when agencies release data containing individual names (or addresses) associated with exposures or disease. Such violations of privacy are fortunately uncommon.

2. *Indirect identification of individuals.* These more typical violations of privacy are generally related to small numbers and result from how agencies provide and display data. Many of the GIS studies described in this book, especially the studies related to rare diseases and unique environmental exposures, involve small numbers of individuals. Such small population studies typically involve small geographic areas. When small numbers (numerator or denominator) are involved, especially in small geographic areas, the possibility exists that data without names or addresses could still be ascribed to individuals. For example, a geographic analysis of teen births in a small, rural town with few teenagers could identify individual teen mothers. Even when large populations are involved, as the number of data items available in a data set increases, so does the likelihood that data analysis could identify individuals. This occurs when GIS users stratify their analyses by multiple demographic variables, such as age, gender, ethnicity, and income. Such analyses can result in small numbers of easily identified individuals within each stratified category. For example, additionally stratifying teen births by ethnicity and income in a large community can potentially identify individuals. Skewed data distributions can also lead to individual identification. For example, survey results can lead to identification of individuals with rare occupations or unusual incomes.

3. *Group disclosure.* Even if GIS studies do not identify individuals, group disclosure, especially in studies of environmental exposure, can lead to financial risk for individuals in an exposed community, including decreased property values and increased insurance cost.[8]

Governmental agencies and other data collectors and producers have an interest in protecting the confidentiality of individuals for several reasons. First, it is standard ethical statistical practice. Second, statutes and organizational policies may prohibit disclosure of personal health information. Third, individuals are unlikely to provide personal health information if they believe that their privacy could be violated.[8]

To protect confidentiality and maintain the public's trust, public health officials must develop safeguards, built into the software, that restrict analyses, reporting, and depiction of very small numbers.[4] Potential standards could prohibit release of health statistics, such as teen births and teen birthrate, if the population denominator (teenage females) were lower than 50. If the denominator were a cohort defined by an event, such as all births, a standard could prohibit release of percentage of outcomes (e.g., first-trimester care) for a community with fewer than 10 events (births). Another alternative, data modification, is to release the data but round the counts of events (e.g., to a base five) to mask low counts.[8] In addition, GIS applications could restrict access to the complete data set and confine stratified analyses to certain specified variables.[8]

Another possible solution is to provide aggregated data only. State and federal agencies have traditionally reported data aggregated at the county, state, and federal levels. Public health officials can do the same for geocoded community level data by aggregating it into any selected community definition. For example, public health officials could share GIS "Data Wizard" software with hospitals unwilling to release discharge data. Local hospitals could use the wizard to geocode the personal health data and aggregate the data by legislative district boundaries. Then they could remove the personal identifiers such as name and address and release the aggregated data to the public health officials for incorporation into the Web-based GIS. Public users would view only data aggregated at the legislative district level. Besides geographic aggregation, GIS applications could allow users to analyze data aggregated over two or more years.

Obviously, aggregated data contain less information than raw data and often may not be adequate to address many public health issues, such as local environmental hazard exposures and localized disease clusters.[10] This is especially true when the geographic area involving the potential cluster is smaller than the geographical level of aggregation or when environmental exposure data are available for different areas than the aggregated health data. Fortunately, researchers are developing new methods, such as geographic masking, that permit detailed geographical analysis of raw data while protecting individual confidentiality. Although a description of such methods is beyond the scope of this book, readers can consult Armstrong et al.[10] for additional information.

One other development contributing to concerns about confidentiality is the Health Insurance Portability and Accountability Act of 1996 (HIPAA). HIPAA has set new requirements protecting the confidentiality of health-related data. These requirements extend to transmission, maintenance, and security of electronic information, all of which can affect potential GIS applications. GIS technology is just one more reason to develop a nationally uniform framework of information sharing that protects privacy while permitting public health practice.[2]

MISINTERPRETATION OF RESULTS

Ironically, the strength of GIS technology may also be its biggest drawback. The elegance of GIS technology is that it integrates many complex data sets into an easily understandable picture, a map. Its simplicity is such that it provides this ability to an ever-expanding array of diverse users. The consequence is a setup for misunderstanding and misuse. Most health determinants—age, ethnicity, socioeconomic status, and education being only the most common examples—cluster geographically. Most GIS analyses assessing whether there is an association between geography and a health outcome will find one. Usually, however, outcomes will cluster geographically because of underlying population characteristics, not because of the geography itself. In the hands of inexperienced users, the temptation will be to leap too quickly to inferences about why geographic clustering is occurring—to use a GIS-produced picture as proof of one's own favored hypothesis.[2]

Geographic analysis of the clustering of cholera deaths in London proved to John Snow that the Broad Street pump was contaminated, but to the England General Board of Health it proved that the Thames was emanating deadly nocturnal vapors. The science of epidemiology is designed to identify associations between exposures and disease and then to assist in determining whether and how these associations represent causal linkages. As GIS technology becomes more widely available, inexperienced users, including those in policy-making positions, may be tempted to make individual-level inferences from ecologic data[1,2] and to make false assumptions about the nature of associations between exposure and health.

The job of public health officials is to reinsert the science and ensure that potential confounders and modifiers of the exposure/disease association have been assessed carefully in the analysis and considered in the conclusions. Any interpretation of geographically referenced health data must look beyond maps to a wider range of analytic tools. For example, a superficial analysis of the geographic variation in childhood asthma hospitalization rates in northern New England (see Figure 2–5) could have led to the conclusion that different populations had different burdens of illness. Closer study revealed that geographic variation in hospital bed supply,

hospital proximity, and possibly the proclivity of physicians to prescribe the most effective medications, not asthma itself, were independent predictors of admission.[11]

Another potential cause of misinterpretation occurs whenever studies involve small populations. Population denominators can be small for a couple of reasons. First, the area studied may contain small numbers of people. Alternatively, as mentioned during the discussion on confidentiality, the entire population may be large, but the denominator may shrink when the GIS user stratifies the analysis by several demographic variables, such as age, gender, ethnicity, and income. In studies involving small denominators, only one or two additional or fewer cases or events can cause large swings in calculated rates, leading map viewers to conclude falsely that such areas or populations have suddenly vastly improved or deteriorated in the particular measure of health status.[12]

Public health officials can help prevent these mistakes by building safeguards into Internet-based GIS applications. For example, they can build epidemiology tutorials into the application for those unfamiliar with epidemiologic concepts. Besides providing instructions on how to use the system, screens could provide easily understood explanations of concepts such as incidence rates, prevalence, confidence intervals, and the need for age adjustment when evaluating certain health outcomes such as mortality rates. Public health officials could have their GIS applications prohibit release of data for very small population denominators and instead create labels for these areas, explaining that the areas were not shown due to statistically unstable rates.[12] Pop-up help screens could contain messages discussing the ecologic fallacy and the need for caution about drawing conclusions when cause-and-effect relationships have not been established previously.[7,13] In addition, built-in links to appropriate county health officials would allow inexperienced users to obtain consultation.

The examples in this book illustrate the many uses and benefits of GIS technology. For GIS technology, as for other new analytic tools, the greatest promise may lie in raising additional questions rather than in coming up with answers. The map should begin or advance, but not end, the investigative process. While GIS technology has the potential to improve epidemiologic research by making some steps quicker, easier, and cheaper to accomplish, its primary value is as an enhancement rather than an alternative to traditional epidemiologic methods and approaches.[1] Epidemiologists and other public health officials will realize this value fully only through collaboration and communication with nontraditional disciplines outside of epidemiology, including medical anthropology, biostatistics, medical geography, and environmental sciences.

CHAPTER REVIEW

1. Like any other new technology, GIS come with limitations and potential for problems. Limitations include data availability, data quality, trained workforce, and costs. Potential problems include community definitions, confidentiality, and misinterpretation of results.

2. Many important data sets are not available, and when they are, users must be careful to evaluate their completeness and quality.
   - Inaccuracies may exist in denominator data and in the spatial data file, leading to low match rates. Low match rates lead to selection bias in subsequent analyses.
   - Public health professionals need to ensure that GIS users carefully assess and account for these limitations in their analyses. Unmatched records often need to be evaluated one at a time.
   - Public health and other users of data should not use data sets without details on their source, quality, currency, and reliability. Data producers and users will need to develop and adhere to standards for currency, quality, and completeness of data incorporated into GIS.
   - Encouraging data producers to geocode their data could facilitate the incorporation of the data into effective GIS applications.

3. GIS researchers can improve the accuracy of their environmental exposure studies in a couple of ways:
   - They should account for the time subjects spend in different locations with varying levels of exposure.
   - They can use GIS technology to develop better estimates of exposure. One way to do this is to measure exposures directly at different locations and then estimate the exposure levels between the points. Another way is to use the modeling techniques. However, models are only as accurate as the data used to create them, they consider only some of the conditions related to exposure, and they become less accurate as the distance increases from the source of exposure.

4. NACCHO case studies have shown that successful GIS applications require six components: hardware, software, trained staff, data, methods, and partnerships. Large or midsized agencies may have sufficient resources to train and dedicate one or more staff members to develop the GIS application and perform relatively sophisticated analyses. Smaller and rural local health departments with fewer resources may consider several other alternatives, such as vertical partnerships, horizontal partnerships, and off-the-shelf applications.

5. Public health officials and their partners will need to be both careful and flexible in defining community. How to portray a community will be constrained by the quality of the data and the perceptions of those within the depicted community.

6. The balance between the public's right to health-related information and the individual's right to privacy poses a significant limitation for public health officials intending to share health-related data with community partners or place data on the Internet. Improvements in GIS technology and attendant improvements in the accessibility of health-related data increase the risk of violating confidentiality. Data containing personal addresses can be as identifying as data with names. Without appropriate, clear laws, guidelines, and standards regarding confidentiality and data release, health agencies and consumers may be unwilling to provide needed information. Those responsible for maintaining the data files should assure appropriate precautions to prevent unauthorized access.

7. There are three ways that data release can identify individuals:
   - Direct release of individual information
   - Indirect identification of individuals, generally related to small numbers
   - Group disclosure

8. Governmental agencies and other data collectors and producers have an interest in protecting the confidentiality of individuals for several reasons:
   - It is standard ethical statistical practice.
   - Statutes and organizational policies may prohibit disclosure of personal health information.
   - Individuals are unlikely to provide personal health information if they believe that their privacy could be violated.

9. To protect confidentiality and maintain the public's trust, public health officials could develop safeguards restricting analyses, reporting, and depiction of very small numbers or could provide aggregated data only.

10. The Health Insurance Portability and Accountability Act of 1996 set new requirements protecting the confidentiality of health-related data. These requirements extend to transmission, maintenance, and security of electronic information, all of which can affect GIS applications.

11. The strength of GIS technology may also be its biggest drawback. The elegance of GIS technology is that it integrates many complex data sets into an easily understandable picture, a map. Most health determinants cluster geographically. Most GIS analyses assessing whether there is an association between geography and a health outcome will find one. Usually, however, outcomes will cluster geographically because of underlying population characteristics, not because of the geography itself. In the hands of inexperienced users, the temptation will be to leap too quickly to inferences about why geographic clustering is occurring.

12. The job of public health officials is to reinsert the science and ensure that potential confounders and modifiers of the exposure/disease association have been assessed carefully in the analysis and considered in the conclusions. Any interpretation of geographically referenced health data must look beyond maps to a wider range of analytic tools.

13. Another potential cause of misinterpretation occurs whenever studies involve small populations. In studies involving small denominators, only one or two additional or fewer cases or events can cause large swings in calculated rates, leading map viewers to conclude falsely that such areas or populations have suddenly vastly improved or deteriorated in the particular measure of health status.[12]

14. Public health officials can help prevent these mistakes by building safeguards into Internet-based GIS applications such as
     - Epidemiology tutorials
     - Pop-up screens that provide easily understood explanations of concepts such as incidence rates, prevalence, confidence intervals, and the need for age adjustment when evaluating certain health outcomes such as mortality rates. The screens could contain messages discussing the ecologic fallacy and the need for caution about drawing conclusions when cause-and-effect relationships have not been established previously.
     - The prohibition of data release for areas with very small population denominators. Labels for these areas could explain that the areas were not shown due to statistically unstable rates.
     - Links to appropriate county health officials allowing inexperienced users to obtain consultation.

REFERENCES

1. M.F. Vine et al. "Geographic Information Systems: Their Use in Environmental Epidemiologic Research." *Environmental Health Perspectives* 105, no. 6 (1997): 598–605.

2. A.L. Melnick and D.W. Fleming. "Modern Geographic Information Systems: Promise and Pitfalls." *Journal of Public Health Management and Practice* 5, no. 2 (1999): viii–x.

3. M.F. MacDorman and G.A. Gay. "State Initiatives in Geocoding Vital Statistics Data." *Journal of Public Health Management and Practice* 5, no. 2 (1999): 91–93.

4. M.Y. Rogers. "Getting Started with Geographic Information Systems (GIS): A Local Health Department Perspective." *Journal of Public Health Management and Practice* 5, no. 4 (1999): 22–33.

5. P.H. Bouton and M. Fraser. "Local Health Departments and GIS: The Perspective of the National Association of County and City Health Officials." *Journal of Public Health Management and Practice* 5, no. 4 (1999): 33–41.

6. A. Melnick et al. "Clackamas County Department of Human Services Community Health Mapping Engine (CHiME) Geographic Information Systems Project." *Journal of Public Health Management and Practice* 5, no. 2 (1999): 64–69.

7. A. Melnick et al. "GIS in Community Health Assessment and Improvement," in *Geographic Information Systems in Public Health: Proceedings from the Third National Conference*, eds. R.C. Williams et al.: U.S. Department of Health and Human Services, Agency for Toxic Substances and Disease Registry, 1998; San Diego, CA: 593–606.

8. L.H. Cox. "Protecting Confidentiality in Small Population Health and Environmental Statistics." *Statistics in Medicine* 15 (1996): 1895–1905.

9. C.M. Croner et al. "Geographic Information Systems (GIS): New Perspectives in Understanding Human Health and Environmental Relationships." *Statistics in Medicine* 15 (1996): 1961–1977.

10. M.P. Armstrong et al. "Geographically Masking Health Data To Preserve Confidentiality." *Statistics in Medicine* 18 (1999): 497–525.

11. D.C. Goodman and J.E. Wennberg. "Maps and Health: The Challenges of Interpretation." *Journal of Public Health Management and Practice* 5, no. 4 (1999): xiii–xvii.

12. T.B. Richards et al. "Geographic Information Systems and Public Health: Mapping the Future." *Public Health Reports* 114 (July/August 1999): 359–361.

13. H. Morgenstern. "Ecologic Studies," in *Modern Epidemiology*, 2d ed., eds. K.J. Rothman and S. Greenland. Philadelphia: Lippincott-Raven, 1998: 459–480.

CHAPTER 10

Getting Started with GIS:
Hardware, Operating Systems, and Software

Before a local health department or other agency invests in a GIS application, it should determine whether it really needs the application or if cheaper alternatives might suffice.[1] For example, a small jurisdiction with limited resources and small numbers of residents may not benefit much from an expensive, detailed geographic analysis. At a minimum, any agency considering adding a GIS application should

- Determine community health priorities that could be amenable to GIS analysis
- Carefully consider how GIS technology would be helpful in addressing these priorities
- Identify whether alternative methodologies could perform the same function at lower cost
- Evaluate the agency's capacity to implement and maintain a GIS application, including staff training, knowledge, skills, and abilities

In many cases, other local government or private agencies may have already developed a GIS application and would welcome partnership with the local health department. Although interagency partnerships involving combinations of hardware, software, and trained staff can produce benefits by saving costs and setting standards around a single GIS product, they can also present coordination challenges.[1]

Once an agency has decided (after a comprehensive needs assessment) to invest in GIS technology, the next steps are to decide on hardware and software. While hardware selection is relatively easy, choosing software is more difficult due to the variety of software available. Because both hardware and software continue to improve rapidly, this chapter will provide suggestions on where to obtain the latest offerings. In addition, this chapter will provide information for public health agencies interested in making their GIS software applications accessible to community partners on the Internet.

HARDWARE

In the 1970s, the early GIS computer applications required a large central computer surrounded by memory and storage disks. By the mid- to late 1980s, further developments of minicomputers resulted in commercially successful GIS applications for the desktop personal computer.[2] Table 10–1 is a summary of the minimum hardware components needed for basic GIS applications. Readers should be aware that continued rapid changes in computer technology might make some of these outdated by the time this book is published.

Large hard drives are necessary for a few reasons. First, attribute and spatial data sets needed to create maps take up a large amount of storage space. Second, most GIS users will want to save maps they create in electronic format, and the maps themselves require a large amount of storage space. (In addition to hard drives, backup devices can also provide storage space.) Third, many data sets and software applications are now available for purchase on CD-ROMs or available for download off the Internet. Copying the CD-ROM contents onto a hard drive can significantly increase the speed of data flow. Fortunately, nearly all personal computers sold today have several-gigabyte or larger hard drives.

Rapid processing speeds and an adequate amount of random access memory (RAM) are essential. Typical GIS software applications perform large amounts of sophisticated mathematical manipulations on huge data sets, impossible without enough RAM. Computers with slow processors can take an inordinate amount of time to create maps, leading to inefficiencies. In general, faster processing speeds lead to

Table 10–1 Minimum Hardware Needed for Basic GIS Applications

Device	Speed or Capacity
Hard drive	At least 4 GB, preferably 10 GB or more
CD-ROM	24 × or faster
Backup capability (Iomega ZIP drive, tape backup, CD-ROM writer or LAN (local area network) backup	
Pentium II or III processor	At least 266 MHZ, preferably 500 MHZ or above
Random access memory (RAM)	At least 64 MB, preferably 128 or above
Video card	4 MB RAM
Color monitor	17 inches; minimum of 1,024 × 768 pixels resolution
Color printer (laser or inkjet)	At least 300 × 300 dots per inch (dpi) resolution
Internet connection	
Optional: Color scanner with optical character recognition (OCR) capability	
Optional: Digital video disk (DVD) and jazz drives	

improved productivity and reduced staff frustration.[1] GIS applications demanding rapid graphics drawing to make maps necessitate video cards that provide enhanced image display and redraw capabilities.[1]

GIS applications create visual products, maps, that look better on large monitors with a minimum of 1,024 × 768 pixels resolution. After viewing several maps and charts, most GIS users will want to print some. Just as the quality of on-screen map images is dependent on the quality of the monitor, the quality of printed maps is dependent on the quality of the printer. Compared to maps and charts printed in color, black and white maps and charts convey less information, are less legible, and certainly provide a less striking visual display. Fortunately, color ink jet printers with a minimum of 300 × 300 dpi resolution are universally available and inexpensive. Somewhat more expensive color laser printers produce somewhat higher-quality maps. For most desktop applications in local agencies, both types of color printers are adequate and will print beautiful maps reproducible by color photocopy machines.[1]

Most GIS users will appreciate having a color scanner for several reasons. First, using some GIS software products, users can link scanned images to objects on a map, such as dots representing the residences of children with reported lead poisoning. By clicking on a specific dot, users can view a scanned photograph of the apartment building or house tagged to that dot. In addition to the photo, users can also view tagged information on the building such as the condition of the paint and construction materials. Second, scanned photographs can serve as backgrounds or base layers on a map. For example, GIS software can display points, lines, and polygons of a map over a scanned picture, such as a photo of a mosquito, to create interesting visual displays. Third, GIS users can scan documents and other information,

including signatures and handwritten notations, and link these to map objects.

Rapid Internet connections, through at least a fast modem, and preferably a DSL or cable hookup, are indispensable. Many attribute data sets and some GIS software products are available for downloading off the Internet. Like processing speed, the faster the Internet condition, the faster the download, the higher the level of productivity, and the lower the degree of staff frustration. In the future, most software products now available on CD-ROM will be available primarily through the Internet. In addition to data and software, the Internet is a repository for GIS resources, including e-mail lists, links to governmental agencies, literature search engines, GIS tutorials,[3] GIS chat rooms, and other GIS information, including "Public Health GIS News and Information." This last resource is a bimonthly electronic report published at <www.cdc.gov/nchs/about/otheract/gis/gis_publichealthinfo.htm>. The report, which began in 1994, is "dedicated to scientific excellence and advancement in disease control and prevention through the use of GIS technology." It provides timely information on a variety of GIS topics, including technical and outreach assistance, notification of relevant professional meetings, events and conferences, communications from GIS users, Web developments, public health GIS literature, and updates on the latest GIS software products. Upcoming reports are available free of charge through the Public Health GIS Users Group listserv and the Web site. To become a listserv member, e-mail listserv@listserv.cdc.gov and type subscribe GIS-STATES-OTHER in the body of the message. The current report, as well as several past issues, can be viewed or downloaded at the Web site, and in the near future, all of the issues will be available on this site.

OPERATING SYSTEMS

Most agencies investing in GIS technology will want to use Microsoft Windows operating systems, either Windows 98 or above, or Windows NT for network-based systems. Although some users favor other systems, such as UNIX, software written for the Windows environment is much more affordable than software written for other operating systems. Although these other systems may be more powerful than Windows-based systems, this power does not justify the cost. In fact, the processing speed and power of contemporary personal computers operating with Windows approaches the speed and power of UNIX-based workstations.[1]

SOFTWARE

Chapter 3 and other chapters described the important functions performed by GIS software. These functions include

- Geocoding: Although desktop GIS products have geocoding capability, nearly all professional users will probably need ancillary products. Fortunately, most GIS software vendors also sell special purpose geocoding software.[1]
- Data display, including dot density maps, chart/graph maps, choropleth maps, and overlays
- Querying, including buffers and distance
- Simple statistical operations

Contemporary GIS software products contain toolbars and menus that allow users to perform the spatial analysis tasks listed in Chapter 3 easily. Menus supply structured query language (SQL) that facilitates queries. For example, by clicking on a specified command, users can select records for houses within the boundaries of a specific polygon. Alternatively, those interested in typing in their own commands can use common-language expressions, such as "Select data records for houses (or other map point objects) that are located within the boundaries of a census tract (or other polygon)."[1] SQL allows users to perform additional steps. After selecting the houses, users interested in childhood lead poisoning could click on commands to retrieve the age of each house and average the age of the houses within each polygon. GIS software contains geographical operators that can identify whether objects on a map, such as childhood lead-poisoning cases or census tracts, lie within, lie outside, intersect, or contain other map objects.[1]

Another useful feature of modern desktop GIS software is its scripting language capability. If a sequence of commands becomes standard and repetitive, users can script the sequence to play automatically as a unit on command. By combining multiple scripts together, advanced users with programming skills can create modules that unsophisticated users can employ by simply entering a few start-up commands. For example, local health department GIS programmers could create childhood lead-poisoning modules containing multiple embedded scripts that could allow community users without programming skills to create sophisticated maps on demand without additional programming. The scripting language capability is one GIS feature that has the potential to increase access to mapping technology.[1]

Over the past few years, the variety of GIS software products has markedly increased. Each easily obtainable product has its own advantages and disadvantages (see Table 10–2).[1] The major producers of desktop GIS software and their products include

- Environmental Systems Research Institute (ESRI; Redlands, CA): ArcView GIS Version 3.2a
- MapInfo Corporation (Troy, NY): MapInfo
- Caliper Corporation (Newton, MA): Maptitude

Several other large software manufacturers have recently begun marketing GIS products, including

- Autodesk, San Rafael, California: Autodesk World
- Intergraph, Huntsville, Alabama: GeoMedia

Joint ventures between commercial software vendors and governmental agencies produce some additional GIS software products, such as Community 2020 (see Chapter 8), produced through collaboration between the Caliper Corporation and the U.S. Department of Housing and Urban Development. Although the first group of software vendors has more experience with GIS software, products from newer producers can have advantages of new approaches to user-software interface and can sometimes perform new functions.

Environmental Systems Research Institute, Inc., producer of ArcView GIS, probably has the most dominant presence in the public health/GIS software arena.[1] Many non–public health governmental agencies already use another ESRI GIS product, UNIX-based ARC/INFO, and ArcView GIS is compatible with ARC/INFO data files. For this reason alone, local public health agencies should strongly consider purchasing ArcView GIS software.[1] Another advantage of ArcView is ESRI's extensive documentation and support for its product. For example, ESRI produces CD-ROM tutorials and learning guides for ArcView GIS. On the downside, ArcView can be quite expensive, considering a base price of $1,195. In addition, to perform some functions, users must purchase additional "extensions." For example, public health GIS users who were interested in finding the most efficient travel routes from patients' homes to the nearest health care facili-

Table 10–2 Selected GIS Software Products: Advantages and Disadvantages

GIS Software	Advantages	Disadvantages
ArcView GIS	Works with ARC/INFO Excellent tutorials and documentation	Modules priced separately
Autodesk World	Reads/writes popular GIS and database formats Scripting language is Visual BASIC	Very limited documentation No geographic or demographic data included
Community 2020	Links with HUD data Web forum for users	Based on older *Maptitude 3.0* rather than more recent, enhanced *Maptitude 4.0* Data templates limited to HUD data
EpiMap	Public domain Simple to use Written by CDC	Very limited GIS features DOS based, but work is underway on a Windows-based version
Geomedia	Open GIS Enterprise solution Scripting language is Visual BASIC	Open GIS functionality does not support all popular GIS formats Very limited documentation No geographic or demographic data included
MapInfo	Excellent documentation Many established users Much after-market data	Few branch offices Quality of resellers may vary greatly
Maptitude	Excellent price Bundled with abundance of data Exports data in variety of GIS formats	Small user base Limited sources of documentation

ties would have to purchase an extension, the ArcView Network Analyst, at an additional cost of $1,495. More information on ESRI software, including purchasing options, can be found at their Web site at <www.esri.com>.

MapInfo Professional 6.0 has established users all over the world, which is particularly helpful for international public health applications.[1] MapInfo has several additional advantages. Like ESRI, it provides extensive documentation for its product and an international network of for-fee seminars. Users familiar with Microsoft Windows will find MapInfo's standard graphical user interface easy to use. Significant disadvantages are MapInfo's company policy of not selling their product directly to consumers and the scarcity of regional company representatives. Those interested in purchasing MapInfo must purchase the software and receive service from a local MapInfo software reseller, whose quality can vary greatly. For more information on MapInfo, and for the location of a local reseller, consumers can contact the MapInfo Web site at <www.mapinfo.com>. The price is competitive with that of ArcView GIS.

Maptitude 4.1, produced by the Caliper Corporation <www.caliper.com> is much more affordable and comes bundled with spatial and attribute data. For $395, purchasers receive the software on three CDs containing the complete set of TIGER line files (although only down to the cen-

sus tract level) and geocoded data with over 600 attributes from the U.S. Census of Population and Housing. Users interested in analyzing data below the census tract level can purchase the DVD version for $595. The DVD version adds census block groups, block centroids, county subdivisions, telephone exchanges, U.S. and World Digital Elevation Models, and congressional districts. Maptitude can read and export data in other formats, including ArcView GIS and MapInfo, and it can perform relatively sophisticated analyses, such as determining the most efficient travel routes, without additional expenditures. One significant drawback to Maptitude is the lack of support for its users. There are not many sources of information on how to use the product, and its accompanying tutorial does not cover all of its functions. Compared to ArcView GIS and MapInfo, with their large network of users, Maptitude purchasers will find few other users they can call for answering questions. Community 2020 combines Maptitude software with Department of Housing and Urban Development (HUD) data. Local health agencies interested in housing data might consider purchasing this product. HUD offers workshops in major cities and a Web forum of Community 2020 users. For more information on Community 2020, including price, advantages, and disadvantages, please see Chapter 8.

A significant advantage to Autodesk World, a relatively new GIS product, is its scripting language, Microsoft Visual BASIC. Many GIS software products, such as ArcView GIS and MapInfo, rely on their own proprietary programming language for scripting. Programmers using these products need to learn the specific programming language. In contrast, users already familiar with the nearly universal Microsoft Visual BASIC can immediately begin writing programs with Autodesk World. Another Autodesk World advantage is its ability to read data files in many formats, including ARC/INFO, ArcView GIS, AutoCAD, AtlasGIS, MapInfo, Microstation design files, dBase Files, Lotus 1–2–3, Access, Excel, FoxPro, Paradox, and ASCII text files.[1] Autodesk World users don't have to worry about the format of databases they choose to analyze because Autodesk World can read just about all of them.

Like other GIS software products, Autodesk World has some specific limitations. First, users needing assistance must use Autodesk World's on-line help system, which may not be very helpful for inexperienced users. For example, the help system includes explanations of Autodesk World functions but frequently omits specific instructions on how to solve problems with the software.[1] Second, Microsoft Visual BASIC, while universal, can be difficult to master. Third, the software does not come with spatial or attribute data.[1] These three deficiencies—minimal support, sophisticated programming language, and the requirement to obtain data sets after purchasing the software—pose a significant problem for small and rural health agencies that may not have access to experienced programmers. Autodesk World is compatible in price with ArcView GIS and MapInfo. More information on Autodesk World is available at the Autodesk Web site at <www.autodesk.com>.

Intergraph Industries, one of the largest international geographic technology corporations, produces GeoMedia 4.1. Like Autodesk World, GeoMedia uses Visual BASIC as its scripting language. GeoMedia is an open GIS in that it can operate on GIS data files in other formats without first translating them into its own format. Another advantage of GeoMedia is that it is open database compliant (ODBC). Computer applications that have an ODBC driver can access data in any database. Unfortunately, few database drivers are available for gaining access to geographic data, so GeoMedia cannot read MapInfo and some other data files. In addition, GeoMedia has limited ability to create data files because Intergraph designed it to be chiefly a data viewer and analyzer. Like Autodesk World, GeoMedia is probably not suited to isolated, small local health agencies because it lacks hardcopy documentation, comes without spatial and attribute data, and requires programmers to know Visual BASIC language. Its price is compatible with that of the other major GIS software products. Additional information on Intergraph software can be found at the Intergraph Web site at <www.intergraph.com>.

One special feature of Intergraph GIS software is that it has the capacity to serve as an enterprise GIS. Enterprise GIS applications feature a large, central database providing access to many users at remote sites.[1] The software resides on the central computer server, avoiding the need to install the software at each remote terminal. In these enterprise applications, most of the users can read the database or view already made maps, but they cannot manipulate the data. Typically, a few employees at the central location have the responsibility to maintain the database and the authority to change the database. Intergraph has two products that contribute to a Web-based enterprise GIS. GeoMedia Web Map allows users to distribute and view geographic data on the Internet. With the second product, GeoMedia Web Enterprise, agencies can create Web-based GIS applications that allow multiple users to view, analyze, and manipulate geographic data on the Internet (see <www.intergraph.com>). Such capacity is essential for future community-based GIS applications that allow the public to analyze data and view and create maps from the comfort of local library computer Internet connections. We will discuss Internet applications later in this chapter.

A Less Expensive Alternative: Epi Info 2000 and Epi Map

Many local health agencies interested in getting involved with GIS technology but with limited resources may want to consider the free, public domain products Epi Info and Epi Map. Since 1985, many state and local public health departments have used these CDC software products for epidemiologic analyses.[4–6] The CDC distributed the first, MS DOS–based version of Epi Info in 1985. Over the years, with input from epidemiologists all over the world, the CDC repeatedly refined the software, which eventually permitted complex epidemiological analyses of common public health problems, such as foodborne illness. By 1997, the CDC had distributed nearly 145,000 copies of the popular software to users in 117 countries, with translations of the manual and software into 13 non-English languages.[5,6] Epi Info, first as a MS DOS version, and now as a Windows-based version called Epi Info 2000, provides data entry, data management, graphic, and statistical analysis functions.[4] In addition, the software can create data sets exportable in several formats, including dBASE. Users can then import these data sets into all leading commercial GIS software products or into Epi Map to make maps.[5]

The MS DOS versions of Epi Info and Epi Map can run on older, relatively unsophisticated personal computers. Staff with little training or computer experience can learn to do simple but useful analyses within several hours.[5] With the MS DOS–based version of Epi Map, users can create custom map polygons on the computer screen. This feature is particularly valuable in disaster situations, hospital infection surveillance, and other local situations where spatial data may not be readily available. To construct the custom maps, users simply tape a transparency or a map over the screen and trace the outline. Users can import boundaries from other GIS software programs, including Atlas, MapInfo, ArcView, and ARC/INFO, if available. Version 2 of Epi Map for DOS provides programming language to create customized point-and-click information systems that allow users to bring up other maps, text, or hypertext.[5] In addition, Epi Map can display several different maps on a computer screen simultaneously. With this feature, health officials can create map presentations comparing disease rates and disease counts by different geographic areas or in the same area by several time periods.[5]

Compared to commercial, Windows-based GIS products, the MS DOS versions of Epi Info and Epi Map have several significant drawbacks. First, their graphic and printing capabilities are limited. Second, their files have unique formats, although available utilities can convert the files into other common formats. Third, because Epi Info and Epi Map are two stand-alone programs, users must transfer any data they prepare in Epi Info to Epi Map to create map displays. To do this, they can use DOS batch file commands or the configurable Epi Info menu.[5]

Figure 10–1 shows two maps displayed on a single computer screen using MS DOS–based Epi Map, Version 2. The map on the right side of the figure is an event or dot-density map, showing reported salmonella cases in Michigan over a four-week period ending in week 52 of 1996. On the left side of the figure, choropleth map polygon shades represent salmonella case rates over the entire year for counties within the state. The two maps in Figure 10–1 are simple, unenhanced versions that are printable with common word-processing software. With additional graphics programs, users can print enhanced versions of the maps. As examples of the capability of MS DOS versions of Epi Info and Epi Map, public health practitioners have used them to create maps displaying[5]

- Rates and counts for hospital surgical wound infections by operating room, recovery room, and hospital room or floor
- Rates of community risk factors
- A series of maps on the same screen showing the change in reportable disease rates over time
- Injuries by type or location

- Well water tests and results
- Refugee camp rates and cases of cholera, malnutrition, and available resources, such as food supplies
- Health-related events occurring during mass gatherings, such as overnight, outdoor concerts

Recently, the CDC released Epi Info 2000, an entirely new version of Epi Info and Epi Map. Like the previous versions, Epi Info 2000 is a public domain product, available without charge for downloading from the CDC Web site. In addition, Epi Info 2000 uses the same strategy as the older versions: users prepare data in Epi Info and then display it using Epi Map. Despite these similarities, Epi Info 2000 is a significant improvement to the MS DOS versions for several reasons. First, the Map command within the analyses program integrates the Epi Info features with Epi Map. Second, the CDC used MS Visual BASIC language to write the software, and the program uses MS Access database tables. These features make the software compatible with many other software products. Third, ESRI, providers of Arc/Info and ArcView software described earlier, developed the mapping functions within Epi Info 2000, making it compatible with ARC/INFO coverages, ESRI shape files, and many bitmap image formats, such as BMP, TIFF, SUN, ERDAS, BIL, BIP, and BSQ.[5]

Compared to commercial software products, Epi Info 2000 has limited GIS functions. However, the CDC is developing features to facilitate geocoding, drawing or editing maps, and incorporating images. Available boundary files for the United States go down only as far as census tract and ZIP code levels, with files that have even less detail available for the rest of the world. Despite its limitations, Epi Info 2000 may provide a way for smaller agencies to become involved in GIS technology. For example, state agencies could make Epi 2000 files, including map boundaries and data files, and training available to small health departments. Using the Internet, they could easily send data files to even the most remote health department. Those interested in downloading the program can go to the CDC Web site, <www.cdc.gov> and click on Products and Publications, Software, and finally Epi Info/Epi Map.[5,7] The CDC provides manuals in electronic format, but those interested in purchasing hard-copy versions can contact vendors referenced on the Web site.

Raster-Based Software

Most of the commercially available desktop software products that we have discussed allow users to display images as backgrounds on maps, with vector information displayed against the background.[1] Public health practitioners inter-

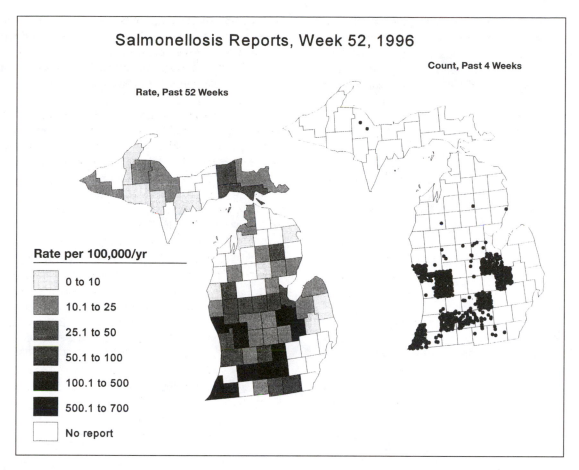

Salmonellosis Reports, Week 52, 1996

Count, Past 4 Weeks

Rate, Past 52 Weeks

Rate per 100,000/yr

- 0 to 10
- 10.1 to 25
- 25.1 to 50
- 50.1 to 100
- 100.1 to 500
- 500.1 to 700
- No report

Figure 10–1 Two maps from the same screen in Epi Map, Version 2 for DOS, at week 52 of observation, based on cumulative (provisional) data in a public health surveillance system: a choropleth map summarizing disease rates for the past 52 weeks and a dot-density map displaying case counts during the past four weeks, by county

ested in performing analyses that are more extensive using raster-based data files should consider Idrisi, a raster-based product produced by Clark University Department of Geography. Available by download, Idrisi has good documentation and support and is popular with raster-based GIS users.[1] Its cost varies from $525 for academic users to $925 for governmental agencies. For more information, potential users should go to the Idrisi Web site at <www.clarklabs.org>. Alternative raster-based software products, produced by vendors like Earth Resource Mapping (ERM), of San Diego, California, can provide more advanced raster processing functions, such as analysis of three-dimensional landscapes. These functions can be useful for health resource planning. For example, in planning construction of health care facilities, three-dimensional analyses can help exclude construction sites that could result in facilities with access limitations due to steep slopes or other terrain features.[1]

Additional information is available at the ERM Web site at <www.ermapper.com>.

GIS ON THE INTERNET

Public health practitioners committed to engaging communities in partnerships for community health assessment and planning will have to make their GIS applications accessible. The best way to do this is to place the GIS applications on a Web site, accessible to multiple users at multiple community locations, including libraries. At this time, technological limitations pose barriers and challenges to making fully functional GIS applications available on the Internet. The remainder of this chapter will discuss how public health practitioners should consider these limitations and challenges in designing Web-based GIS applications.

One of the biggest challenges to realizing the potential of Web-based GIS technology is the technological difficulty associated with enabling full GIS mapping capabilities on the Web.[8] The GIS mapping Web sites depicted in Table 10–3 illustrate the degree of technological sophistication currently available on the Internet. These Web sites have several features in common:

- They are designed for the general public: for example, they can help individuals plan travel routes of the closest location of hotels to meeting sites.
- Most importantly, they do not provide full GIS spatial analysis capabilities. For example, their mapping capabilities are usually limited to only a few functions, such as address matching and census data displays.

Table 10–3 Examples of Interactive Internet Mapping Sites

Site	Intended Use/Application	Features	Other Mapping Functionality
EnviroMapper www.epa.gov/enviro	General mapping. Additional data layers are displayed as the map scale increases	S, C, I, Z, H, L, U	Customizable scalebars; provides users with a query tool; EPA also provides the following mapping applications: SiteInfo, County Info, BasinInfo, and ZipInfo. These sites are for creating site, county, basin, and ZIP-based map areas respectively
Yahoo Maps http://maps.yahoo.com/yahoo	Address matching by street address, business	A, S, Z, N, E, H, U	Driving directions
Xerox PARC Map Viewer http://pubweb.parc.xerox.com/map	General mapping. First Internet mapping site (created in 1993) Maintenance was stopped in 1997	Z, N, H, L, W	Can look at different projections, data layers of borders and rivers that can be added or removed (only U.S. for address matching)
Maps On Us www.mapsonus.com	Address matching by street address	A, S, Z, E, C, H, U	Driving directions, more pan and zoom options that others offer, shows latitude and longitude numbers, weather
MapBlast www.mapblast.com	Address matching	A, S, Z, N, E, C, H, U, D	Advanced location search, data layers: home and health, office/computer, fashion/sports, auto/transportation, finance/banks, travel/lodging, other
MapQuest www.mapquest.com	Worldwide address matching, additional data layers	A, S, I, Z, N, E, C, H, W	Can add data layers as follows: attractions, automotive, banking, civic, dining, education, entertainment, health care, lodging, recreation, services, shopping, transportation, Web sites
Tiger Mapping Service http://tiger.census.gov	Distribute census data	S, Z, N, L, C, H, U	21 Census data layers
CIESIN www.ciesin.org	Distribute census data	S, I, Z, C, L, H, U	JAVA interface, most dynamic site, can change colors and lots of layers

Key to Codes:

A =	Address matching	I =	Identify by point and click	E =	E-mail functionality	W =	Worldwide maps
S =	Scalebar	Z =	Zoom/pan	H =	Help or frequently asked questions	U =	USA maps
C =	Customizable	N =	North arrow	L =	Legend	D =	Canada maps

- Their design does not consider public health issues, such as confidentiality.

There are a couple of reasons for these limitations. First, most GIS software programs developed independently from Internet hypertext markup language (HTML). Fortunately, newer versions of GIS software are beginning to use Web-accessible software, such as JAVA or ActiveX. In the meantime, most statistical packages are adapted primarily for desktop GIS use, not for the Web. Internet Explorer, produced by ESRI, allows only basic statistical functions on the Web, while statistical software products that are more powerful are not yet adapted to the Internet. For example, a GIS add-on statistics module, produced by a popular statistical software vendor, SAS, cannot run over the Web. Currently available technology, such as the Smart Viewer Web Server developed by SPSS, enables only viewing of reports, graphics, and tables on the Web. Consequently, public health agencies cannot currently provide Web-based tools that would allow community partners to perform their own statistical analyses. Instead, they are limited to publishing outputs of statistical analyses on their Web sites, such as the report on hospital performance, patient profiles, and length of stay, published by SPSS with its Smart Viewer.

A second limitation to the development of full Web-based GIS applications is the size of most GIS data files, especially maps. The large file size tends to slow access and display functions, especially with relatively slow modem connections available at remote sites. In addition, the large data sets require significant computer computational power at both server and user ends. Fortunately, a couple of developing technological strategies promise to improve the speed of data access, analysis, and display. GIS servers can change the data format of images requested by users automatically into compressible formats, such as a Graphics Interchange Format (GIF) or Joint Photographic Experts Group (JPEG). The compressed formats travel more quickly over modem and other Internet connections. The user's computer can then uncompress the file automatically for analysis and/or display. In addition, as computers become faster and Internet access speeds increase, especially through modem and DSL connections, Internet-GIS applications will improve.

Although the basic elements of desktop and Web-based GIS applications are similar, their organization is quite different. Desktop GIS applications contain the components and functions entirely within an individual computer, whereas Web-based applications distribute the GIS components and functions between the client (individual user) and the Web-based server (the GIS program provider, such as a state or local public health agency).[8] Our lead-poisoning example depicted in Chapter 3 illustrates the server/user relationship (see Figure 10–2). In this case, the state health department houses the server, which contains the attribute database (the lead case report file), the spatial data, and the GIS software. The server performs several functions, including collecting, storing, updating, and geocoding the lead case report files. The client, in this case local health department staff, simply focuses on querying the database, performing analyses, and creating map displays.[8] A local analogous relationship could have the local health agency housing the server, while the client, a community-based organization, queried the database from a personal computer with an Internet connection.

Several models, ranging in levels of complexity, illustrate how these Web-based relationships could work. Model 1, the simplest example, is the most common application currently in use (see Figure 10–3).[8] At the client end, the required components of this model are a personal computer (PC) with mapping software, a commercially available Web browser, such as Microsoft Internet Explorer or Netscape, and an Internet connection. The local or state public health agency maintains a Web server containing the database and accessible at its Uniform Resource Locator (URL) Internet address and a GIS server containing the GIS software. Sitting at the PC (which could be available at home or at a local library), the client sends a request for a map over the Internet to the Web server, which in turn sends the request to the GIS server. The GIS server responds to the query by preparing the digital map image and sends the image to the Web server, which in turn sends the image to the client's Web browser and onto the client's computer. Finally, the client uses the mapping software to display the image. Advantages of this model are its simplicity, ease of use, and low cost. The major disadvantages of this model include the limited ability to analyze data, the limited ability to create customized maps, and the limit to one request at a time, resulting in slow performance speeds.[8]

The next level of complexity, model 2, permits the client to perform more sophisticated analyses (such as query, analyze, and summarize) and to create more customized maps using browser-based and server-based programming (see Figure 10–4).[8] Other advantages of model 2 include its capacity to process more transactions, to bring data files from different sites together, and to allow multiple users to work with these data on multiple desktop computers. A significant limitation to this model is that it requires the client to have sophisticated programming skills.

Model 3 is the most advanced Web-based GIS model (see Figure 10–5).[8] This model comes closest to providing GIS functionality comparable to a full-function desktop GIS. To optimize the output speed for data transfer, it uses multiple servers working together. Using specially scripted JAVA or ActiveX browser programs, the client sends a request to the Web server, which forwards the request to the GIS server. Next, the GIS server responds to the request by retrieving selected layers from the database servers either through the Web (if the database servers are maintained by other organi-

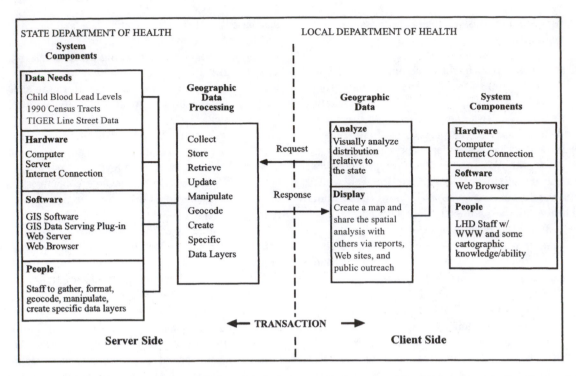

Figure 10–2 Client and server relationships in a Web-based GIS environment where a local health department is the client and state health department is the server

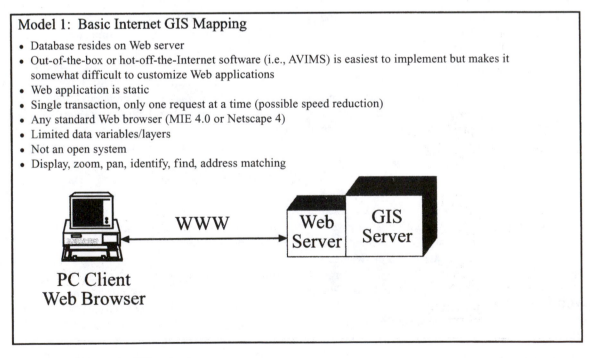

Figure 10–3 Model 1 for Internet GIS technology

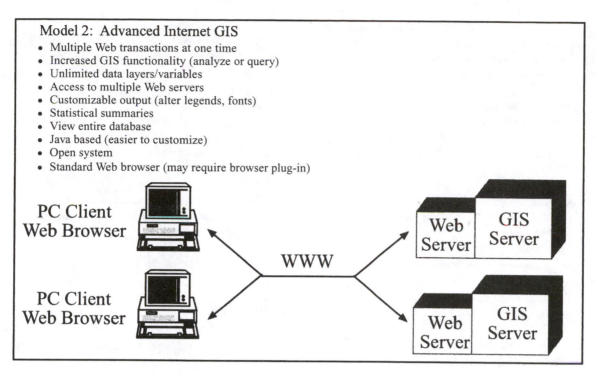

Model 2: Advanced Internet GIS
- Multiple Web transactions at one time
- Increased GIS functionality (analyze or query)
- Unlimited data layers/variables
- Access to multiple Web servers
- Customizable output (alter legends, fonts)
- Statistical summaries
- View entire database
- Java based (easier to customize)
- Open system
- Standard Web browser (may require browser plug-in)

Figure 10–4 Model 2 for Internet GIS technology

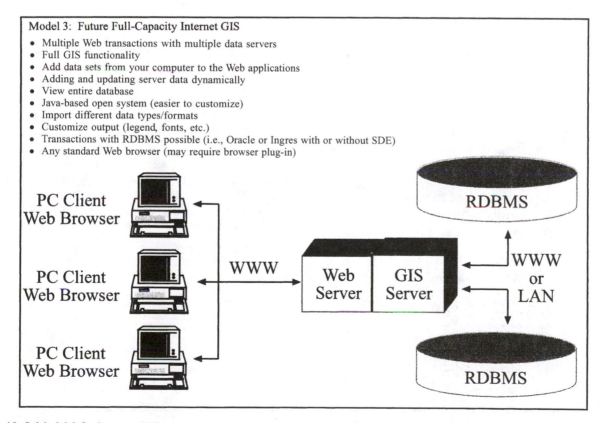

Model 3: Future Full-Capacity Internet GIS
- Multiple Web transactions with multiple data servers
- Full GIS functionality
- Add data sets from your computer to the Web applications
- Adding and updating server data dynamically
- View entire database
- Java-based open system (easier to customize)
- Import different data types/formats
- Customize output (legend, fonts, etc.)
- Transactions with RDBMS possible (i.e., Oracle or Ingres with or without SDE)
- Any standard Web browser (may require browser plug-in)

Figure 10–5 Model 3 for Internet GIS technology

zations) or through a local area network (if the database servers are maintained by the same agency). A significant advantage to this model is that it permits clients to select and display the layers they want when they want, much like a full-function desktop GIS.

Before investing in Internet GIS technology based on these or other models, public health agencies should use the same type of evaluative process they would use before making any other investment in new technology. At a minimum, they should consider

- Financial resources available
- Staffing capabilities, including staff time, skills, knowledge, and abilities
- Physical facilities
- Available hardware and software
- Data resources
- Whether conventional desktop GIS is adequate for the agency and its users

Outside consultants can help agencies decide whether to invest, and once they decide to do so, help them organize their Internet-based GIS cheaply and efficiently. After deciding to invest in an Internet application, additional considerations should include

- How to incorporate remote users with different software platforms and operating systems
- How GIS objects (data layers and health features within the data layers) communicate with each other in a dynamic system
- How selection of programming language can influence system design
- How to ensure accuracy of data and maintain metadata
- The distribution of system overhead for data creation, data storage, and data security[8]

Once a public health agency addresses these and other considerations,[8] it will need to invest in the following components:

- A server—Microsoft's New Technology (NT) servers can work well with most commercially available software, which are often available free of charge from the large software manufacturers (including Microsoft)
- An Internet connection, as fast as possible
- GIS software plus interface programs (or plug-ins) for both the server and the browser
- HTML programming software for the Web pages— HTML software is inexpensive, and much of it is available free of charge for downloading off the Web
- A Web browser—system designers should test multiple browsers to make sure they are compatible with the planned GIS application
- Data—before incorporating data into the Internet application, agency staff must check the data for formatting and accuracy.

Finally, the public health agency must assemble these components, test them, and maintain them.[8]

At present, most public health agencies interested in displaying maps on a Web site will find options similar to model 1 suitable for their needs. For smaller agencies with few users and resources, this model permits clients with a desktop personal computer to create a static GIF or JPEG file of a final GIS map and insert the static image on a Web page. On the other hand, larger agencies, and collaborations of agencies with large numbers of users desiring more complex analyses, will be interested in systems based on more advanced technology, as reflected in models 2 and 3.

These models reflect the current state of Internet GIS technology. Internet GIS applications are a very new development: GIS software that allowed programmers to geographically enable their Web sites became available only in the last five years.[9] As we proceed into the twenty-first century, advances in technology will make these complex, difficult-to-understand models much more simple. Public health agencies will find well-trained information technology professionals available to maintain their servers. Future public health professionals using GIS technology with a personal computer and Web browser will not need sophisticated programming skills. With similar desktop personal computers, Web browsers, and Internet connections, available in local libraries, community residents without any programming skills should be able to perform relatively sophisticated GIS analyses.

CHAPTER   REVIEW

1. Before a local health department or other agency invests in a GIS application, it should determine whether it really needs the application or if cheaper alternatives might suffice. At a minimum, any agency considering adding a GIS application should
   - Determine community health priorities that could be amenable to GIS analysis
   - Carefully consider how GIS technology would be helpful in addressing these priorities
   - Identify whether alternative methodologies could perform the same function at lower cost
   - Evaluate the agency's capacity to implement and maintain a GIS application, including staff training, knowledge, skills, and abilities

2. Once an agency has decided (after a comprehensive needs assessment) to invest in GIS technology, the next steps are to decide on hardware and software. Minimum hardware components include
   - Large hard drives
   - Rapid processing speeds
   - Adequate random access memory (RAM)
   - Large monitors with sufficient resolution
   - Color printers with sufficient resolution (ink jet or laser)
   - Color scanners
   - A rapid Internet connection

3. Most agencies investing in GIS technology will want to use Microsoft Windows operating systems, either Windows 98 or above, or Windows NT for network-based systems.

4. The important functions performed by GIS software include
   - Geocoding: Although desktop GIS products have geocoding capability, professional users will probably need ancillary products. Fortunately, most GIS software vendors sell special purpose geocoding software.[1]
   - Data display, including dot density maps, chart/graph maps, choropleth maps, and overlays
   - Querying, including buffers and distance
   - Simple statistical operations

5. Contemporary GIS software products contain toolbars and menus that allow users to perform the spatial analysis tasks easily. Menus supply structured query language (SQL) that facilitates queries.

6. Another useful feature of modern desktop GIS software is its scripting language capability. If a sequence of commands becomes standard and repetitive, users can script the sequence to play automatically as a unit on command. By combining multiple scripts, advanced users with programming skills can create modules that unsophisticated users can employ by simply entering a few start-up commands.

7. Over the past few years, the variety of GIS software products has markedly increased. Each easily obtainable product has its own advantages and disadvantages. The major producers of desktop GIS software and their products include
   - Environmental Systems Research Institute (ESRI; Redlands, CA): ArcView GIS Version 3.2a
   - MapInfo Corporation (Troy, NY): MapInfo
   - Caliper Corporation (Newton, MA): Maptitude
   - Autodesk (San Rafael, CA): Autodesk World
   - Intergraph (Huntsville, AL): GeoMedia
   Joint ventures between commercial software vendors and governmental agencies produce some additional GIS software products, such as Community 2020.

8. Many local health agencies interested in getting involved with GIS technology but with limited resources may want to consider the free, public domain products Epi Info and Epi Map. Epi Info includes data entry, data management, graphic, and statistical analysis functions. The MS DOS versions of Epi Info and Epi Map can run on older, relatively unsophisticated personal computers. Staff with little training or computer experience can learn to do simple but useful analyses within several hours. Compared to commercial, Windows-based GIS products, the MS DOS

versions of Epi Info and Epi Map have some limitations.

9. Public health practitioners interested in performing complex analyses using raster-based data files should consider Idrisi, a raster-based product produced by the Clark University Department of Geography. Alternative raster-based software products, produced by vendors like Earth Resource Mapping (ERM), of San Diego, California, can provide more advanced raster processing functions, such as analysis of three-dimensional landscapes. These functions can be useful for health resource planning.

10. Public health practitioners committed to engaging communities in partnerships for community health assessment and planning will have to make their GIS applications accessible. The best way to do this is to place the GIS applications on a Web site, accessible to multiple users at multiple community locations, including libraries. At this time, technological limitations pose barriers and challenges to making fully functional GIS applications available on the Internet.

11. Although the basic elements of desktop and Web-based GIS applications are similar, their organization is quite different. Desktop GIS applications contain the components and functions entirely within an individual computer, whereas Web-based applications distribute the GIS components and functions between the client (individual user) and the Web-based server (the GIS program provider, such as a state or local public health agency).

12. Before investing in Internet GIS technology, public health agencies should consider
   - Financial resources available
   - Staffing capabilities
   - Physical facilities
   - Available hardware and software
   - Data resources
   - Whether conventional desktop GIS is adequate for the agency and its users

13. Outside consultants can help agencies decide whether to invest, and, once they decide to do so, help them organize their Internet-based GIS cheaply and efficiently. Essential components include
   - A server
   - An Internet connection, as fast as possible
   - GIS software plus interface programs (or plug-ins) for both the server and the browser
   - HTML programming software for the Web pages
   - A Web browser
   - Data—before incorporating data into the Internet application, agency staff must check the data for formatting and accuracy

The public health agency must assemble these components, test them, and maintain them.

REFERENCES

1. S.E. Thrall. "Geographic Information System (GIS) Hardware and Software." *Journal of Public Health Management and Practice* 5, no. 2 (1999): 82–90.

2. H.J. Scholten and M.J.C. de Lepper. "The Benefits of the Application of Geographical Information Systems in Public and Environmental Health." *World Health Statistics Quarterly* 44 (1991): 160–170.

3. G. Rushton and M.P. Armstrong. "Improving Public Health through Geographical Information Systems. An Instructional Guide to Major Concepts and Their Implementation." Web Version 1.0. December 1997. <www.uiowa.edu/~geog/health/index.html>.

4. A.G. Dean et al. "Epi Info: A General-Purpose Microcomputer Program for Public Health Information Systems." *American Journal of Preventive Medicine* 7, no. 3 (1991): 178–182.

5. A.G. Dean. "Epi Info and Epi Map: Current Status and Plans for Epi Info 2000." *Journal of Public Health Management and Practice* 5, no. 4 (1999): 54–57.

6. B. Harbage and A.G. Dean. "Distribution of Epi Info Software: An Evaluation Using the Internet." *American Journal of Preventive Medicine* 16, no. 4 (1999): 314–317.

7. Centers for Disease Control and Prevention. Epi Info–Epi Map. <www.cdc.gov/epiinfo/>.

8. T.W. Foresman. "Spatial Analysis and Mapping on the Internet." *Journal of Public Health Management and Practice* 5, no. 4 (1999): 57–63.

9. G.I. Thrall. "The Future of GIS in Public Health Management and Practice." *Journal of Public Health Management and Practice* 5, no. 4 (1999): 75–82.

CHAPTER 11

The Future of GIS and the Role of Public Health Officials

FACILITATING PUBLIC HEALTH FUNCTIONS

This book has presented examples of how GIS technology already facilitates public health planning, management, and practice. One way to understand how the use of this technology could improve public health practice in the future is to examine it in relation to traditional public health functions of the past. In 1945, a report by Haven Emerson for the American Public Health Association Committee on Administrative Practice described six basic functions of local health departments:[1-3]

1. Vital statistics
2. Communicable-disease control
3. Sanitation
4. Laboratory services
5. Hygiene of maternity, infancy, and childhood
6. Health education of the general public

These six functions, known as the "Basic Six," became the cornerstone for public health practice in the postwar United States. More than 40 years later, in 1988, after a thorough assessment of the public health system, the Institute of Medicine (IOM) issued a report, *The Future of Public Health.*[4] Even though the public health system had grown over the preceding decades and the nation's health status had improved, the Institute found that the public health system was in disarray. The report identified several problems facing the public health system, including the AIDS epidemic, limited resources due to competition with the medical care system, dissipation of public appreciation and support for public health, and other intractable health and social issues. To solve these problems, the IOM determined that the nation needed

a new vision for public health, based on three core public health functions:[4,5]

1. Assessment
2. Policy development
3. Assurance

The IOM defined assessment as collecting, analyzing, and making available information on the health of a community. On the basis of the assessment, public health agencies work with their community partners to develop scientifically based policies aimed at improving community health. In their third core role, public health agencies assure their constituents that services based on these policies are available and effective, either by encouraging or requiring others to act or by providing services directly.

By 1994, six years after the IOM report, the United States was in the midst of a debate on health care reform. Public health leaders were concerned that any comprehensive health care reform plan might omit public health services, mainly because policy makers and the public did not understand the core functions of public health. To convey the public health message, they began to reformulate the core functions into lists of services and functions more meaningful to the public. Many public health organizations participated, including the National Association of County and City Health Officials (NACCHO), the Association of State and Territorial Health Officials (ASTHO), and the Office of Assistant Secretary of Health. Although the lists were similar, public health leaders decided that a single list would be more conducive to conveying the public health message to the nation.

In early 1994, a working group on the core functions of public health, composed of representatives from public health

241

agencies at the local, state, and federal levels, charged a subgroup to develop a consensus list of the "essential services of public health." Led by the CDC's Public Health Program Practice Office (PHPPO) and the Office of Disease Prevention and Health Promotion, a subgroup named the Essential Public Health Services Work Group (EPHSWG) first stated that the mission of public health was to "promote physical and mental health and prevent disease, injury and disability."[3]

Members of the subgroup included representatives from ASTHO, NACCHO, IOM, the Association of Schools of Public Health (ASPH), the Public Health Foundation, the National Association of State Alcohol and Drug Abuse Directors, the National Association of State Mental Health Program Directors, and the Public Health Service. Next, the workgroup developed two lists, one describing what public health does (the purpose of public health) and the other describing how public health carries out its responsibilities (the practice of public health). The "what" list identified six fundamental obligations of agencies responsible for population-based health[1,4] as a framework to measure and improve the core functions. GIS technology can help public health agencies at all levels, local, state, and federal, to perform their functions and meet these obligations.

Undoubtedly, GIS technology supports commonly accepted public health functions described by earlier or more contemporary lists. Table 11–1 provides just a few examples[1–3,6–8] illustrating how existing GIS technology could facilitate the public health functions and obligations defined in the Emerson and the EPHSWG reports.

A 1994 Georgia Division of Public Health Study, done in collaboration with the Georgia March of Dimes Birth Defects Foundation and the Centers for Disease Control and Prevention (CDC), shows how GIS technology can facilitate the performance of maternal and child health programs to improve birth outcomes.[9] Risk factors for poor birth outcomes include maternal drug and alcohol use, including tobacco use, and inadequate prenatal care. For example, maternal cocaine use during pregnancy is associated with intrauterine growth retardation, placental abruption, preterm delivery, congenital anomalies, and other adverse health effects for the mother and child.[10] Historically, it has been difficult to measure the prevalence of perinatal exposure to substances like cocaine because mothers fearing prosecution are less likely to seek prenatal care and, if they do get care, are less likely to report drug use.

The original goal of the Georgia study was to find out whether public health officials could use dried blood spots routinely collected from all newborn infants to determine the prevalence of perinatal exposure to cocaine. Study participants were infants born during a two-month period in 1994 and for whom an adequate dried blood sample was still available after routine metabolic screening. The study tested the dried blood anonymously because investigators had not obtained informed consent and were concerned about the mothers' fear of prosecution. Investigators excluded newborns younger than 31 weeks' gestation or with birth weights under 1,500 g (3 pounds, 5 ounces) because half of these infants were routinely tested seven days after birth, beyond the time period for reliable detection of cocaine metabolites in the dried blood specimen. The study also excluded multiple births and all other newborns tested after seven days of age. As a result, 14,968 (91 percent) of the 16,470 eligible infants born during the two-month period submitted dried blood specimens for testing by the CDC for the cocaine metabolite.

Investigators gathered data about maternal characteristics from the birth certificate. To protect the mothers' anonymity, they ensured that personal identifying information, such as maternal name, was not present in the database at the same time as the laboratory results. In addition, the design of the analysis files avoided including any information that, when combined, could permit identification of any person.

Dried blood specimens from 73 infants in the study tested positive for benzoylecognine (BE), a chemical resulting from metabolism of cocaine in the body. These results represented a statewide prevalence rate of 4.9 cases of perinatal cocaine exposure per 1,000 newborns. Investigators found evidence of perinatal exposure to cocaine throughout the state: mothers of BE-positive newborns resided in 17 of the 19 health districts in Georgia. Figure 11–1 shows the distribution of newborns testing positive for BE by ZIP code of mother's residence during the two-month period in 1994. To preserve anonymity, investigators excluded ZIP codes containing fewer than 50 births during the time period.

Maternal characteristics associated with perinatal cocaine exposure (see Table 11–2) included

- Older age (over 25)
- No father's name on the birth certificate
- Education of less than 13 years
- Self-reported cigarette smoking, alcohol drinking, or both during pregnancy
- Inadequate weight gain during pregnancy
- Black race
- Having had three or more previous live-born infants
- Having a short period between pregnancies
- Maternal residence in large standard metropolitan statistical areas (population greater than or equal to 1,000,000)

Although 74 percent of the mothers of BE-positive newborns had some prenatal care, and 34 percent began their care in the first trimester, these mothers were more likely to

Table 11–1 Possible GIS Roles in Facilitating Public Health Functions and Obligations

	Functions/Obligations	*Example of GIS Supporting Role*
Emerson[2]:	*Vital statistics*, or the recording, tabulation, interpretation, and publication of the essential facts of births, deaths, and reportable diseases	State and local health departments can maintain health statistics by geographic area, such as census block group approximations to high school attendance areas or legislative districts Using GIS maps, they can present the data for comparison between geographic areas, such as between high school attendance areas and the state or county, assisting the interpretation and publication of community health information
Emerson[2]: EPHSWG[2]:	*Control of communicable diseases*, including tuberculosis, venereal diseases, malaria, and hookworm disease Prevention of epidemics and the spread of disease	Disease risk is associated with behaviors and environmental factors. Using GIS technology, health officials can identify the location of populations at risk for specific diseases by • Overlaying disease incidence data, such as communicable-disease reports, with behavioral data, such as the Youth Risk Behavior Survey (YRBS; see Chapter 8)[6] or lifestyle cluster groups (see Chapter 7).[7,8] • Mapping geographic areas where populations are at risk for disease related to exposure to potential physical, chemical, and biological factors, such as radiation, lead, and mosquito vectors (see Chapters 4 and 5). On the basis of these maps, health officials can target preventive measures while educating communities about potential risks.
Emerson[2]: EPHSWG[3]:	Environmental *sanitation*, including supervision of milk and milk products, food processing, and public eating places and maintenance of sanitary conditions of employment Protection against environmental hazards	Health officials can use GIS to map the location of facilities they inspect, such as restaurants and other food-processing facilities, pools, and septic systems. With this information, they can • Efficiently assign staff to inspect facilities based on facility performance, geographic location, and travel time • Evaluate the impact of failing septic systems on drinking water sources (see Chapter 4)
EPHSWG[3]:	Prevention of injuries	Health officials can use GIS to document the risk of injuries due to naturally occurring events, such as earthquakes, and "manmade" events, such as automobile accidents (see Chapter 6).
Emerson[2]:	Public health *laboratory services*	State public health laboratories can geocode their data, facilitating surveillance of communicable disease (see Chapter 5).
Emerson[2]: EPHSWG[3]:	*Hygiene of maternity, infancy, and childhood*, including supervision of the health of the school child (this includes prenatal and postpartum care and immunization of children)[4] Assurance of the quality and accessibility of health services	GIS can provide information on maternal and child health, such as • Residence location of newborns • Communities with high rates of teen births (see Chapter 7)[6] • Communities with high infant mortality rates • Communities with concentrations of old housing and children with reported high lead levels (see Chapter 4) • Communities with children at risk for being underimmunized (see Chapter 5) • Adequacy of prenatal care for vulnerable locations • Locations of community assets, such as community health centers (see Chapter 7)

continues

Table 11–1 continued

Functions/Obligations	Example of GIS Supporting Role
Emerson[2]: *Health education* of the general public, so far as this is not covered by the functions of departments of education EPHSWG[3]: Promotion and encouragement of healthy behaviors and mental health	Health officials can use GIS to promote healthy behaviors in their communities by • Documenting the locations of populations with the greatest need for specific health information, using data such as lifestyle cluster groups (see Chapter 7)[7,8] • Targeting tailored educational messages to these populations • Providing GIS-enabled Internet sites containing health information, accessible through personal computers
EPHSWG[3]: *Response to disasters* and assistance to communities in recovery	In responding to natural disasters, such as hurricanes, floods, and earthquakes, health officials can assist in recovery efforts by using GIS to • Document the predisaster environment, including information such as the location of buildings at risk for damage • Assess the likelihood of a particular environmental event at any location

Note: EPHSWG, Essential Public Health Services Work Group.

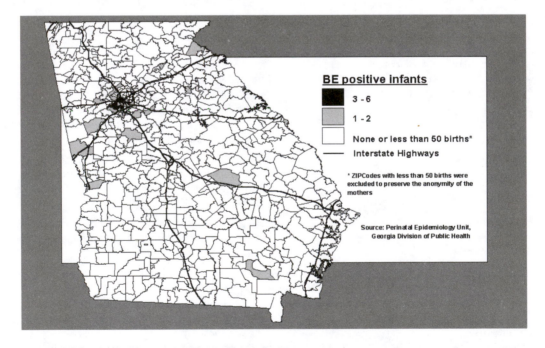

Figure 11–1 Geographic distribution of cases of benzoylecognine (BE)—a cocaine metabolite—in newborn infants, by ZIP code of mother's residence; Georgia, February 22 through April 23, 1994

have received late or no prenatal care compared to mothers of negative-testing infants. Mothers of BE-positive newborns were more likely to have given birth in large hospitals with specialized perinatal services (level III) and in hospitals with no obstetric services or outside of hospitals (level 0) than in hospitals with intermediate obstetric services (levels I and II).

Figure 11–2 is a map of ZIP codes containing mothers at high risk for using cocaine during pregnancy, based on the residence of mothers having at least five of eight risk factors

Table 11–2 Number and Rate* of Detection of Benzoylecognine (BE) in Residual Dried Blood Spots of Newborns, by Selected Maternal Characteristics—Georgia, 1994

Maternal Characteristic	Sample Size	BE-positive infant				
		No.	Rate	(95% CI[†])	OR[§]	(95% CI)
Age group (yrs)						
<25	7,143	17	2.4	(1.4–3.8)	1.0	referent
≥25	7,824	56	7.2	(5.4–9.3)	3.0	(1.8–5.1)
Education (yrs)						
≤12	8,855	59	6.7	(5.1–8.6)	2.9	(1.6–5.0)
≥13	5,993	14	2.3	(1.3–3.9)	1.0	referent
Cigarette smoking and drinking during pregnancy						
Cigarette smoking only	1,584	28	17.7	(11.7–25.5)	8.1	(5.2–12.6)
Drinking only	111	3	27.0	(5.6–79.0)	12.5	(4.9–31.9)
Both	106	13	122.6	(65.3–209.7)	63.1	(43.6–91.3)
Neither	13,117	29	2.2	(1.5–3.2)	1.0	referent
Weight gain during pregnancy (lbs)						
<15	996	13	13.1	(6.9–22.3)	3.7	(2.1–6.8)
15–24	3,001	18	6.0	(3.6–9.5)	1.7	(1.0–3.0)
≥25	9,955	35	3.5	(2.4–4.9)	1.0	referent
Unknown	1,016	7	6.9	(2.8–14.2)	2.0	(0.9–4.4)
Race/Ethnicity[@]						
Black, non-Hispanic	5,049	61	12.1	(9.2–15.5)	9.3	(5.6–15.5)
White, non-Hispanic	9,139	12	1.3	(0.7–2.3)	1.0	referent
Hispanic	491	0	—	—	—	—
Other	287	0	—	—	—	—
Previous births						
0	6,520	6	0.9	(0.3–2.0)	1.0	referent
1–2	7,277	30	4.1	(2.8–5.9)	4.5	(2.0–10.0)
≥3	1,171	37	31.6	(22.2–43.6)	35.4	(20.7–60.8)
Interpregnancy interval (mos)						
0–6	675	15	22.2	(12.4–36.7)	3.9	(2.2–6.7)
≥7	7,542	44	5.8	(4.2–7.8)	1.0	referent
No previous birth	6,520	6	0.9	(0.3–2.0)	0.2	(0.1–0.3)
Unknown	231	8	34.6	(15.0–68.2)	6.1	(3.1–12.0)
Residence						
Large SMSA**	7,471	48	6.4	(4.7–8.5)	2.2	(1.2–4.1)
Other SMSA	3,003	12	4.0	(2.1–15.6)	1.4	(0.6–3.0)
Non-SMSA	4,493	13	2.9	(1.5–5.0)	1.0	referent
Month of pregnancy at initiation of prenatal care						
0–3	12,080	25	2.1	(1.3–3.1)	1.0	referent
4–6	2,139	21	9.8	(6.1–15.0)	4.8	(2.8–8.1)
7–9	447	8	17.9	(7.7–5.3)	8.8	(4.5–17.1)
No prenatal care	167	15	89.8	(50.3–148.1)	47.6	(32.4–69.8)
Unknown	135	4	29.6	(8.1–75.9)	14.5	(6.6–33.0)
Hospital services received						
Specialized perinatal	7,152	45	6.3	(4.6–8.4)	2.2	(1.3–3.6)
Intermediate obstetric	7,661	22	2.9	(1.8–4.3)	1.0	referent
No obstetric services	149	6	40.3	(14.8–87.6)	14.6	(7.3–29.2)
Total [++]	**14,968**	**73**	**4.9**	**(3.8–6.1)**		

* Per 1,000 live-born infants.
† Confidence interval.
§ Odds ratio.
@ Numbers for racial/ethnic groups other than blacks, whites, and Hispanics were too small for meaningful analysis.
** Standard metropolitan statistical area. Large SMSAs have populations ≥ 1,000,000.
++ Some numbers do not total to 14,968 because of missing data: age (one); education (120); smoking and drinking during pregnancy (50); race and ethnicity (two); SMSA (one); and hospital services received (six).

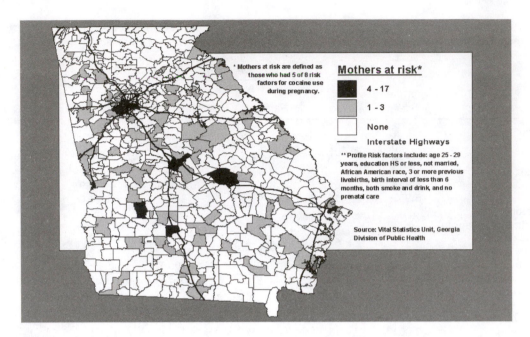

Figure 11–2 Areas with mothers at high risk for using cocaine during pregnancy (as defined by a risk profile developed from the study), by ZIP code of mother's residence; Georgia, February 22 through April 23, 1994

found during the study. Figure 11–3 combines the information in the previous two maps by depicting these "high-risk" ZIP codes simultaneously with the ZIP codes showing confirmed cases of infants testing positive for the cocaine metabolite, BE. These maps illustrate that although infants throughout the state are at risk for perinatal exposure to cocaine, infants in urban areas are more likely to test positive.

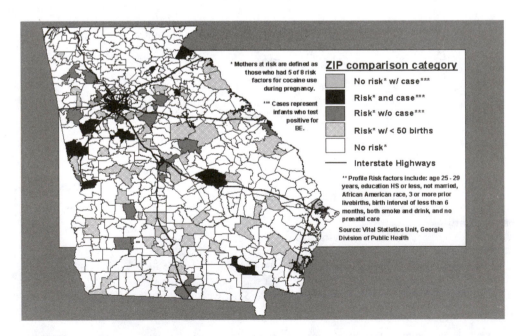

Figure 11–3 Comparison of high-risk ZIP codes identified by a risk profile developed from the study and ZIP codes with confirmed cases of infants testing positive for benzoylecognine (BE), by ZIP code of mother's residence; Georgia, February 22 through April 23, 1994

Certainly, these finding have limitations. The results probably underestimated the true prevalence of cocaine exposure during pregnancy in Georgia for several reasons. First, the laboratory test is unreliable seven days after exposure. Screening newborns only at birth undoubtedly missed exposures that may have come much earlier in pregnancy. Second, the study design created selection bias by excluding from the sample newborns at higher risk for cocaine exposure, such as low–birth weight and premature newborns and newborns in intensive care units. In addition, dried blood samples were not collected for fetal deaths and may not have been collected for newborns dying soon after birth.

Besides evaluating perinatal cocaine exposure, Georgia investigators used GIS technology to evaluate other pregnancy risk factors and pregnancy outcomes by ZIP code of mother's residence. These maps were easy to create because the data were available in the birth (vital statistics) database. Some of them are based on data aggregated over one or more years; others are based on data from the two-month period of the study. Figure 11–4 shows the geographic distribution of congenital syphilis cases reported in 1994; Figure 11–5 shows the geographic distribution of newborns with very low birth weight born during the two-month period of the study; Figure 11–6 shows the geographic distribution of newborns identified as having fetal alcohol syndrome from 1990 through 1994; Figure 11–7 shows the geographic distribution of mothers who had received no prenatal care and who gave birth during the two-month period of the study; Figure 11–8 shows the geographic distribution of mothers reporting heavy alcohol use during pregnancy and giving birth from 1990 through 1994; and Figure 11–9 shows the geographic distribution of mothers reporting heavy smoking during pregnancy and giving birth during the two-month study period.

While these maps are useful, public health officials must ensure that they and others interpret them with caution. As discussed in Chapter 2, our perinatal database relies on self-reports. Physicians filling out birth certificates may not accurately report maternal behaviors such as tobacco, alcohol, and drug use. Other unreliable information may include APGAR scores and gestational age. In addition, some congenital conditions, including fetal alcohol syndrome and congenital syphilis, may not become apparent until some time after birth, making the birth data incomplete and less reliable for geographic analysis of these conditions.

Although public health officials must recognize the limitations of these data sets, the information is still useful for targeting preventive programs. We do not need to know the location of specific individuals with risk factors in designing and targeting population-based prevention programs such as mass education. In addition, having information on areas where women may be at increased risk for behaviors affecting birth outcomes can help officials determine the best location for treatment programs aimed at reducing or preventing such behaviors.

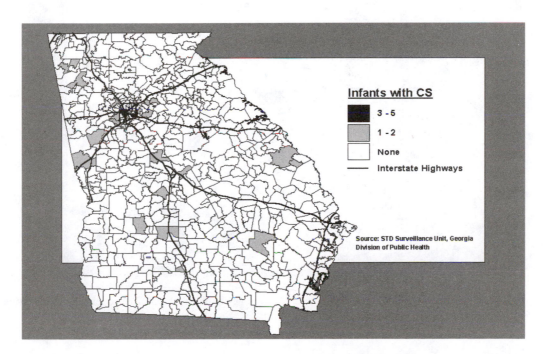

Figure 11–4 Geographic distribution of cases of congenital syphilis (CS) in newborn infants, by ZIP code of mother's residence, Georgia, 1994

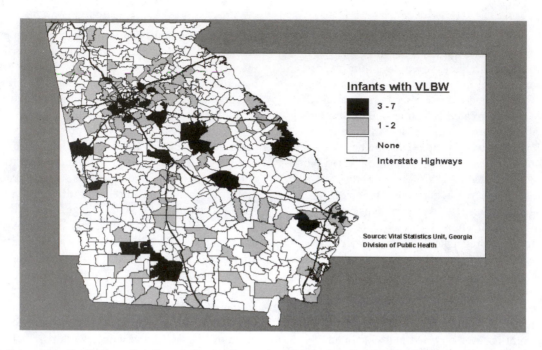

Figure 11–5 Geographic distribution of newborn infants with very low birth weight (VLBW), by ZIP code of mother's residence, Georgia, February 22 through April 23, 1994

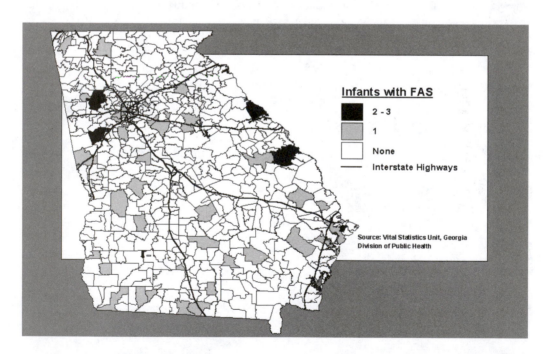

Figure 11–6 Geographic distribution of fetal alcohol syndrome (FAS) in newborn infants, by ZIP code of mother's residence, Georgia, 1990 through 1994

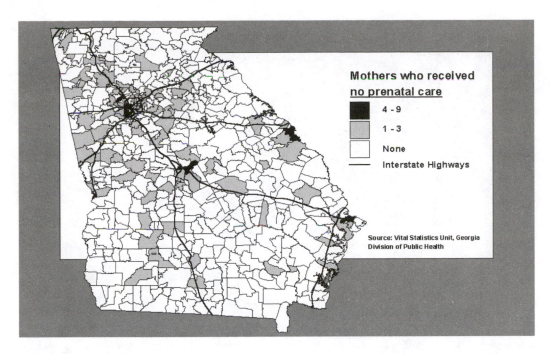

Figure 11–7 Geographic distribution of mothers who received no prenatal care during pregnancy, by ZIP code of mother's residence, Georgia, February 22 through April 23, 1994

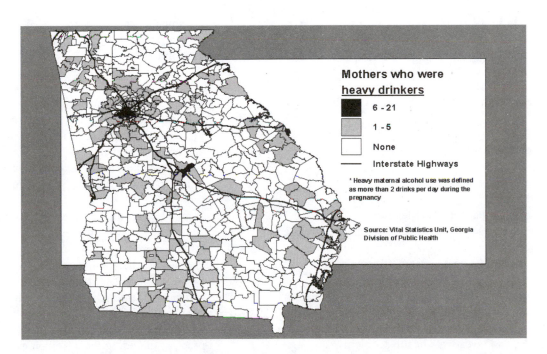

Figure 11–8 Geographic distribution of heavy maternal alcohol use during pregnancy, by ZIP code of mother's residence, Georgia, 1990 through 1994

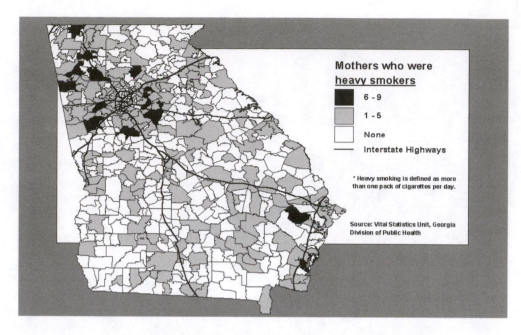

Figure 11–9 Geographic distribution of heavy maternal smoking during pregnancy, by ZIP code of mother's residence, Georgia, February 22 through April 23, 1994

FACILITATING PUBLIC HEALTH PERFORMANCE

Besides facilitating what public health does, GIS technology can facilitate how public health performs its functions. The EPHSWG's second list, the "how" list, described 10 essential services as the practice of public health. These services are:

1. Monitor health status to identify and solve community health problems.
   - Accurate ongoing assessment of the community's health status
   - Identification of threats to health
   - Determination of the needs for personal health care services
   - Attention to the health status of groups that are at higher risk than the total population
   - Collaboration to manage integrated information systems with private providers and health benefit plans
2. Diagnose and investigate health problems.
   - Epidemiologic identification of emerging health threats
   - Access to a public health laboratory capability to conduct rapid screening and high-volume testing
   - Active infectious disease epidemiology programs

   - Technical capacity for epidemiologic investigation of disease outbreaks and patterns of chronic disease and injury
3. Inform, educate, and empower people about health issues.
   - Social marketing and targeted media public communication
   - Provision of accessible health information resources at community levels
   - Active collaboration with personal health care providers to reinforce health promotion messages and programs
   - Joint health education programs with schools, churches, and Web sites
4. Mobilize community partnerships and action to identify and solve health problems.
   - Convening and facilitating community groups and associations (including those not typically considered health related)
   - Undertaking defined health improvement planning process, including the development of preventive, screening, rehabilitation, and support programs
   - Skilled coalition building for community health
5. Develop policies and plans that support individual and community health efforts:
   - Leadership development at all levels of public health

–Systematic community-level and state-level planning for health improvement in all jurisdictions

–Development and tracking of measurable health objectives as a part of continuous quality improvement strategies

–Joint evaluation with the medical health care system to define consistent policy regarding prevention and treatment services

–Development of codes, regulations, and legislation to guide the practice of public health

6. Enforce laws and regulations that protect health and ensure safety.

–Full enforcement of sanitary codes, especially in the food industry

–Full protection of drinking-water supplies

–Enforcement of clean air standards

–Timely follow-up of hazards, preventable injuries, and exposure-related diseases identified in occupational and community settings

–Monitoring of quality of medical services

–Timely review of new drug, biologic, and medical device applications

7. Link people to needed personal health services and ensure the provision of health care when otherwise unavailable (outreach or enabling services).

–Ensuring effective entry for socially disadvantaged people into a coordinated system of clinical care

–Ensuring linkage to services for special population groups through culturally and linguistically appropriate materials and staff

–Ongoing care management

–Transportation services

–Targeted health information to high-risk population groups

–Technical assistance for effective work site health promotion/disease prevention programs

8. Ensure a competent public and personal health care workforce.

–Education and training for personnel to meet the needs for public and personal health service

–Efficient processes for licensure of professionals and certification of facilities with regular verification and inspection follow-up

–Adoption of continuous quality improvement and lifelong learning within all licensure and certification programs

–Active partnerships with professional training programs to ensure community-relevant learning experiences for all students

–Continuing education in management and leadership development programs for those charged with administrative/executive roles

9. Evaluate effectiveness, accessibility, and quality of personal and population-based health services.

–Ongoing evaluation of health programs, based on analysis of health status and service utilization data

–Provision of information necessary for allocating resources and reshaping programs

10. Conduct and support research for new insights and innovative solutions to health problems.

–Continuous linkage with appropriate institutions of higher learning and research

–Internal capacity to mount timely epidemiologic and economic analyses and conduct needed health services research

A thorough review of this list and the examples in this book suggests that GIS technology can facilitate the performance of virtually all of these services. As GIS technology evolves and becomes more widely available, the role of public health officials will undoubtedly evolve with it. Many more data sets, containing information on a broad range of social, demographic, and health-related data, will be available on the Web. The same information now available only to public health officials will be available to the public.[1] On a community level, GIS technology will be essential in evaluating health outcomes, community well-being, and quality of life.[1] On an individual level, GIS technology will be helpful in managing patient care: for example, by facilitating the development of portable health records containing information on clinic visits and preventive services.[1]

Table 11–3 provides some examples of how GIS technology could affect public health practice in the early twenty-first century[1] based on the IOM core functions and the 10 essential services. Underlying these examples is the assumption that data, information, and resources currently available to governmental officials will be available to the public. For example:

- Geographically referenced data will be available to the public on the Internet.
- Data analysis performed by public health officials, including their interpretation of data, will be available to the public.
- Policy decisions made by public health officials will be publicly available.
- Community activists and other "watchdog" groups will have access to the same technological tools, including epidemiologic software, as public health officials. They will use these tools to scrutinize decisions made by public health officials.

Rather than posing a threat, the new technology poses incredible opportunities for public health officials and their

Table 11–3 Examples of Potential GIS Applications in Public Health Management and Practice That May Become Routine in the 21st Century

IOM Core Function	Essential Service	GIS Example	Description of Activity
Assessment	Monitoring health status to identify community health problems	Monitoring crime reports	The law enforcement agency shares data on crime reports. Using GIS, the agency or the local health director prepares maps showing reported teen male arrest rates for violent crime by neighborhood of residence over the past 90 days. Maps also indicate rates or events by weapon used, and the setting of crime occurrence, such as school or home. The maps are available on the Internet for download by the general public, including concerned parents.
Assessment	Diagnosing and investigating health problems and health hazards in the community	Diagnosing health problems	Working in partnership, and using inpatient and outpatient medical records, the local health department (LHD) and hospitals and managed care organizations create maps showing the location of patients with health problems. The health department epidemiologist analyzes the data to determine whether there is geographic clustering of specific health problems that suggest the possibility of natural or manmade environmental causes. The public and the media have access to the same data, but it is in aggregated form, preventing identification of individuals. Pop-up screens and help windows direct the public to local health officials to answer questions and provide additional information.
Policy development	Informing, educating, and empowering people about health issues	Educating on behaviorally based health problems	The LHD has made GIS and data, including the Youth Risk Behavior Survey data, available on the Internet. The software allows parents to map rates of teen smoking by high school attendance areas or any other geographic area. Parents in the Hispanic community, concerned that their children have increased rates of tobacco use, work with the health department and the local board of health to develop a targeted media campaign.
Policy development	Mobilizing community partnerships and action to identify and solve health problems	Mobilizing community partnerships	Local African American leaders are concerned about the incidence of untreated hypertension in their community. In partnership with the LHD and the faith community, they use GIS to map the location of community assets such as churches, and they estimate the demographic composition of each congregation. Community leaders, with support from the local health department, organize a community planning meeting, inviting leadership from the predominantly African American churches. At this meeting, the partners join in developing appropriate health education and health promotion materials and programs.
Policy development	Developing policies and plans that support individual and community health efforts	Conducting joint or competing geographic analyses	The LHD is concerned about health care access. Using available data, the LHD prepares maps showing the residence of patients using safety net agencies and the market share for hospitals and health plans. The LHD estimates and maps the locations of people without health insurance. Two competing local managed care organizations have prepared maps using data available over the Internet. Each set of maps is different. This leads to a debate on data quality and the appropriateness of assumptions and models used in each analysis. The results of this debate will lead to policies aimed at improving access to health care in the community.

continues

Table 11–3 continued

IOM Core Function	Essential Service	GIS Example	Description of Activity
Assurance	Enforcing laws and regulations that protect health and ensure safety	Enforcing regulations	The state environmental agency has cited a factory for violating an ordinance requiring the installation of a filtering device to prevent air pollution. Six months after the citation, an agency inspector uses raster imagery to determine whether the factory installed the filter and to evaluate the amount of environmental damage. The public has access to a Web site maintained by the LHD showing the location of restaurants with significant food code violations.
Assurance	Linking people to needed personal health services and ensure the provision of health care when otherwise unavailable	Linking services to populations in need	An LHD determines that a non–English-speaking immigrant tuberculosis patient also has significant heart disease. Using GIS, an LHD outreach worker finds the location of the nearest physician who speaks the same language as the patient and gives the patient a map with directions to the physician's office in the patient's language.
Assurance	Ensuring a competent public and personal health care workforce	Conducting GIS training for public health employees	The CDC provides GIS educational seminars for LHD employees over the Internet. These seminars allow interaction so that LHD staff can ask questions specific to their community. CDC and LHD staff can quickly construct maps for the discussion. Successful completion of the educational seminar series can lead to public health/GIS certification of the employee.
Assurance	Evaluating effectiveness, accessibility, and quality of personal and population-based health services	Evaluating access	An LHD determines that it needs to open an additional clinic to improve access for WIC and immunization services. Using GIS software and a database with the demographics of current and potential patients, LHD staff determine the location of new clinics that minimize clinic market overlap while maximizing access for vulnerable populations. A state Medicaid agency uses hospitalization data to compare the rates of coronary artery bypass grafts versus angioplasty in different communities within the state. The agency shares the results of the analysis with health care providers and participating hospitals for further study and consideration of practice changes.
Assurance	Conducting and supporting research for new insights and innovative solutions to health problems	Producing serendipitous discoveries and new insights	A researcher in a university geography department maps the water table recharge zone for the water well fields that supply a city's drinking water supply. When adding overlays of a rezoning proposal, the researcher discovers that the proposed high population density, multiple family dwellings, and an industrial park are within the water table recharge zone, threatening the drinking water supply.

communities. Table 11–3 illustrates that GIS technology is eminently compatible with the core public health functions of assessment, policy development, and assurance. Several of the newest public health practice tools, such as Assessment Protocol for Excellence in Public Health (APEXPH)

and its latest version, Mobilizing for Action through Planning and Partnerships (MAPP),[11] are not only compatible with GIS but enhanced through GIS technology.

In the early 1990s, NACCHO, in collaboration with other public health organizations, developed APEXPH as an instrument to enhance the practice of local health departments within their communities. For many health departments and their communities, a major issue had been how to assess community health given the chaotic location of health-related data. The original version of APEXPH, and later APEXPH'98, provided tools to organize the process of community health assessment. The development of MAPP (designed by collaboration between NACCHO and the CDC) further enhanced the process of community health assessment by requiring a strategic approach, tying it to the essential services and engaging communities.[5] The vision for MAPP is "communities achieving improved health and quality of life by mobilizing partnerships and taking strategic action."[11(p.1)] One element of MAPP requires a comprehensive community health status assessment, involving indicators in multiple domains. These domains include asset mapping and quality-of-life, environmental health, socioeconomic, demographic, behavioral risk factors, infection diseases, sentinel events, social and mental health, maternal and child health, health resource availability, and health status indicators. Unquestionably, through its capacity to integrate multiple data sets, GIS technology can enhance the MAPP community health assessment. For jurisdictions containing multiple or diverse communities, GIS tools such as the Community Health Mapping Engine (CHiME) described in Chapter 7 can facilitate the assessment both for the entire jurisdiction and at the subcounty, community level. MAPP and GIS tools are complementary. Future versions of MAPP should include a geospatial component.

The DeKalb County Board of Health (DCBOH), in the Atlanta metropolitan area, has used GIS technology to take the APEXPH process to the subcounty level.[12] In developing its GIS application, the DCBOH decided to use ArcView GIS software for several reasons:

- The state public health agency, the Georgia Division of Public Health, has used ArcView GIS in its Georgia Information Network for Public Health Officials (INPHO) project. To ensure that local GIS applications would be compatible with INPHO, the state has recommended that all 19 health districts in Georgia use ArcView GIS. Although the DCBOH serves as a county health department, it is one of the 19 state administrative areas, also known as health districts. The head of the state agency for public health, the commissioner of the Georgia Department of Human Resources, appoints the director of the DCBOH, subject to approval by the county board of health.
- All environmental health offices in the state had already been using ArcView GIS because the state distributed the software for use in a flood recovery project in 1995.

- The official planning agency for the Atlanta metropolitan area, the Atlanta Regional Commission, has provided a basic course in using ArcView GIS, with discounts for local government agency staff. In addition, to encourage collaboration, the commission has sponsored regular regional meetings for GIS users from different agencies.
- The Atlanta Regional Commission has also provided a spatial database, the Economic Development Information System (EDIS), compatible with ArcView GIS. For only $245, the EDIS CD-ROM contains data on streets, census tracts, and ZIP codes in the region. Compared with a match rate of 60 percent using TIGER, the DCBOH can achieve an 85 percent match rate using EDIS. Trained staff can increase the rate to 95 percent by geocoding records individually using hard-copy city maps.

The DeKalb County Board of Health decided to define communities for analysis based on high school districts. Using the high school districts as a guide, the board used the GIS software to combine contiguous census tracts to form 13 community health assessment areas. Attribute data included birth and death data obtained from state vital records. Using GIS, board staff created maps for each community health assessment area showing five-year averages for

- Infant mortality
- Years of potential life lost (YPLL) for HIV/AIDS, unintentional injuries, cancer, homicide, heart disease, suicide, and stroke

The board of health included these maps in its community health assessment report, *The Status of Health in DeKalb: Opportunities for Prevention and Community Service, 1997.* In addition, since 1997, the DeKalb County Board of Health has been using GIS to display the residences of newborns based on

- Risk for exposure to lead-based paint due to proximity to pre-1950 housing
- Service areas for the five health centers providing primary medical care within the health district

On the basis of this information, the Children First program provides each health center a report helping them follow up and screen children in their service area who are at risk for lead poisoning.

The DeKalb County Board of Health is a large local health department, with an annual budget of over $20 million and approximately 400 staff, serving a population of around

600,000. The department has assigned two staff in their epidemiology office to GIS activities. In addition, a staff member within the environmental health program uses GIS technology. However, only one of the staff does primarily GIS work. The other staff member involved in the project is a data analyst cross-trained in GIS, allowing for support when the primary staff person is unavailable. The DeKalb County Board of Health does not have line-item budget for GIS. GIS activities are included within the Epidemiology program budget.[12]

In addition to APEX and MAPP, GIS technology is compatible with other recently developed public health tools such as PATCH (Planned Approach to Community Health) and the Healthy Communities Model Standards. PATCH, developed by the CDC, includes a process for community needs assessment that is flexible enough to be compatible with GIS.[5] Likewise, the Model Standards steps of community organizational structure assessment, community health needs assessment, determination of local priorities and community health resources, and continuous monitoring and evaluation of effort, lend themselves to GIS analyses.[5,13]

EVALUATING PUBLIC HEALTH AGENCY PERFORMANCE

Besides providing health agencies with a tool to enhance their performance, GIS technology can also help measure public health agency performance. The United States contains approximately 3,000 local health departments. On the basis of local and state factors, these health agencies vary by composition, level of available resources, and the assortment of services they provide.[14–16] The first step in evaluating performance is to determine the jurisdiction served by the health agency. A 1996 survey performed by NACCHO,[13,14] mailed to all 2,834 local health departments within the United States, with a response rate of 88 percent, identified six major categories of local health agency jurisdictions (Table 11–4).

By mapping these jurisdictions (and their attributes), which vary even within states, GIS technology can help evaluate public health performance, as illustrated by several examples. The first example, depicted in Figure 11–10, shows how GIS can identify populations served by health departments with varying types of jurisdiction within a state. Figure 11–10 is a map of North Dakota, with polygons depicting the mix of single-county and multicounty local public health units, known in North Dakota as health districts. Local governments operate these health districts. Counties outside a district are not necessarily without public health services; in such counties, the state health agency may provide local public health services. Without GIS, assessing the health status

Table 11–4 Types of Local Health Department by Jurisdiction

Jurisdiction Type	Number	% of Total Responses
Single county	1,524	61
Multicounty	168	7
Multidistrict	38	2
City-county	257	10
City	200	8
Township	256	10
Other	49	2
Total responders	2,492	100
Nonresponders	293	

of populations served by each district health department would take two steps. One would have to process single-county health data and denominator data, one county at a time, and then aggregate these into each multicounty district. GIS technology facilitates this process by creating the appropriate single- or multicounty polygons representing the health district jurisdictions, geocoding the relevant data, and then incorporating the geocoded data automatically into these jurisdictions on the basis of the latitude/longitude coordinates for each polygon.

Figure 11–11 shows how GIS can help distinguish local health departments not only by jurisdiction, but also by type of services. Wyoming has three types of health agencies:

1. Five multicounty state health department "districts" or administrative regions designed for health planning and delivery
2. Two city-county local health departments operated through an agreement by a city and county government to fund a combined city-county program
3. Twenty-one county health departments operated by a single local government

The polygons depicted in the choropleth map in Figure 11–11 quickly identify the state planning district and local public health agency responsible for services anywhere within the state.

Many states have city health districts providing a variety of services within a county also served by a county health department. Frequently the city health department provides public health services within the city limits, while the county health agency provides services within the county but outside the city. In some cases the county provides some services within the city, with the city agency providing other services. Before the development of GIS, it was possible to display only the jurisdiction served by the city health de-

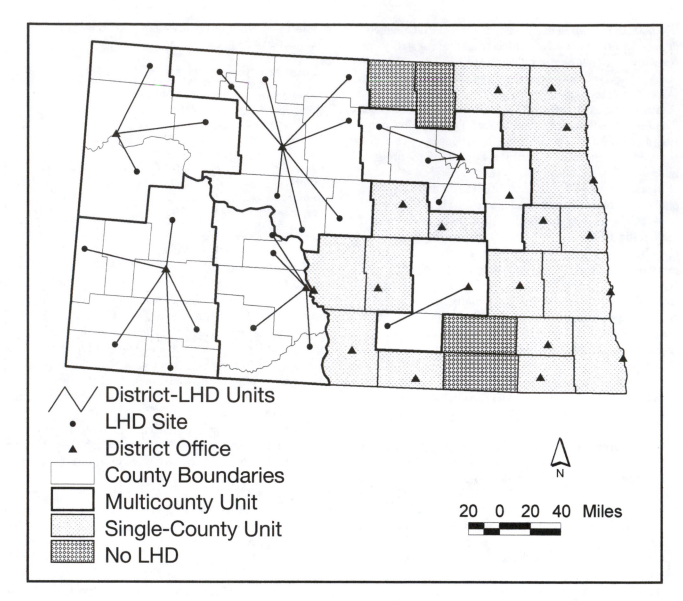

Figure 11–10 Single-county and multicounty local health districts in North Dakota, June 1997. LHD, local health department.

partments or other subcounty health agencies as dots on a map. Figure 11–12, a map of three counties in Ohio, illustrates how GIS technology can map the boundaries of county and coexisting subcounty public health agencies within a state. In Summit County, the Akron City Health district and the city of Baberton provide public health services within their city limits, depicted as clear polygons. The remaining cross-hatched area of the county shows where the Summit County Health District provides public health services. Similar arrangements exist in the neighboring two counties on the map. In addition to depicting these arrangements, GIS technology permits assessment of health status by area served by the city, the county, or both.

In some states, like New Jersey, the arrangements are even more complex, with township and multitownship local health departments providing varying, and in some cases, overlapping public health services. Figure 11–13, a map of local health agencies in Middlesex County, New Jersey, illustrates how easily GIS can portray these relationships. Middlesex County contains seven local health departments. Four are located in single townships (Edison, Piscataway, South Plainfield, and Woodbridge), while multiple township units (Middlebrook Regional Health Commission, Middlesex County Health Department, and South Brunswick Health Department) operate the other three. As with the county-city relationships in Ohio, the boundaries of some of these health

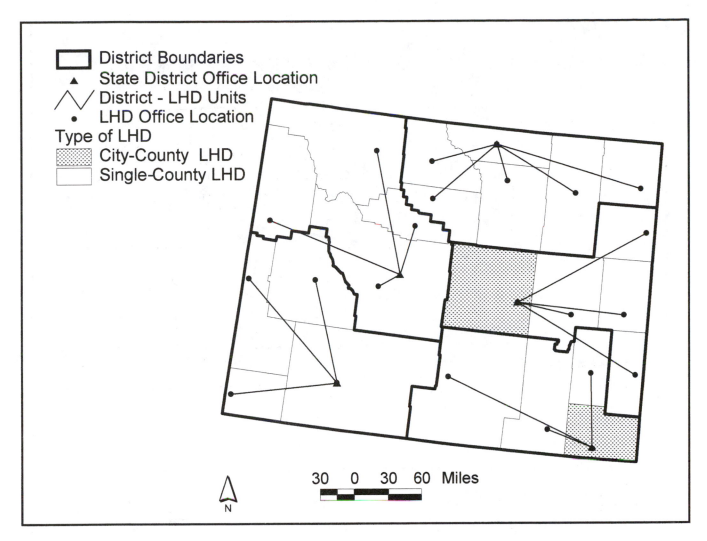

Figure 11–11 City-county and single-county local health departments (LHDs) and the five state public health districts in Wyoming, June 1997

departments may lie within a region served by another public health agency. For example, the Edison Township Health Department is doughnut shaped, completely encircling Metuchen, a township served by another health department. In addition, within New Jersey a single health department may serve noncontiguous areas. For example, the choropleth map shows that the Middlesex County Health Department serves four outlying areas: Dunellen, Metuchen, Perth Amboy, and Carteret. The map illustrates another level of complexity in New Jersey, that local health departments can serve areas located in different political jurisdictions, including different counties. For example, the Middlebrook Regional Health Commission has public health responsibility for one area in Middlesex County (Middlesex Boro) and five areas in neighboring Somerset County (Bound Brook, Green Brook Township, South Bound Brook, Warren Township, and Watchung). Besides portraying these relationships, by linking with other data sources, GIS technology can also analyze and portray community health status by each local agency's jurisdiction, facilitating community health planning.

In addition to the 3,000 local public health departments, the United States contains over 3,000 local boards of health. In most states the boundaries of these entities are the same, but in some there is quite a bit of variation. For example, while New Jersey has four times the number of local boards of health as local health departments, Mississippi has 81 local health departments but no local board of health. GIS technology can not only illustrate these arrangements, including overlap, but also evaluate the delivery of essential services based on these arrangements.[16]

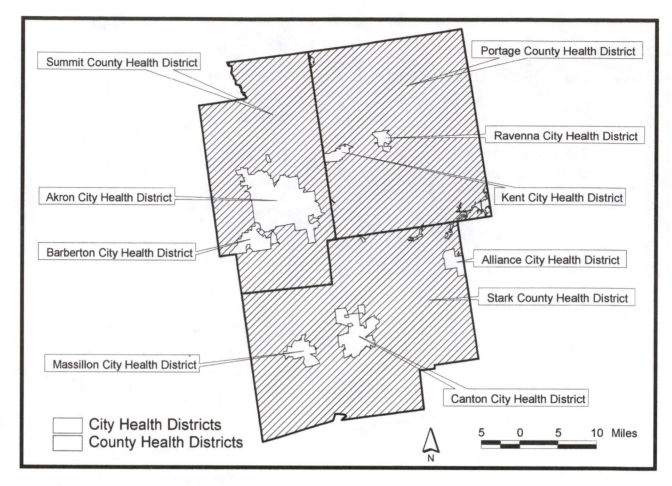

Figure 11–12 City and county local health districts in three counties in Ohio, June 1997

Besides making these complex arrangements understandable, GIS technology has several other applications in evaluating and improving local public health agency performance. First, by classifying public health agencies, by identifying the population they serve, and by linking these data to other attribute data sources, GIS can help select representative health agency samples for surveys evaluating performance of specific essential services. Figure 11–14, from a study in Montana, illustrates this by showing how GIS can help evaluate the performance of one of the 10 essential services. The Montana map contains polygons of county and local health department boundaries and polygons of specific census tracts and block groups. Shaded polygons represent areas designated as medically underserved populations (MUPs) and health professional shortage areas (HPSAs). The Health Resource Services Agency within the U.S. Department of Health and Human Services created these designations based on problems with access to health care for vulnerable populations. Factors considered in these designations include

- The ratio of available health care workforce to the number of people in an area or population group
- Infant mortality or other health status indicators within the area
- Health care access for people living within the area, including ability to pay and accessibility of services

Figure 11–14 illustrates that using GIS to simply overlay health department jurisdiction data with HPSA and MUP data can identify a subset of local health departments containing medically underserved populations within their jurisdiction. By identifying these health departments ahead of time, GIS can help investigators efficiently target appropriate health departments with surveys on their performance of essential service #7: "Link people to needed personal health services and assure the provision of health care when otherwise unavailable."

A second GIS application related to public health performance is its use in evaluating whether surveys of local

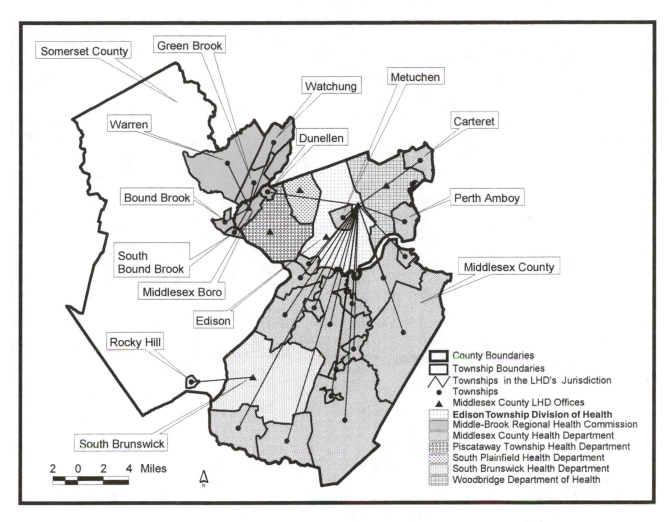

Figure 11–13 Township and multitownship local health departments (LHDs) in Middlesex County, New Jersey, June 1997

health agency performance are representative and valid. By linking survey results to other data sources, GIS can help investigators compare local health agency responders and nonresponders in association with other attribute data, such as demographic data. Figure 11–15, based on a study in Wyoming, illustrates how this might work. The polygons on the Wyoming map represent boundaries of local health departments, with the shading indicating whether the health department responded to the 1997 NACCHO survey of local health department activities. Dots overlaying the polygons represent the population distribution of Native Americans throughout the state, based on U.S. Bureau of the Census demographic data. The map (and underlying tables developed with the GIS application) clearly shows that most (approximately two-thirds) of the Native American population in Wyoming lived in jurisdictions that did not respond to the survey. Obviously, if the survey had included questions about

public health services and activities for Native Americans, the results for Wyoming would not have been representative or valid.[16]

A third potential GIS application related to public health performance is its use in selecting groups of jurisdictions with similar characteristics. These groupings are useful for comparing health outcomes (and therefore performance). One project already underway, the Community Health Status Indicators Project (CHSI), illustrates how GIS technology could facilitate this work. The CHSI, funded by the Health Resources and Services Administration (HRSA), was developed through a collaborative effort by ASTHO, NACCHO, and the Public Health Foundation (PHF).[17] The goal of the CHSI was to present county-level data in a user-friendly format for communities interested in health assessment and planning. Three essential characteristics of the CHSI are its inclusion of multiple data sources, the presentation of multiple

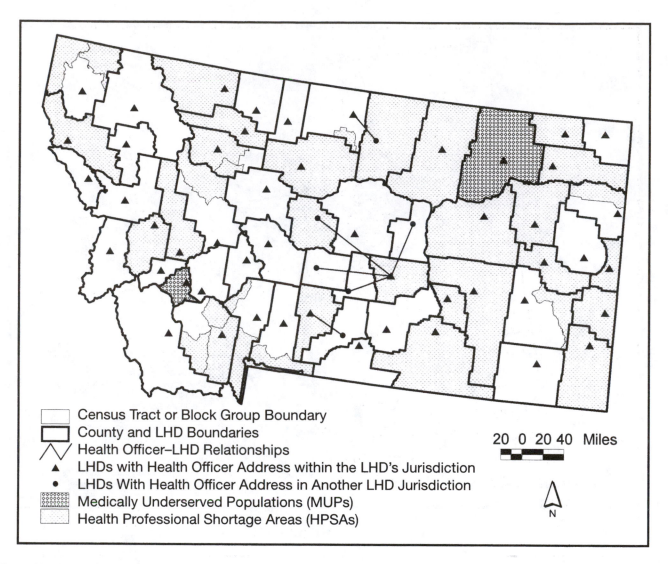

Figure 11–14 LHD boundaries superimposed over the boundaries of census tracts and block groups that were federally designated HPSAs or MUPs in Montana, June 1997

health status indicators for all 3,082 counties across the United States, and comparisons with "peer" counties and other standards. Agencies providing data included

- Centers for Disease Control and Prevention, including the National Center for Health Statistics
- U.S. Bureau of the Census
- U.S. Environmental Protection Agency
- Health Resources and Services Administration
- Substance Abuse and Mental Health Services Administration

Data presentations for each county contained

- Population characteristics
- Four summary measures of health
- Leading causes of death
- Birth and death measures
- Vulnerable populations
- Environmental health measures
- Use of preventive services
- Behavioral risk factors for premature death
- Access to health care

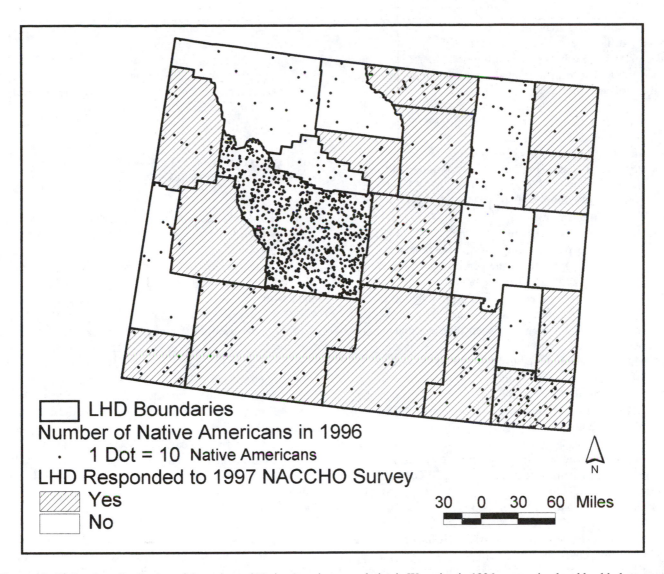

Figure 11–15 Random distribution of the estimated Native American population in Wyoming in 1996, comparing local health department (LHD) jurisdictions that responded and did not respond to the national LHD profile survey conducted in 1997 by the National Association of County and City Health Officials (NACCHO)

For some of the health indicators, no county-level data were available, and project staff substituted state-level data. Reported rates are age adjusted. Readers interested in CHSI reports for specific counties can obtain them in printed or electronic format by contacting the CHSI Web site at <www.communityhealth.hrsa.gov/>.[17] The Web site also contains a link to a companion document, the "Community Health Status Report: Data Sources, Definitions and Notes," containing additional information on data sources and methodology.

The unique feature of the CHSI reports is their inclusion of health measure comparisons for each county with 1997 U.S. rates, *Healthy People 2010* targets, and peer counties. Peer counties are counties sharing several characteristics, such as population size, density, age distribution, and poverty. Each county's CHSI report includes typical (e.g., median) demographic and health status measures for their peer communities. These measures allow communities to compare their health status indicators with other similar communities across the United States.[17,18] Through these comparisons, communities may be able to account for factors that make a difference in their health status.[17,18] To identify the peer groups, an advisory committee of federal, state, and local public health professionals and academics used several factors as criteria:

- Frontier status (the National Committee on Rural Health recommended this classification if the county had fewer than seven persons per square mile)[17–19]
- Population size, using NACCHO's population categories (less than 25,000; 25,000–49,999; 50,000–99,999; 100,000–249,999; 250,000–499,999; 500,000–999,999; 1,000,000 or more)
- Poverty quartiles (less than or equal to 10.55 percent; 10.56–14.15 percent; 14.16–19.25 percent; more than 19.26 percent), based on the percentage of individuals in the county living below the poverty level
- Median age categories, based on the percentage of children (percentage of persons younger than 18 years less than 26.13 percent or greater than or equal to 26.13 percent) and elderly (percentage of persons age 65 or older less than or equal to 14.70 percent or greater than 14.70 percent) in the county
- Population density, as measured by half deciles (e.g., CHSI stratum 45 ranges between 42 and 157 persons per square mile)

Using these criteria in a stepwise process, project staff developed 88 groupings (strata) of 20 to 50 counties, providing several peers for each county. They grouped counties first by frontier status and then population size. Next, depending on the number of counties resulting in each grouping, they used the remaining criteria until they reached an optimum grouping size. As a result, while all county groupings use the first two criteria, only some used the other variables of poverty, age, and population density. Because of the large number within each group, counties can choose a few peer counties that they believe to be most like them for comparison. For more information on the strata determination, readers should consult the HRSA Web site; the site includes a link to a document containing tables showing the characteristics of all 88 strata.[18]

The tables and the reports on the Web site illustrate the project's first attempt at forming peer groupings of counties, but other methods and criteria might prove more useful. GIS technology can help this process in several ways. First, its capacity to incorporate multiple sources of data, including geospatial and attribute data, can help automate the process of peer county selection. After helping select the peer county groupings, GIS technology can provide much more than mere comparisons of summary indicators. It can facilitate comparisons of health status of jurisdictions to each other and to standards such as *Healthy People 2010* using the original raw data sets. In addition, GIS technology is not limited to using counties as the geographic base. The technology can create many other polygons for other types of jurisdictions, such as health districts, cities, towns, and other subcounty jurisdictions for peer comparison purposes and for evaluation of local public health agency performance.

LIMITATIONS OF GIS IN EVALUATING PUBLIC HEALTH PERFORMANCE

As we gain experience using GIS technology to measure community health status and evaluate public health performance, we will need to address several challenges. First, how do we define local health agencies and local boards of health? Figure 11–16, a choropleth map of local health departments and health officers in Montana, illustrates this potential problem. While every Montana county has a local board of health (LBOH) and a health officer, there are six local health departments (LHDs) where the health officer's mailing address is in another jurisdiction. Fifteen LHDs have less than a full-time employee. Cartographers could create very different maps depending on the source they use to define LHDs. If they used the NACCHO and CDC definition, "an administrative or service unit of the local or state government, concerned with health, and carrying some responsibility for the health of a jurisdiction smaller than a state,"[15(p.1)] all 15 counties with less than a full-time person in Montana would appear on the map as LHDs. On the other hand, if they used the ASTHO definition, which requires each LHD to employ at least one full-time person, none of the counties would appear as a LHD.[15] One advantage of GIS technology is that once it contains the attribute data on local health departments, it can instantly create maps based on a variety of definitions.[16]

An additional problem related to LHD definition occurs when states and/or communities establish public health agencies that do not meet the "administrative or service unit of local government" definition. If we are to evaluate and compare performance of different entities, we will need to include these types of public health agencies. South Dakota, with 66 counties but only two LHDs, provides an example of this "alternative" type of public health provider. Before 1966, public health nurses employed by the state provided preventive services from clinics across the state. Beginning in 1966 with a few selected counties, the South Dakota Health Department, local county commissioners, and local health care providers, such as hospitals, formed alliances that moved these clinical services from state responsibility to a local health care entity. The alliances formed community health councils in each county and assigned state public health nurses to assist the councils and coordinate population-based

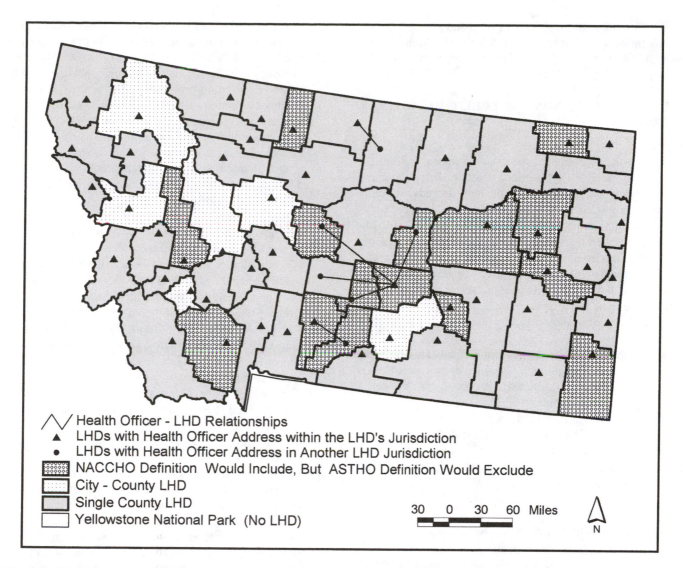

Figure 11–16 Differences in jurisdictions that would be designated as local health departments (LHDs) in Montana in June 1997, comparing the LHD definition recommended by the National Association of County and City Health Officials (NACCHO) with the LHD definition recommended by the Association of State and Territorial Health Officials (ASTHO).

activities. By 1998, 11 counties had established these alternative public health delivery systems.[16]

The variation of roles and responsibilities of different LHDs across and within states in delivering public health services presents a second challenge to GIS evaluation of public health performance. Different LHDs, even within a state, frequently provide different services. For example, some LHDs do not provide environmental services, leaving this responsibility to the state or another local entity. Even if they have the responsibility for a given service, some LHDs choose to contract with another LHD or other entity for delivery of the service. GIS-enhanced evaluations of LHD per-

formance will need to account for these variations when linking community health status and other performance measures to LHD services.[16]

Many performance measures require data for which LHDs have traditionally not had access. As mentioned in earlier chapters, the third challenge to GIS evaluation will be to develop data registries from multiple government and private sources at the local, state, and federal levels. Finally, as mentioned in Chapter 9, confidentiality concerns and statistically unstable rates inherent in small-area analysis present the fourth challenge to GIS analysis of public health performance. To meet this challenge, we will need to develop small-area GIS applications that contain valid and reliable statistical methods while protecting individual and group confidentiality and privacy.[16]

A RESEARCH AGENDA FOR PUBLIC HEALTH GIS

This book has discussed the uses, promises, and limitations of GIS technology in public health practice and management, including how it could evaluate and advance public health performance in the twenty-first century. Considering its value for our communities, public health officials have the responsibility to continue to ensure that promise of this wonderful new tool is realized. To do so, we will need a national public health research agenda aimed at identifying new public health GIS applications and addressing barriers to their successful implementation. Several items for future research must include[1]

- Development of guidelines and methods for data sharing so that governmental agencies at all levels (local, state, and federal) can share and access data collected by their sister agencies
- Guidelines and new methodologies for improving the currency of this data so that policy decisions can be based on analysis of up-to-date information; these guidelines and methodologies must address the timeliness of data sharing
- Development of guidelines and methodology to protect confidentiality and privacy of individuals and groups while presenting information useful for communities conducting health assessments
- Development of standards for monitoring and verifying the quality of data, including data from commercial sources, such as demographic projections; these will include standards for metadata
- Creation of guidelines, recommendations, and perhaps even requirements for data sources on making their data geographically referenced (such as requiring geocoding of vital records or hospital discharge data)
- The identification of additional data, currently not collected or not accessible, that could be useful for public health management and policy decisions
- The development of complementary software, such as Data Wizards, that allow automated incorporation of new data sets into the GIS application
- The evaluation of the role of public health managers and practitioners in providing health information to their communities and the prioritization of this health information

- The development of processes to identify benchmarks or other indices of the quality of health in rural and urban areas
- The design of user-friendly community health planning software, based on prototypes such as the Clackamas County Community Health Mapping Engine (CHiME); this research should develop GIS applications that could help communities perform community health assessments and evaluate community health improvement programs. In addition, this research should address standards for these applications, including epidemiology tutorials, safeguards, and help links to avoid misinterpretation of results
- The design and standards for Internet-enabled GIS to be used by local and regional public health managers and community members (through home or library-based personal computers); these standards should result in applications that look the same anywhere in the United States (or perhaps globally)
- The development of GIS applications useful in planning health services delivery, such as the placement of clinics, hospitals, emergency medical services, and other health care providers
- The creation of "expert systems technology"[1] so that governmental agencies automatically (perhaps over the Internet) check with each other before making policy decisions in order to avoid conflict and improve collaboration
- The institution of policy and funding to ensure the development of local public health GIS technology infrastructure, including data and methodology, especially for LHDs in rural communities lacking technological resources. Development of this GIS infrastructure in resource-depleted areas would be analogous to rural electrification efforts early in the twentieth century, which brought essential infrastructure to areas of need.[1]

THE FUTURE OF GIS AND THE ROLE OF PUBLIC HEALTH OFFICIALS

As we enter the twenty-first century, the development of GIS and other technologies may very well revolutionize the practice of public health. Governments and academics will no longer have exclusive capacity to use analytical technology; the technology will be available and easy to use for everyone.[1] In addition, data sets will become near universally available, with data access constrained only by privacy and confidentiality concerns. One likely role (and responsibility) for public health officials will be provider of community (and individual) health data over the Internet. Health departments will develop Web-based GIS applications allowing any individual, with a minimum of technological ability, to access, analyze, and disseminate an ever-increasing number of health-related data sets. As a result, we will see changes in the organization of public health management and practice as a service industry and changes in ways that public and private organizations at the community level operate and share health-related information.[1]

DIFFUSING THE TECHNOLOGY, SERVING AS RESOURCES, AND INSERTING THE SCIENCE

Although communities will have access to the same tools, data, and technologic resources as public health officials, public health managers will still have many important roles to play. Potential roles include building data systems, mobilizing community partnerships, serving as resources, inserting (and teaching) science, and ultimately facilitating community health improvement. Rather than a traditional "top-down" approach, concerned community residents and organizations will identify community health problems and approach local public health agencies for assistance, either financial or programmatic, to address these problems.[1] Public health officials wanting dialogue and strengthened relationships with local communities, and wanting to develop policy through collaboration, will have to make health information readily available. Through such dialogue with their public health partners, communities will decide what data are relevant for community health improvement. Public health officials will then help obtain the data sets and incorporate them into an effective assessment system. They will essentially create a "one-stop shopping" data system, eliminating the need for users to search for data from multiple sources.

The information will have to be high quality and adequately referenced. Health officials, at all levels, local, state, and federal, will have to work with their public and private partners to develop guidelines for metadata. These guidelines will include standards for geocoding and data quality. In addition, health officials at all levels will have a responsibility, with their public and private partners, to develop guidelines on data sharing and confidentiality. Adequate guidelines should lead to the development of new and improved data sets, such as morbidity data, that will be relevant to every community. Once data become readily available, public health officials will have an additional responsibility to work with their partners in teaching them basic concepts in epidemiology and ensuring that they use the data appropriately.

Like other analytic tools, the greatest promise of GIS technology lies in raising additional questions rather than in coming up with answers. The maps we create will begin or advance, but not end, the process of community health improvement. In this way, the development of GIS and other new technologies may change the fundamental role of public health officials. Public health professionals of the twenty-first century will work closely with their community partners to ask questions about community health at the neighborhood level. Together, we will use the new technology to develop neighborhood-based programs that rely on community strengths and meet community needs. Public health officials will serve as resources and facilitators in gathering data, ensuring data quality, and inviting their partners to the community health improvement table. As the technology and information become more available, public health officials will lead the way in promoting assessment, policy development, and assurance as community responsibilities rather than government responsibilities.

CHAPTER   REVIEW

1. The core functions of public health, as defined by the Institute of Medicine, are assessment, policy development, and assurance. Assessment is collecting, analyzing, and making available information on the health of a community. On the basis of the assessment, public health agencies work with their community partners to develop scientifically based policies aimed at improving community health. Public health agencies then assure their constituents that services based on these policies are available and effective, either by encouraging or requiring others to act or by providing services directly.

2. In early 1994, a working group on the core functions of public health, composed of representatives from public health agencies at the local, state, and federal levels, charged a subgroup to develop a consensus list of the "essential services of public health." The Essential Public Health Services Work Group (EPHSWG) stated that the mission of public health was to "promote physical and mental health and prevent disease, injury and disability." The work group developed two lists, one describing what public health does (the purpose of public health) and the other describing how public health car-

ries out its responsibilities (the practice of public health).

3. The "what" list identified six fundamental obligations of agencies responsible for population-based health as a framework to measure and improve the core functions. GIS technology can help public health agencies at all levels, local, state, and federal, perform their functions and meet these obligations:

   - Prevent epidemics and the spread of disease.
   - Protect against environmental hazards.
   - Prevent injuries.
   - Ensure the quality and accessibility of health services.
   - Promote and encourage healthy behaviors and mental health.
   - Respond to disasters and assist communities in recovery.

4. Besides facilitating what public health does, GIS technology can facilitate how public health performs its functions. The "how" list described 10 essential services as the practice of public health. These services are as follows:

   - Monitor health status to identify and solve community health problems.
   - Diagnose and investigate health problems.
   - Inform, educate, and empower people about health issues.
   - Mobilize community partnerships and action to identify and solve health problems.
   - Develop policies and plans that support individual and community health efforts.
   - Enforce laws and regulations that protect health and ensure safety.
   - Link people to needed personal health services and ensure the provision of health care when otherwise unavailable.
   - Ensure a competent public and personal health care workforce.
   - Evaluate effectiveness, accessibility, and quality of personal and population based health services.
   - Conduct and support research for new insights and innovative solutions to health problems.

5. Several of the newest public health practice tools, such as Assessment Protocol for Excellence in Public Health (APEXPH) and its latest version, Mobilizing for Action through Planning and Partnerships (MAPP), are not only compatible with GIS but enhanced through GIS technology.

6. GIS technology is not just a tool for enhancing public health agency performance. It can also help measure health department performance. The United States contains approximately 3,000 local health departments, which vary by composition, level of avail-

able resources, and the assortment of services they provide. The first step in evaluating performance is to determine the jurisdiction served by each health agency. Many geographic areas receive different services from overlapping county, city, and township health departments. GIS mapping can help by displaying complex arrangements in an easily understood visual format.

7. Besides making complex arrangements understandable, GIS technology has several other applications in evaluating and improving local public health agency performance:

   - It can help select representative health agency samples for surveys evaluating performance of specific essential services.
   - It can evaluate whether surveys of local health agency performance are representative and valid by comparing local health agency responders and nonresponders in association with other attribute data.
   - GIS technology is helpful for selecting groups of jurisdictions with similar characteristics. These groupings are useful for comparing health outcomes (and therefore performance). One project already underway, the Community Health Status Indicators Project (CHSI), allows communities to compare their health status indicators with those of other similar communities across the United States. Through these comparisons, communities might be able to account for factors that make a difference in their health status.

8. As we gain experience using GIS technology to measure community health status and evaluate public health performance, we will need to address several challenges related to

   - The definition of local health agencies and local boards of health
   - The variation of roles and responsibilities of different local health departments across and within states in delivering public health services
   - The need for additional data previously not available to local health departments but required to adequately measure performance
   - Confidentiality concerns and statistically unstable rates inherent in small area analysis

9. To ensure that we make maximal use of GIS technology, we need a national public health research agenda aimed at identifying new public health GIS applications and addressing barriers to their successful implementation. Items for future research should include the development of guidelines, methods, and standards for

   - Data sharing, ensuring that different agencies use data collaboratively

- The identification and automatic incorporation of new data that could be useful for public health management and policy decisions
- Internet-enabled GIS
- Ensuring data currency and quality
- Ensuring the confidentiality and privacy of individuals and groups
- Ensuring that data are geographically referenced
- Ensuring that user-friendly community health planning software includes safeguards to prevent misinterpretation of results

In addition, future research should address

- The evaluation of the role of public health managers and practitioners in providing health information to their communities
- The development of processes to identify benchmarks or other indices of the quality of community health

- The development of GIS applications useful in planning health services delivery
- Policies that ensure the development of local public health GIS technology infrastructure, especially in rural communities lacking technological resources

10. Public health professionals of the twenty-first century will work closely with their community partners to ask questions about community health at the neighborhood level. Public health officials will serve as resources and facilitators in gathering data, ensuring data quality, and inviting their partners to collaborate in improving community health. As GIS technology and data become more accessible, public health officials will lead the way in promoting assessment, policy development, and assurance as community responsibilities rather than government responsibilities.

REFERENCES

1. G.I. Thrall. "The Future of GIS in Public Health Management and Practice." *Journal of Public Health Management and Practice* 5, no. 4 (1999): 75–82.

2. H. Emerson. *Local Health Units for the Nation: A Report of the Subcommittee on Local Health Units, Committee on Administrative Practice, American Public Health Association.* New York: Commonwealth Fund, 1945.

3. J.A. Harrell et al. "The Essential Services of Public Health. Leadership in Public Health." *University of Illinois at Chicago* 3, no. 3 (fall 1994): 27–31.

4. Committee for the Study of the Future of Public Health. Institute of Medicine, Division of Health Care Services. *The Future of Public Health.* Washington, DC: National Academy Press, 1988.

5. B. Turnock. *Public Health: What It Is and How It Works.* Gaithersburg, MD: Aspen Publishers, Inc., 2001.

6. A. Melnick et al. "Clackamas County Department of Human Services Community Health Mapping Engine (CHiME) Geographic Information Systems Project." *Journal of Public Health Management and Practice* 5, no. 2 (1999): 64–69.

7. M.Y. Rogers. "Using Marketing Information To Focus Smoking Cessation Programs in Specific Census Block Groups along the Buford Highway Corridor, DeKalb County, Georgia, 1996." *Journal of Public Health Management and Practice* 5, no. 2 (1999): 55–56.

8. Claritas PRIZM Lifestyle Cluster data sets were licensed through Claritas, Inc., by the Georgia Department of Human Resources, Division of Public Health, for local public health planning.

9. M.D. Brantley et al. "Population-Based Prevalence of Cocaine in Newborn Infants: Georgia 1994," in *Geographic Information Systems in Public Health: Proceedings from the Third National Conference,* eds. R.C. Williams et al. San Diego, CA: U.S. Department of Health and Human Services, Agency for Toxic Substances and Disease Registry, 1998: 509–523.

10. Centers for Disease Control and Prevention. "Population-Based Prevalence of Perinatal Exposure to Cocaine: Georgia 1994." *Morbidity and Mortality Weekly Report* 45, no. 41 (1996): 887–891.

11. National Association of County and City Health Officials. "Mobilizing for Action through Planning and Partnerships." Washington, DC, 2000. <www.naccho.org/PROJECT77.cfm>.

12. M.Y. Rogers. "Getting Started with Geographic Information Systems (GIS): A Local Health Department Perspective." *Journal of Public Health Management and Practice* 5, no. 4 (1999): 22–33.

13. American Public Health Association. *Healthy Communities 2000: Model Standards.* Washington, DC: American Public Health Association, 1991.

14. National Association of County and City Health Officials. *1992–1993 National Profile of Local Health Departments.* Washington, DC: NACCHO, 1995.

15. National Association of County and City Health Officials. *Preliminary Results from the 1997 Profile of U.S. Local Health Departments.* Research Brief No. 1. Washington, DC: NACCHO, 1998.

16. T.B. Richards. "Toward a GIS Sampling Frame for Surveys of Local Health Departments and Local Boards of Health." *Journal of Public Health Management and Practice* 5, no. 4 (1999):65–75.

17. National Association of County and City Health Officials. "Community Health Status Indicators Project (CHSI)." Washington, DC. <www.naccho.org/PROJECT2.cfm>.

18. Health Resources and Services Administration. "Community Health Status Indicators Project." <www.communityhealth.hrsa.gov/>.

19. F.J. Popper. "The Strange Case of the Contemporary American Frontier." *Yale Review* 76, no. 1 (1986): 101–121.

Glossary

SOURCES

Definitions are from the following sites:

- <www.census.gov/geo/www/tiger/glossary.html>
- <http://nhresnet.sr.unh.edu/granitNet/granit/glossary.html>
- <www.esri.com/library/glossary/glossary.html>
- <www.env.gov.bc.ca/gis/glosstxt.html>
- <www.atsdr.cdc.gov/glossary.html>
- <http://giswww.pok.ibm.com/glosstext.html>
- <www.cdc.gov/nchs/icd9.htm>
- <www.hcfa.gov/stats/medpar.htm>

Address
The number or other designation assigned to a housing unit, business establishment, or other structure for mail delivery, emergency services, etc.

Aggregate
To combine records in a data file by geographic area or by attribute. For example, GIS software can combine birth records for analysis on the basis of whether they share a common location, such as census block group, census tract, county, or state, or whether they share an attribute, such as mother's age or ethnicity.

Aggregation, baseline
The baseline aggregation is the smallest geographic level of aggregation for which data are available.

Aggregation, higher-level
The aggregation of the data available at lower baseline levels into larger geographic areas. For example, a higher level of aggregation results when assigning records with information on census block group into census tracts, counties, or states for analysis.

Attribute data
Data containing information on any theme of interest. Attribute data can include morbidity and mortality information as well as social, demographic, economic, and environmental data.

Average daily traffic flow (ADT)
The average number of cars traveling on a road per weekday, generally calculated from a minimum of 48 hours of weekday traffic flow.

Base map
A digital map containing data on the fundamental features that will contribute to the final map, such as county boundaries, census tract and census block group boundaries, streets, and environmental features such as rivers. The base map is the foundation for later adding health-related data for geographic analysis.

Biologic plausibility
How consistent a proposed disease cause is with what is known about the biology of the disease process.

Block group (BG)
A combination of census blocks that is a subdivision of a census tract or block numbering area (BNA). A BG consists of all blocks whose numbers begin with the same digit in a given census tract or BNA: for example, BG 3 within a census tract or BNA includes all blocks numbered between 301 and 399. The BG, generally consisting of between 300 and

3,000 people, is the lowest level of geography for which the U.S. Bureau of the Census has tabulated sample data in the 1990 census. It was used to tabulate sample data in the 1970 and 1980 censuses only for those areas that had block numbers.

Block number
A three-digit number, which may have a one- or two-letter alphabetic suffix for the census, identifying a specific census block.

Block numbering area (BNA)
An area delineated by state officials or the U.S. Bureau of the Census, following bureau guidelines, for grouping and numbering census blocks in counties or equivalent entities in which census tracts have not been established. A BNA is equivalent to a census tract in the bureau's geographic hierarchy.

Buffer
A geographic area, created using GIS software, of designed width around a point, line, or area. For example, GIS software can draw a 25 m zone around main roads to identify areas with potentially high levels of lead. Then the software can calculate the number of events, such as the number of children with reported high lead levels, or the size of a denominator population, such as the number of children aged birth to six years living within the buffer area.

Census (decennial)
The enumeration of population and housing, taken by the U.S. Bureau of the Census in years ending in zero. Article 1 of the U.S. Constitution requires that a census be taken every 10 years for reapportioning the U.S. House of Representatives. The first census was taken in 1790; the census of housing began in 1940.

Census block
The smallest entity for which the U.S. Bureau of the Census collects and tabulates decennial census information; bounded on all sides by visible and nonvisible features shown on bureau maps.

Census-designated place (CDP)
The U.S. Bureau of the Census defines a CDP as an entity comprising a densely settled concentration of people outside of an incorporated place but locally identified by a name. State and local officials and the U.S. Bureau of the Census cooperatively delineate CDPs following bureau guidelines. For the 1940 through the 1970 censuses, CDPs were called unincorporated places.

Census division
A grouping of states within a census region established by the U.S. Bureau of the Census. Currently, the nine divisions (East North Central, East South Central, Middle Atlantic, Mountain, New England, Pacific, South Atlantic, West North Central, and West South Central) represent relatively homogeneous areas within each region.

Census region
Four groupings of states (Northeast, South, Midwest, and West) established by the U.S. Bureau of the Census in 1942. The bureau subdivides each region into divisions. (See **Census division**.)

Census tract
A small, relatively permanent statistical subdivision of a county in a metropolitan area (MA) or a selected nonmetropolitan county, delineated by a local committee of census data users (a CSAC) for presenting decennial census data. Census tract boundaries normally follow visible features but may follow governmental unit boundaries and other nonvisible features in some instances; they always nest within counties. Designed to be relatively homogeneous units with respect to population characteristics, economic status, and living conditions at the time the CSAC established them, census tracts usually contain between 1,000 and 8,000 inhabitants. They may be split by any subcounty geographic entity.

Census tract number
A four-digit number, sometimes with a two-digit suffix, identifying a census tract. Census tract numbers are unique within a county and usually unique within a metropolitan area (MA). Almost all census tract numbers range from 0001 to 9499, but the leading zeros are not shown on U.S. Bureau of the Census maps or printed reports.

Central place
The core incorporated place(s) or census-designated place(s) of an urbanized area, usually consisting of the most populous place(s) in the urban area. If a central place also is defined as an extended city, only the portion of the central place contained within the urbanized area is recognized as the central place.

Centroid
The central location within a specified geographic area.

Chart/graph map
A type of map that displays bar charts, line charts, or pie charts instead of symbols.

Choropleth map

Type of map in which given geographic areas, or polygons, such as census tracts or counties, are shaded to depict the value of an attribute, such as the percentage of older housing stock within each geographic area.

Chronic diseases

Illnesses that are prolonged, do not resolve spontaneously, and are rarely cured completely.

City

A type of incorporated place in 49 states and the District of Columbia. In 20 states, some or all cities are not part of any minor civil division (MCD). The U.S. Bureau of the Census treats these as county subdivisions, equivalent to MCDs.

Cluster

A disease cluster of any kind is the occurrence of a greater than expected number of cases of a particular disease within a group of people, a geographic area, or a period of time.

Comprehensive Environmental Response, Compensation and Liability Act (CERCLA)

Enacted in 1980, the Comprehensive Environmental Response, Compensation and Liability Act (CERCLA) created the EPA Superfund Program. Amended by the 1986 Superfund Amendments and Reauthorization ACT (SARA), the Superfund Program has broad authority to respond to uncontrolled releases of hazardous substances from inactive hazardous waste sites that endanger public health.

Conformal projection

A map projection that preserves shapes but, in doing so, distorts distances and size (area).

Congressional district (CD)

An area established by state officials or the courts for electing a person to the U.S. House of Representatives. Each CD within a state must contain, as nearly as possible, an equal number of inhabitants. Following each decennial census, the number of CDs within each state may change, and the boundaries may change more than once during a decade.

Consolidated metropolitan statistical area (CMSA)

The U.S. Office of Management and Budget (OMB) designates a geographic area as a CMSA on the basis of the following criteria: it must qualify as a metropolitan statistical area (MSA), it must contain a population of at least one million, it must contain components recognized as primary metropolitan statistical areas (PMSAs), and local opinion must favor the designation. Outside of New England, whole counties are components of CMSAs; within New England, cities and towns are components. (See **Metropolitan area, Metropolitan statistical area, Primary metropolitan statistical area**.)

Contiguous

A descriptive term for geographic areas adjacent to one another, sharing either a common boundary or a common point.

Contour lines

Lines on an isopleth map connecting points having the same attribute, such as elevation or a rate or proportion (e.g., the proportion of people without health insurance).

Coordinate system

References used to display the locations of points in space in either two or three dimensions. With a vector database, points, lines, and polygons are generally expressed on a two-dimensional (planimetric) map using x and y coordinates. In a raster database, row and column numbers of cells are considered coordinates.

County

A type of governmental unit that is the primary legal subdivision of every state except Alaska and Louisiana. In Alaska, the corresponding unit is called a borough; in Louisiana, a parish.

County subdivision

A legal division of a county recognized by the U.S. Bureau of the Census for data collection. Examples include, but are not limited to, cities, towns, townships, minor civil divisions, and villages.

Decennial census

See **Census (decennial)**.

Diagnosis-related grouping (DRG) system

In 1982, the U.S. Congress passed the Tax Equity and Fiscal Responsibility Act (TEFRA) to control hospital costs. On the basis of TEFRA, effective October 1, 1983, Medicare implemented a prospective payment system (PPS) for reimbursing inpatient hospital operating costs. This system replaced the existing retrospective cost reimbursement system whereby interim rates were paid on each bill and end-of-year adjustments were made on the basis of the information contained in hospital cost reports. Most hospitals are now paid a fixed amount, determined in advance, for the operating costs of each case according to one of approximately

500 diagnosis-related groups (DRGs). A discharge is assigned to a DRG on the basis of diagnosis, surgery, patient age, discharge destination, and sex. Each DRG has a weight established for it, based primarily on Medicare billing and cost data. Each weight reflects the relative cost, across all hospitals, of treating cases classified in that DRG. Medicaid now also uses the DRG PPS. Hospitals receive a flat fee for the hospitalization of a patient with a diagnosis within a DRG, regardless of the actual costs incurred in the patient's course of treatment. If incurred costs are higher than the prospective payment, the hospital absorbs the loss; if the costs are lower, the hospital retains the difference.

Digital map
In contrast to an analog (paper) map, a digital map is stored, displayed, and analyzed on a computer.

Digitize
To convert analog map data into digital data for use in a computer. (See **Scanning**.)

Dose-response relationship
The association between exposure to increasing doses of a chemical or other environmental agent, such as radiation, and a subsequent disease outcome, such as cancer. A positive relationship strengthens the likelihood, but does not prove, that exposure to the agent caused the disease.

Ecologic fallacy (ecologic bias)
An erroneous conclusion of a causal relationship between a suspected risk factor and a disease outcome based on associations found at the population level. An example of the ecologic fallacy would be concluding that coffee consumption increases the risk for heart disease on the basis of a comparison of coffee consumption and heart disease incidence rates in different countries. Ecologic fallacy can be avoided by using study designs, such as cohort and case-control studies, that evaluate risk factors and disease status of individuals.

Enterprise GIS
A GIS serving as a centralized assessment tool for use by several agencies and their partners.

Environmental justice
The fair treatment and meaningful involvement of all people regardless of race, color, national origin, or income with respect to the development, implementation, and enforcement of environmental laws, regulations, and policies. Fair treatment means that no group of people, including a racial, ethnic, or socioeconomic group, should bear a disproportionate share of the negative environmental consequences resulting from industrial, municipal, and commercial operations or the

execution of federal, state, local, and tribal programs and policies. The goal of environmental justice is to ensure that all people, regardless of race, national origin, or income, are protected from disproportionate impacts of environmental hazards. To be classified as an environmental justice community, residents must be a minority and/or low-income group; excluded from the environmental policy setting and/or decision-making process; subject to a disproportionate impact from one or more environmental hazards; and experiencing a disparate implementation of environmental regulations, requirements, practices, and activities in their communities.

Equal-area projection
A map projection that maintains areas accurately but, in doing so, distorts distances and shapes.

Equidistant projection
A map projection that measures distances accurately but, in doing so, distorts size (area) and shape.

Exposure
The dose of a substance reaching an individual.

Feature
Features define any part of the landscape, whether natural or manmade, visible or nonvisible. Maps can display all kinds of features. (See **Natural feature, Nonvisible feature,** and **Visible feature.**)

Geocoding
The process by which GIS software matches each record in an attribute database with the geographic files. By using the address information in an attribute database and comparing this with the address information in a stored spatial database, the geocoding process assigns each record in the attribute database to a point location on a map.

Geographic hierarchy
A system of relationships among geographic areas, in which each area (except the smallest) is subdivided into smaller areas that in turn may be subdivided further. For example, from largest to smallest: nation, region, division, state, county, census tract, block group, block.

Global Positioning System (GPS)
The GPS relies on a network of satellites originally developed by the U.S. military for navigational purposes. Now civilians using hand-held ground instruments that receive signals from these satellites can precisely calculate their own location with a high degree of accuracy. Investigators in the field can use these devices to identify the location of spe-

cific events and risk factors and can incorporate these data into their GIS for mapping.

Governmental unit
A geographic entity established by legal action for implementing administrative or governmental functions.

Graduated symbol map
See **Proportional symbol map**.

Health district
A governmental unit specifically providing public health services representing multiple counties or city-county combinations.

Hospital referral regions
Three hundred six tertiary care regions made up of groups of hospital service areas based on hospitalization for major cardiovascular procedures.

Hospital service areas (HSAs)
Health care markets where most Medicare beneficiaries receive inpatient care.

Incorporated place
Within the United States, a type of governmental unit, incorporated under state law as a city, town (except in New England, New York, and Wisconsin), borough (except in Alaska and New York), or village, having legally prescribed limits, powers, and functions.

International Classification of Disease (ICD) codes
International Classification of Disease (ICD) codes, published by the World Health Organization, refer to two related ways to classify diseases, the ICD-9 (International Classification of Diseases, Ninth Revision) and the ICD-9-CM (The International Classification of Diseases, Ninth Revision, Clinical Modification). The ICD-9 is the classification used to code and classify mortality data from death certificates. The latest revision, the ICD-10, is replacing the ICD-9. The ICD-9-CM is used to code and classify morbidity data from inpatient and outpatient records, physician offices, and most National Center for Health Statistics surveys. The ICD-9-CM consists of a tabular list containing a numerical list of the disease code numbers in tabular form; an alphabetical index to the disease entries; and a classification system for surgical, diagnostic, and therapeutic procedures. The ICD coding system is designed to promote international comparability in the collection, processing, classification, and presentation of mortality statistics. This includes providing a consistent format for reporting causes of death on the death certificate. More information on the ICD-10 classification

system is available at the World Health Organization Web site at <www.who.int/whosis/icd10/index.html>.

Isopleth map
A map that displays attribute data, such as the proportion of adults without health insurance, by lines or contours that connect points having the same value of the attribute.

LANDSAT
A program developed by the National Aeronautics and Space Administration (NASA) using U.S.–launched satellites to produce images of the earth's surface.

Latitude
Based on a spherical reference system, latitude is the angular distance north and south of the equator on the earth's surface.

Legislative district
An area from which resident voters elect a person to serve in a state legislative body.

Linear feature
A geographic entity, such as a street, waterway, boundary, or railroad, that can be represented by a line in a vector database.

Lines
Features, such as streets, connecting two or more points on a vector map.

Longitude
Based on a spherical reference system, longitude is the angular distance east and west of the prime (Greenwich) meridian.

Map objects
Data layers and health features within the data layers.

Match rate
The proportion of records containing an address in a data file that are matched with a point on a digital map.

Matching
The ability to match data containing an address with a point on a map.

Mean
The mean is equal to the sum of all quantities or values in a group of measurements divided by the number of quantities or values in the group.

Media

An environmental term encompassing soil, water, air, plants, animals, or any other parts of the environment that can contain contaminants.

Median

The quantity or value dividing a group of quantities or values into two equal groups, so that half of the quantities or values are greater than the median and half are less than the median.

Meridian

A line drawn on the earth's surface connecting the shortest distance between the poles.

Metadata

Data about data, including details on the data source, quality, timeliness, and reliability.

Metropolitan area

An inclusive term, established by the U.S. Office of Management and Budget (OMB), that refers to metropolitan statistical areas (MSAs), consolidated metropolitan statistical areas (CMSAs), and primary metropolitan statistical areas (PMSAs). Before 1983, the OMB defined these areas as standard metropolitan statistical areas (SMSAs). For New England, the OMB has defined an alternative set of areas, New England County Metropolitan Areas (NECMAs).

Metropolitan statistical area (MSA)

A geographic entity defined by the U.S. Office of Management and Budget (OMB) for use by federal agencies, based on a core area containing a large population with contiguous communities having significant social and economic integration with the core. To be qualified as an MSA, an area must contain a city with a population of at least 50,000 or an urban area with a total population of at least 100,000 (75,000 in New England). The county or counties containing the largest city and surrounding densely populated areas are central counties of the MSA. To be included in the MSA, additional outlying counties must meet other criteria of metropolitan character, such as a specified minimum population density or percentage of the population that is urban. In New England, the OMB defines MSAs in terms of cities and towns, following rules concerning commuting and population density.

Minor civil division (MCD)

A type of governmental unit that is the primary legal subdivision of a county in 28 states, created to govern or administer an area rather than a specific population. Towns, townships, and districts are examples of MCDs.

Modeling

A procedure for testing hypotheses about causes of disease and the nature and processes of disease transmission. Investigators can use GIS to identify geographic areas where suspected risk factors for a disease exist. Because GIS technology can consider a large number of risk factors, investigators can create models based on different combinations of risk factors and can test these models in relation to how well they predict disease outcomes.

Municipality

A generic term for a general-purpose local government, such as a minor civil division.

National Priorities List (NPL)

The Environmental Protection Agency's listing of hazardous sites that have undergone preliminary assessment and site inspection to determine which locations pose immediate threat to persons living or working near the hazardous release. These sites are most in need of cleanup.

Natural feature

Any part of the landscape resulting from natural processes in contrast to manmade features. Streams, rivers, and ridges are examples of natural features.

Nonvisible feature

Any feature on a map that is not visible, such as a political boundary (city or county line), a property line, or an imaginary extension of a street or road.

Office of Management and Budget (OMB)

The OMB is part of the Executive Branch of the U.S. government. It is responsible for evaluating, formulating, and coordinating management procedures and program objectives within and among federal departments and agencies. It also controls the administration of the federal budget and routinely gives U.S. presidents recommendations regarding budget proposals and relevant legislative enactments.

Overlay

An overlay displays more than one attribute or theme on a map at a time. For example, an overlay can portray housing data and reported cases of high lead levels on one map.

Parcel

A particular piece of land, or lot.

Pixel

A cell in a raster-format spatial database.

Place

A concentration of population with legal boundaries (an incorporated place) or a concentration of population delineated by the U.S. Bureau of the Census as a census-designated place (CDP).

Planimetric maps

Maps that show land features in a two-dimensional representation and do not include topographical or relief data.

Plume

An area of chemicals in a particular medium, such as air or groundwater, moving away from its source in a long band or column. A plume can be a column of smoke from a chimney or chemicals moving with groundwater.

Points

Exact location on the earth (e.g., location of alcohol-serving outlets) with specific x and y coordinates (latitude and longitude).

Polygons

Specific two-dimensional areas on a map enclosed by boundary lines, such as county boundaries, blocks, block groups, or census tracts.

Population density

A numerical expression of the extent to which people cluster within a specific geographic area, expressed by the number of people per square mile or per square kilometer. To calculate the population density, divide the total population of an entity, such as a city or county, by the total land area of the entity.

Post office box address

An address referring to a box number in a post office building. The post office box address does not refer to the actual physical location of a housing unit or business establishment.

Primary metropolitan statistical area (PMSA)

A geographic entity defined by the U.S. Office of Management and Budget (OMB) for use by federal agencies, consisting of a large urbanized county or a cluster of such counties (cities and towns in New England) having substantial commuting interchange. To meet this definition, a PMSA must exist within a metropolitan statistical area (MSA) containing a population of at least one million. Within such MSAs, the OMB may define two or more PMSAs if they meet statistical criteria and if local opinion is in favor. When the OMB recognizes one or more PMSAs within an MSA, the balance of the original, larger area becomes an additional PMSA, and the OMB then designates the larger area of which the PMSAs are components as a consolidated metropolitan statistical area (CMSA).

Prime meridian

0° longitude (Greenwich meridian), creating a plane on the earth's surface from which angles are measured to establish longitude.

Probability map

A map showing the probability that observed rates in given geographic areas are significantly higher than expected, with p values for each area.

Projection

The mathematical model that transforms three-dimensional features on the earth's curved surface to a two-dimensional map.

Proportional symbol map

An event map in which the size of the symbol is proportional to the number of events at a given location.

Proximate population

In a spatial coincidence study, the population living within the same block group or within a buffer containing a toxic release inventory (TRI) facility or other potential environmental hazard.

Query

The ability to query is a feature of GIS software that allows users to ask questions about geographic data. For example, a user could query a patient database to select all patients living within a specified distance (buffer) of a clinic site. Then the user could perform additional operations on the data, such as determining the proportion of these patients with commercial insurance.

Raster

A regular grid of cells covering a geographic area.

Raster database

A database containing spatial and attribute information in the form of a grid of cells. Cells with the same values represent specific features, such as forests, bogs, or other land uses.

Region (census geographic)

See **Census region**.

Registry

A system for collecting and maintaining, in a structured record, information on specific persons from a defined population. For example, state cancer registries collect and maintain data on state residents diagnosed with cancer.

Remote sensing

The measurement of features on the earth's surface by a sensor (such as a satellite) that is not in direct physical contact with the earth's surface.

Reservation, American Indian

An American Indian entity with boundaries established by treaty, statute, and/or executive or court order. Federal and state governments have established reservations as territory over which American Indians have governmental jurisdiction. The U.S. Bureau of Indian Affairs (BIA), within the U.S. Department of the Interior, identifies for the U.S. Bureau of the Census the federally recognized reservations, their names, and their boundaries. State governments identify the names and boundaries of state reservations.

Resolution

A measure of the accuracy at which a map can show the location and shape of features. The smaller the scale, the larger the area displayed on a map and the smaller the resolution. Maps of large areas with low resolution cannot display as much detail as maps of smaller geographic areas and may not be able to display very small features. On a raster database, resolution is inversely proportional to the size of the cells in the database. The smaller the cells, the greater the degree of resolution, the smaller the land area displayed, and the greater the accuracy.

Route of exposure

The way in which a person may contact a chemical substance. For example, drinking/eating (ingestion) and bathing (skin contact) are two different routes of exposure to contaminants that may be found in water.

Rubber sheeting

A process that transforms spatial data by stretching or compressing the data to fit with other data.

Rural

Within the United States, the population and territory outside any urban area (UA) and the urban part of any place with a decennial census population of 2,500 or more.

Rural address

An address consisting of a delivery route number and a box number, both assigned by the local post office for delivery of mail at a specific physical location.

Rural-urban continuum codes

U.S. Department of Agriculture (USDA) codes that classify all U.S. counties by the degree of urbanization and adjacency to a metropolitan area. The USDA uses these codes in determining eligibility for several federal programs. The codes allow researchers to break county-level data into finer residential groups than the standard metro/nonmetro. The USDA developed these codes on the basis of the June 1993 Office of Management and Budget definition of metropolitan and nonmetropolitan counties.

Sample

A subset of a population, used to estimate information about the population. In the verb form, *to sample* is to select statistically a subset of the total population to estimate information about the population.

Satellite imagery

Digital data obtained from remote sensors on satellites.

Scale

The ratio between the size of an object (or the length of a distance) on a map and the size of the object (or the actual distance) in the real world. On a map with a scale of 1:24,000, a distance of 1 cm is equivalent to a distance of 24,000 cm on the earth.

Scanning

An automatic process (using a device called a scanner) that converts images from a map or photograph into digital form.

School attendance area

A geographic entity designated by state, county, or local officials designating the school(s) that children in that particular area must attend. Although the U.S. Bureau of the Census does not provide separate data for school attendance areas, investigators can use GIS technology to draw census block group approximations to school attendance areas (see Chapter 8).

Scripting language

Scripting language is a feature enabling users to play automatically a frequently used sequence of commands without entering each individual command. If a sequence of commands becomes standard and repetitive, users can script the sequence to play automatically as a unit. By combining multiple scripts together, advanced users with programming skills can create modules that unsophisticated users can employ by simply entering a few start-up commands.

Small-area data

The U.S. Bureau of the Census uses this term to refer to census statistics tabulated at the census block, block group, and census tract level. Most investigators would consider data for areas with fewer than 5,000 inhabitants as small-area data.

Smoothing

A process used to eliminate two problems found in choropleth maps: the uniform display of attributes within geographic boundaries, even when they vary, and the sharp variations in measured attributes across geographic borders, even when the underlying distribution changes gradually and continuously. Smoothing results in an isopleth map.

Spatial coincidence study

In environmental equity research, spatial coincidence analysis is an alternative approach to queries based on buffering. While buffering allows researchers to compare the ethnic/racial composition of populations on the basis of varying the distance from a hazardous facility, the spatial coincidence method compares populations living in geographic areas (such as census tracts or block groups) containing potential environmental hazards with populations living in hazard-free areas.

Spatial data

Electronic data, in raster or vector format, readable by a computer, including geographic codes and coordinates. This digital map contains data on the features that will contribute to the map, such as county boundaries, census tract and census block group boundaries, streets, and environmental features such as rivers. This spatial information is the foundation for later adding health-related data for geographic analysis.

Spatially referenced data

Attribute data containing information on location, such as a street address, census tract, or county.

Spatial filter

A set of overlapping circles of fixed size that are centered on a regular grid of points.

Standardized incidence ratio (SIR)

Calculated by dividing the observed number of cases by an expected number for the investigated population over the time period reviewed.

State

A type of governmental unit that is the primary legal subdivision of the United States.

Structured query language (SQL)

A useful feature of GIS software that facilitates queries. Menus supply specific language that allows users to question the database by clicking on an already specified command. For example, with one click, users can select records for houses within the boundaries of a specific polygon. Alternatively, those interested in typing in their own commands can use common-language expressions, such as "Select data records for houses (or other map point objects) that are located within the boundaries of a census tract (or other polygon)." SQL allows users to perform additional steps. After making their first selection, users can click on additional menu items to retrieve additional information. For example, after selecting the houses, with one click, users could retrieve the mean age of the houses within each polygon.

Superfund

See **Comprehensive Environmental Response, Compensation and Liability Act (CERCLA)**.

Superfund Amendments and Reauthorization ACT (SARA)

See **Comprehensive Environmental Response, Compensation and Liability Act (CERCLA)**.

Surveillance

An activity that evaluates exposure or trends in adverse health effects over a specified period of time. Surveillance refers to the ongoing systematic collection, analysis, and interpretation of health data in the process of describing and monitoring a health event. Health officials use data obtained through surveillance activities to plan, implement, and evaluate public health interventions.

Survey

A collection of information from a sample of people.

Thematic map

A map that displays the geographic distribution of a single attribute or feature, such as teen births or land cover.

TIGER database (TIGER file)

A spatial computer file containing geographic information representing the position of roads, rivers, railroads, and other census-required map features. The file contains attributes associated with each of these features, including names, address ranges, and class codes. In addition, the file contains the position of the boundaries for geographic areas that the U.S. Bureau of the Census uses in its data collection, processing, and tabulation operations and the attributes of these areas, such as names and codes. The file has multiple partitions, such as counties or groups of counties, although it represents the entire U.S. space, including Puerto Rico and other outlying areas, as a single seamless data inventory.

Topography

Landforms, water and other drainage features, and features such as gravel pits and mine tailings. A single feature, such as a mountain or valley, is called a topographic feature.

Town

A type of minor civil division (MCD) found in the New England states, New York, and Wisconsin; a type of incorporated place in 30 states and the Virgin Islands of the United States. In New Jersey, Pennsylvania, and South Dakota, the U.S. Bureau of the Census treats towns as the equivalent of a minor civil division.

Township

A type of minor civil division in 16 states.

U.S. Geological Survey (USGS)

A bureau within the U.S. Department of the Interior that is the main topographic mapping agency for the United States.

U.S. Postal Service (USPS)

An independent corporation of the U.S. government, providing mail processing and delivery services to individuals and businesses within the United States.

Urban

All population and territory within the boundaries of urban areas and the urban portion of places outside of urban areas that have a decennial census population of 2,500 or more.

Urban area

For the purposes of the U.S. Bureau of the Census, the territory within urban areas and the urban portion of places outside of urban areas that have a decennial census population of 2,500 or more. Other federal government agencies may define the term on the basis of different criteria.

Urban fringe

The closely settled territory adjacent to the central place(s) of an urbanized area. The census blocks that constitute the urban fringe generally have an overall population density of at least 1,000 people per square mile of land area.

Urbanized area (UA)

An area consisting of a central place(s) and adjacent urban fringe that together have a minimum residential population of at least 50,000 people and generally an overall population density of at least 1,000 people per square mile of land area. The U.S. Bureau of the Census uses published criteria to determine the qualification and boundaries of urbanized areas.

Vector

Vector has two meanings: (1) an insect or other living carrier that transmits an infectious organism from an infected individual or its wastes to a susceptible individual or its surroundings; (2) a mathematical quantity that has both magnitude and direction.

Vector database

A spatial database in which points, lines, and polygons represent geographic features.

Village

A type of incorporated place in 20 states and American Samoa. The U.S. Bureau of the Census treats all villages in New Jersey, South Dakota, and Wisconsin, and some villages in Ohio, as county subdivisions.

Visible feature

Any feature on a map, manmade or natural, that can be seen on the ground, such as a street or road, railroad track, power line, stream, shoreline, fence, ridge, or cliff.

Volatile organic compounds (VOCs)

Substances containing carbon and different proportions of other elements such as hydrogen, oxygen, fluorine, chlorine, bromine, sulfur, or nitrogen. These substances easily become vapors or gases. VOCs include commonly used solvents such as paint thinners, lacquer thinners, degreasers, and dry cleaning fluids.

ZIP (Zone Improvement Plan) code

A 5-, 7-, 9-, or 11-digit code assigned by the U.S. Postal Service to a section of street, a collection of streets, an establishment, structure, or group of post office boxes, for the delivery of mail.

Table of Sources

Health Planning, *Journal of Public Health Management and Practice*, Vol. 5, No. 4, p. 11, © 1999, Aspen Publishers, Inc.

Table 2–4   *Source:* Reprinted from C.V. Lee and J.L. Irving, Sources of Spatial Data for Community Health Planning, *Journal of Public Health Management and Practice*, Vol. 5, No. 4, p. 12, © 1999, Aspen Publishers, Inc.

Table 2–5   *Source:* Reprinted from C.V. Lee and J.L. Irving, Sources of Spatial Data for Community Health Planning, *Journal of Public Health Management and Practice*, Vol. 5, No. 4, p. 13, © 1999, Aspen Publishers, Inc.

Figure 2–7   *Source:* Data from D.C. Goodman and J.E. Wennberg, Maps and Health: The Challenges of Interpretation, *Journal of Public Health Management and Practice*, Vol. 5, No. 4, p. xv, © 1999, Aspen Publishers, Inc. and State Departments of Health Uniform Hospital Discharge Data Set files.

Figure 2–8   *Source:* Data from D.C. Goodman and J.E. Wennberg, Maps and Health: The Challenges of Interpretation, *Journal of Public Health Management and Practice*, Vol. 5, No. 4, p. xiv, © 1999, Aspen Publishers, Inc. and *The Dartmouth Atlas of Health Care 1999*.

Figure 2–9   *Source:* Reprinted from T.L. Schlenker, R. Sadler, I. Risk, C. Staes, and H. Harris, Incidence Rates of Hepatitis A by ZIP Code Area, Salt Lake County, Utah, 1992-1996, *Journal of Public Health Management and Practice*, Vol. 5, No. 2, p. 18, © 1999, Aspen Publishers, Inc.

Exhibit 2–2   *Source:* Reprinted from Centers for Disease Control and Prevention, Atlanta, Georgia, http://cdc.gov/epo/dphsi/infdis.htm.

Figure 2–10   *Source:* Reprinted from *National Air Quality and Emissions Trends Report, 1997*, QOAQPS, EPA, December 1998.

Exhibit 2–3   *Source:* Reprinted from U.S. Bureau of the Census, TIGER, TIGER/Line, and Census TIGER files.

Exhibit 2–4   Courtesy of Oregon Department of Human Resources, Health Division, *Oregon Birth File MetaData*, Portland, Oregon.

CHAPTER 3

Figure 3–1   *Source:* Reprinted from G. Rushton, Methods to Evaluate Geographic Access to Health

Services, *Journal of Public Health Management and Practice*, Vol. 5, No. 2, p. 94, © 1999, Aspen Publishers, Inc.

Figure 3–2   *Source:* Reprinted from S.M. Lafferty and E. Cromley, Your First Mapping Project on Your Own: From A to Z, *Journal of Public Health Management and Practice*, Vol. 5, No. 2, p. 79, © 1999, Aspen Publishers, Inc.

Figure 3–3   *Source:* Reprinted from S.M. Lafferty and E. Cromley, Your First Mapping Project on Your Own: From A to Z, *Journal of Public Health Management and Practice*, Vol. 5, No. 2, p. 80, © 1999, Aspen Publishers, Inc.

Figure 3–4   *Source:* Data from M.Y. Rogers, Getting Started with Geographic Information Systems (GIS): A Local Health Department Perspective, *Journal of Public Health Management and Practice*, Vol. 5, No. 4, p. 29, © 1999, Aspen Publishers, Inc. and DeKalb County Department of Public Safety and Office of Assessment, Surveillance and Epidemiology, Population Based Services, DeKalb County Board of Health.

Figure 3–5   *Source:* Data from C. Duclos, T. Johnson and T. Thompson, Development of Childhood Blood Lead Screening Guidelines, Duval County, Florida, 1998, *Journal of Public Health Management and Practice*, Vol. 5, No. 2, p. 10, © 1999, Aspen Publishers, Inc. and Florida Bureau of Environmental Epidemiology.

Figure 3–6   *Source:* Data from J. Cai and Q.B. Welch, Age-Adjusted Homicide Rates by ZIP Codes, Kansas City, Missouri, 1991-1995, *Journal of Public Health Management and Practice*, Vol. 5, No. 2, p. 28, © 1999, Aspen Publishers, Inc. and Death Certificates 1991-1995, Kansas City Health Department, Kansas City, Missouri.

Figure 3–7   *Source:* Data from D. Solet, J.R. Allen, C. Talltree and J.W. Krieger, VISTA/PH Software for Community Health Assessment, *Journal of Public Health Management and Practice*, Vol. 5, No. 2, Aspen Publishers, Inc. and Seattle-King County Department of Public Health, and Hospitalization Discharge Data: Washington State Dept. of Health, Office of Hospital and Patient Data Systems.

Figure 3–8   *Source:* Data from M. Rogers, Using Marketing Information to Focus Smoking Cessation Programs in Specific Census Block Groups along the Buford Highway Corridor, DeKalb County, Georgia, 1996, *Journal of Public Health Management and Practice*, Vol. 5, No. 2, p. 56, © 1999, Aspen Publishers, Inc. and Population Based Services, DeKalb County Board of Health, Georgia and Claritas, Inc. by Georgia Department of Human Resources, Division of Public Health.

Figure 3–9   *Source:* Reprinted with permission from G. Rushton and M. Armstrong, GIS in Public Health: GIS Procedures-Mapping, 1997. http://www.uiowa.edu/~geog/health/mapping/num.html. Last update 12 October 1999. Accessed 18 February 2001.

Figure 3–10   *Source:* Reprinted with permission from G. Rushton and M. Armstrong, GIS in Public Health: GIS Procedures-Mapping, 1997. http://www.uiowa.edu/~geog/health/mapping/num.html. Last update 12 October 1999. Accessed 18 February 2001.

Figure 3–11   *Source:* Reprinted from M.F. Vine, D. Degnan and C. Hanchette, Geographic Information Systems: Their Use in Environmental Epidemiologic Research, *Environmental Health Perspectives*, Vol. 105, No. 6, p. 601, 1997.

Figure 3–12   *Source:* Data from P.H. Bouton and M. Fraser, Local Health Departments and GIS: The Perspective of the National Association of County and City Health Officials, *Journal of Public Health Management and Practice*, Vol. 5, No. 4, p. 38, © 1999, Aspen Publishers, Inc. and Lincoln-Lancaster County Health Department, February 1999.

Figure 3–13   *Source:* Data from M. Kulldorff, Geographic Information Systems (GIS) and Community Health: Some Statistical Issues, *Journal of Public Health Management and Practice*, Vol. 5, No. 2, p. 102, © 1999, Aspen Publishers, Inc. and the New Mexico Tumor Registry for the National Cancer Institute's Surveillance, Epidemiology and End Results (SEER) program.

Figure 3–14   *Source:* Reprinted from M. Kulldorff, Geographic Information Systems (GIS) and Community Health: Some Statistical Issues, *Journal of Public Health Management and Practice*, Vol. 5, No. 2, p. 103, © 1999, Aspen Publishers, Inc.

Figure 3–15   *Source:* Data from M. Cheatham, Percent of Adults Without Health Insurance in Ingham County, Michigan, 1994, *Journal of Public Health Management and Practice*, Vol. 5, No. 2, p. 53, © 1999, Aspen Publishers, Inc. and Ingham County Health Department 1997.

Figure 3–16   *Source:* Reprinted with permission from G. Rushton and M. West, Women with Localized Breast Cancer Selecting Mastectomy Treatment, Iowa, 1991-1996, *Public Health Reports* 114, © 1999, pp. 370–371, Oxford University Press, Inc.

Figure 3–17   *Source:* Reprinted with permission from G. Rushton and M. West, Women with Localized Breast Cancer Selecting Mastectomy Treatment, Iowa, 1991-1996, *Public Health Reports* 114, © 1999, pp. 370-371, Oxford University Press, Inc.

Figure 3–18   *Source:* Reprinted with permission from G. Rushton and M. West, Women with Localized Breast Cancer Selecting Mastectomy Treatment, Iowa, 1991-1996, *Public Health Reports* 114, © 1999, pp. 370-371, Oxford University Press, Inc.

Figure 3–19   *Source:* Reprinted from M. Kulldorff, Geographic Information Systems (GIS) and Community Health: Some Statistical Issues, *Journal of Public Health Management and Practice*, Vol. 5, No. 2, p. 104, © 1999, Aspen Publishers, Inc.

Figure 3–20   *Source:* Reprinted from M. Kulldorff, Geographic Information Systems (GIS) and Community Health: Some Statistical Issues, *Journal of Public Health Management and Practice*, Vol. 5, No. 2, p. 105, © 1999, Aspen Publishers, Inc.

CHAPTER 4

Figure 4–1   *Source:* Reprinted from D. Wartenberg, M. Greenberg and R. Lathrop, Identification and Characterization of Populations Living Near High-Voltage Transmission Lines: A Pilot Study, *Environmental Health Perspectives*, Vol. 101, No. 7, p. 629, © 1993, Aspen Publishers, Inc.

Figure 4–2   *Source:* Reprinted from D. Wartenberg, M. Greenberg and R. Lathrop, Identification and Characterization of Populations Living Near High-Voltage Transmission Lines: A Pilot Study, *Environmental Health Perspectives*, Vol. 101, No. 7, p. 629, © 1993, Aspen Publishers, Inc.

Table 4–1   *Source:* Reprinted from D. Wartenberg, M. Greenberg and R. Lathrop, Identification and Characterization of Populations Living Near High-Voltage Transmission Lines: A Pilot Study, *Environmental Health Perspectives*, Vol. 101, No. 7, p. 630, © 1993, Aspen Publishers, Inc.

Figure 4–3   *Source:* Reprinted from W.D. Henriques and R.F. Spengler, Locations Around the Hanford Nuclear Facility Where Average Milk Consumption by Children in 1945 Would Have Resulted in an Estimated Median Iodine-131 Dose to the Thyroid of 10 Rad or Higher, Washington, *Journal of Public Health Management and Practice*, Vol. 5, No. 2, p. vi of Errata, © 1999, Aspen Publishers, Inc. and Center for Disease Control, Hanford Environmental Dose Reconstruction Project.

Figure 4–4   *Source:* Reprinted from P. English et al., Examining Associations Between Childhood Asthma and Traffic Flow Using a Geographic Information System, *Environmental Health Perspectives,* Vol. 107, No. 9, p. 762, 1999.

Table 4–2   *Source:* Reprinted from Centers for Disease Control and Prevention, Screening Young Children for Lead Poisoning: Guidance for State and Local Public Health Officials, Atlanta, Georgia, 1997.

Figure 4–5   *Source:* Reprinted from Centers for Disease Control and Prevention, Screening Young Children for Lead Poisoning: Guidance for State and Local Public Health Officials, Atlanta, Georgia, 1997.

Figure 4–6   *Source:* Reprinted with permission from D. Wartenberg, Screening for Lead Exposure Using a Geographic Information System, *Environmental Research*, No. 59, © 1992, p. 313, Academic Press, Inc.

Figure 4–7   *Source:* Reprinted with permission from D. Wartenberg, Screening for Lead Exposure Using a Geographic Information System, *Environmental Research*, No. 59, © 1992, p. 314, Academic Press, Inc.

Figure 4–8   *Source:* Reprinted with permission from D. Wartenberg, Screening for Lead Exposure Using a Geographic Information System, *Environmental Research*, No. 59, © 1992, p. 315, Academic Press, Inc.

Table 4–3   *Source:* Reprinted with permission from D. Wartenberg, Screening for Lead Exposure Using a Geographic Information System, *Environmental Research*, No. 59, © 1992, p. 315, Academic Press, Inc.

Figure 4–9   *Source:* Reprinted with permission from D. Wartenberg, Screening for Lead Exposure Using a Geographic Information System, *Environmental Research*, No. 59, © 1992, p. 316, Academic Press, Inc.

Table 4–4   *Source:* Reprinted with permission from D. Wartenberg, Screening for Lead Exposure Using a Geographic Information System, *Environmental Research*, No. 59, © 1992, p. 316, Academic Press, Inc.

Figure 4–10   *Source:* Reprinted from W.G. Guthe et al., Reassessment of Lead Exposure in New Jersey Using GIS Technology, *Environmental Research*, No. 59, 1992, p. 320, Academic Press, Inc. and New Jersey Department of Housing.

Figure 4–11   *Source:* Reprinted from W.G. Guthe et al., Reassessment of Lead Exposure in New Jersey Using GIS Technology, *Environmental Research*, No. 59, 1992, p. 321, Academic Press, Inc. and New Jersey Department of Housing.

Figure 4–12   *Source:* Reprinted from W.G. Guthe et al., Reassessment of Lead Exposure in New Jersey Using GIS Technology, *Environmental Research*, No. 59, 1992, p. 322, Academic Press, Inc. and New Jersey Department of Housing.

Figure 4–13   *Source:* Reprinted from W.G. Guthe et al., Reassessment of Lead Exposure in New Jersey Using GIS Technology, *Environmental Research*, No. 59, 1992, p. 323, Academic Press, Inc. and New Jersey Department of Housing.

Figure 4–14   *Source:* Reprinted from W.G. Guthe et al., Reassessment of Lead Exposure in New Jersey Using GIS Technology, *Environmental Research*, No. 59, 1992, p. 324, Academic Press, Inc. and New Jersey Department of Housing.

Figure 4–15   *Source:* Reprinted from C.L. Hanchette, GIS and Decision Making for Public Health Agencies: Childhood Lead Poisoning and Welfare Reform, *Journal of Public Health Management and Practice*, Vol. 5, No. 4, p. 45, © 1999, Aspen Publishers, Inc.

Figure 4–16   *Source:* Reprinted from C. Duclos, T. Johnson and T. Thompson, Development of Childhood Blood Lead Screening Guidelines, Duval County, Florida, Bureau of Environmental Epidemiology, 1998, *Journal of Public Health Management and Practice*, Vol. 5, No. 2, pp. 9-10, © 1999, Aspen Publishers, Inc.

Figure 4–17   *Source:* Reprinted from S. Wilkinson et al., Lead Hot Zones and Childhood Lead Poisoning Cases, Santa Clara County, California, 1995, *Journal of Public Health Management and Practice*, Vol. 5, No. 2, p. 12, © 1999, Aspen Publishers, Inc. and Santa Clara Valley Health & Hospital System, Public Health Department, Disease Control and Prevention and U.S. Census Bureau.

Figure 4–18   *Source:* Reprinted from R. Rao et al., Geographic Distribution of Mean Blood Lead Levels by Year in Children Residing in Communities Near the Bunker Hill Lead Smelter Site, 1974-1983, *Journal of Public Health Management and Practice*, Vol. 5, No. 2, p. 14, © 1999, Aspen Publishers, Inc.

Figure 4–19   *Source:* Data from P.B. Bouton and M. Fraser, Local Health Departments and GIS: The Prospective of the National Association of County and City Health Officials, *Journal of Public Health Management and Practice*, Vol. 5, No. 4, p. 36, © 1999 and Needham BOH Septic System Records, Needham, Massachusetts, January 1999 and the Massachusetts Department of Environmental Protection.

Figure 4–20   *Source:* Data from M. Ralston, Elevated Nitrate Levels in Relation to Bedrock Depth, Linn County, Iowa, 1991-1996, *Journal of Public Health Management and Practice,* Vol. 5, No. 2, p. 40, © 1999, Aspen Publishers, Inc.

Figure 4–21   *Source:* Data from W. Boria et al., Public Notification to Families with Newborns at Risk of Methemoglobinemia from Drinking Water Exposure, Clymer, New York, 1996-1998, *Journal of Public Health Management and Practice*, Vol. 5, No. 2, p. 38, © 1999, Aspen Publishers, Inc. and Chautaugua County, New York.

Figure 4–22   *Source:* Data from J. Pruitt, Monitoring Volatile Organic Compounds in Private Wells Near a Community Landfill by Tax Parcel, Harford County, Maryland, 1986-1998, *Journal of Public Health Management and Practice*, Vol. 5, No. 2, p. 42, © 1999, Aspen Publishers, Inc. and Water Sampling Database of Harford County Health Department, Harford County, Maryland.

Figure 4–23   *Source:* Data from D.L. Partridge and M.D. Mathews, A Computer Simulation of Groundwater Withdrawal Patterns for Public Water Supply Wells, Hutchinson, Kansas, 1998-2003, *Journal of Public Health Management and Practice*, Vol. 5, No. 2, p. 44, © 1999, Aspen Publishers, Inc.

Figure 4–24   *Source:* Reprinted with permission from E. Sheppard et al., GIS-Based Measures of Environmental Equity: Exploring Their Sensitivity and Significance, *Journal of Exposure Analysis and Environmental Epidemiology*, No. 9, p. 21, © 1999, Nature Publishing Group.

Figure 4–25   *Source:* Reprinted from E. Sheppard et al., GIS-Based Measures of Environmental Equity: Exploring Their Sensitivity and Significance, *Journal of Exposure Analysis and Environmental Epidemiology*, No. 9, © 1999, p. 22, Nature Publishing Group.

Table 4–5   *Source:* Reprinted with permission from E. Sheppard et al., GIS-Based Measures of Environmental Equity: Exploring Their Sensitivity and Significance, *Journal of Exposure Analysis and Environmental Epidemiology*, No. 9, p. 22, © 1999, Nature Publishing Group.

Figure 4–26   *Source:* Reprinted with permission from E. Sheppard et al., GIS-Based Measures of Environmental Equity: Exploring Their Sensitivity and Significance, *Journal of Exposure Analysis and Environmental Epidemiology*, No. 9, p. 23, © 1999, Nature Publishing Group.

Table 4–6   *Source:* Reprinted with permission from E. Sheppard et al., GIS-Based Measures of Environmental Equity: Exploring Their Sensitivity and Significance, *Journal of Exposure Analysis and Environmental Epidemiology*, No. 9, p. 24, © 1999, Nature Publishing Group.

Table 4–7   *Source:* Reprinted with permission from E. Sheppard et al., GIS-Based Measures of Environmental Equity: Exploring Their Sensitivity and Significance, *Journal of Exposure*

Analysis and Environmental Epidemiology, No. 9, p. 24, © 1999, Nature Publishing Group.

Figure 4–27   *Source:* Reprinted with permission from E. Sheppard et al., GIS-Based Measures of Environmental Equity: Exploring Their Sensitivity and Significance, *Journal of Exposure Analysis and Environmental Epidemiology*, No. 9, p. 27, © 1999, Nature Publishing Group.

Table 4–8   *Source:* Reprinted with permission from E. Sheppard et al., GIS-Based Measures of Environmental Equity: Exploring Their Sensitivity and Significance, *Journal of Exposure Analysis and Environmental Epidemiology*, No. 9, p. 22, © 1999, Nature Publishing Group.

Table 4–9   *Source:* Copyright (1998) From Improving the U.S. EPA Toxic Release Inventory Database for Environmental Health Research, *Journal of Toxicology and Environmental Health*, Part B, No. 1, p. 262. Reproduced by permission of Taylor & Francis, Inc., http://www.routledge-ny.com.

Table 4–10   *Source:* Reprinted from C.M. Neumann, D.L. Forman and J.E. Rothlein, Hazard Screening of Chemical Releases and Environmental Equity Analysis of Populations Proximate to Toxic Release Inventory Facilities in Oregon, *Environmental Health Perspectives*, Vol. 106, No. 4, p. 220, © 1998.

Figure 4–28   *Source:* Reprinted from C.M. Neumann, D.L. Forman and J.E. Rothlein, Hazard Screening of Chemical Releases and Environmental Equity Analysis of Populations Proximate to Toxic Release Inventory Facilities in Oregon, *Environmental Health Perspectives*, Vol. 106, No. 4, p. 220, © 1998.

Table 4–11   *Source:* Reprinted from C.M. Neumann, D.L. Forman and J.E. Rothlein, Hazard Screening of Chemical Releases and Environmental Equity Analysis of Populations Proximate to Toxic Release Inventory Facilities in Oregon, *Environmental Health Perspectives*, Vol. 106, No. 4, p. 221, © 1998.

Figure 4–29   *Source:* Reprinted from P.B. Bouton and M. Fraser, Local Health Departments and GIS: The Prospective of the National Association of County and City Health Officials, *Journal of Public Health Management and*

Practice, Vol. 5, No. 4, pp. 33-41, © 1999, Aspen Publishers, Inc.

CHAPTER 5

Figure 5–1   *Source:* Data from J. Devine, W. Gallo and H.T. Janowski, Identifying Predicted Immunization "Pockets of Need," Hillsborough County, Florida, 1996-1997, *Journal of Public Health Management and Practice*, Vol. 5, No. 2, p. 16, © 1999, Aspen Publishers, Inc. and Florida Department of Health, Bureau of Immunization, May 1998.

Figure 5–2   *Source:* Data from T.L. Schlenker et al., Incidence Rates of Hepatitis A by ZIP Code Area, Salt Lake County, Utah, 1992-1996, *Journal of Public Health Management and Practice*, Vol. 5, No. 2, p. 18, © 1999, Aspen Publishers, Inc. and Salt Lake City-County Health Department.

Figure 5–3   *Source:* Reprinted with permission from C. Siegel et al., Geographic Analysis of Pertussis Infection in an Urban Area: A Tool for Health Services Planning, *American Journal of Public Health*, Vol. 87, No. 12, p. 2024, © 1997, American Public Health Association.

Figure 5–4   *Source:* Reprinted from R.H. Jenks and J.W. Jollye, Animal Rabies Cases in Central Palm Beach County, Florida, 1994-1998, *Journal of Public Health Management and Practice*, Vol. 5, No. 2, p. 32, © 1999, Aspen Publishers, Inc.

Figure 5–5   *Source:* Data from M. Stefanak, K.A. Vaughn and J.F. Shaheen, Positive Raccoon-Strain Rabies Cases in Mahoning County, Ohio, 1997, *Journal of Public Health Management and Practice*, Vol. 5, No. 2, p. 34, © 1999, Aspen Publishers, Inc. and Mahoning County Board of Health, 1997 Data, Mahoning County, Ohio.

Figure 5–6   *Source:* Reprinted with permission from U. Kitron et al., Geographic Information System in Malaria Surveillance: Mosquito Breeding and Imported Cases In Israel, 1992, *American Journal of Tropical Medicine and Hygiene*, Vol. 50, No. 5, p. 552, © 1994, The American Society of Tropical Medicine and Hygiene.

Table 5–1   *Source:* Reprinted with permission from D.D. Chadee and U. Kitron, Spatial and Temporal Patterns of Imported Malaria Cases and Local Transmission in Trinidad, *American Journal of Tropical Medicine and Hygiene*, Vol. 61, No. 4, p. 514, © 1999, The American Society of Tropical Medicine and Hygiene.

Figure 5–7   *Source:* Reprinted with permission from D.D. Chadee and U. Kitron, Spatial and Temporal Patterns of Imported Malaria Cases and Local Transmission in Trinidad, *American Journal of Tropical Medicine and Hygiene*, Vol. 61, No. 4, p. 515, © 1999, The American Society of Tropical Medicine and Hygiene.

Figure 5–8   *Source:* Reprinted with permission from D.D. Chadee and U. Kitron, Spatial and Temporal Patterns of Imported Malaria Cases and Local Transmission in Trinidad, *American Journal of Tropical Medicine and Hygiene*, Vol. 61, No. 4, p. 516, © 1999, The American Society of Tropical Medicine and Hygiene.

Figure 5–9   *Source:* Reprinted with permission from U. Kitron et al., Spatial Analysis of the Distribution of LaCrosse Encephalitis in Illinois, Using a Geographic Information System and Local and Global Spatial Statistics, *American Journal of Tropical Medicine and Hygiene*, Vol. 57, No. 4, p. 471, © 1997, The American Society of Tropical Medicine and Hygiene.

Figure 5–10   *Source:* Reprinted with permission from U. Kitron et al., Spatial Analysis of the Distribution of LaCrosse Encephalitis in Illinois, Using a Geographic Information System and Local and Global Spatial Statistics, *American Journal of Tropical Medicine and Hygiene*, Vol. 57, No. 4, p. 471, © 1997, The American Society of Tropical Medicine and Hygiene.

Figure 5–11   *Source:* Reprinted with permission from U. Kitron et al., Spatial Analysis of the Distribution of LaCrosse Encephalitis in Illinois, Using a Geographic Information System and Local and Global Spatial Statistics, *American Journal of Tropical Medicine and Hygiene*, Vol. 57, No. 4, p. 472, © 1997, The American Society of Tropical Medicine and Hygiene.

Figure 5–12   *Source:* Reprinted with permission from U. Kitron et al., Spatial Analysis of the Distribution of LaCrosse Encephalitis in Illinois, Using a Geographic Information System and Local and Global Spatial Statistics, *American*

Journal of Tropical Medicine and Hygiene, Vol. 57, No. 4, p. 472, © 1997, The American Society of Tropical Medicine and Hygiene.

Figure 5–13   *Source:* Reprinted with permission from F.O. Richards, Use of Geographic Information Systems in Control Programs for Onchocerciasis in Guatemala, *Bulletin of Pan American Health Organization*, Vol. 27, No. 1, p. 54, © 1993, Pan American Health Organization. To obtain information about PAHO publications, visit their website at http://publications.paho.org or write to the Pan American Health Organization, Publications Program, 525 Twenty-third St., NW, Washington, DC 20037, Fax: (202) 338-3869.

Figure 5–14   *Source:* Reprinted with permission from F.O. Richards, Use of Geographic Information Systems in Control Programs for Onchocerciasis in Guatemala, *Bulletin of Pan American Health Organization*, Vol. 27, No. 1, p. 54, © 1993, Pan American Health Organization. To obtain information about PAHO publications, visit their website at http://publications.paho.org or write to the Pan American Health Organization, Publications Program, 525 Twenty-third St., NW, Washington, DC 20037, Fax: (202) 338-3869.

Figure 5–15   *Source:* Reprinted with permission from G.E. Glass et al., Environmental Risk Factors for Lyme Disease Identified with Geographic Information Systems, *American Journal of Public Health*, Vol. 85, No. 7, © 1995, p. 946, American Public Health Association.

Table 5–2   *Source:* Reprinted with permission from G.E. Glass et al., Environmental Risk Factors for Lyme Disease Identified with Geographic Information Systems, *American Journal of Public Health*, Vol. 85, No. 7, © 1995, p. 947, American Public Health Association.

Figure 5–16   *Source:* Reprinted with permission from M.E. Bavia et al., Geographic Information Systems and the Environmental Risk of Schistosomiasis in Bahia, Brazil, *American Journal of Tropical Medicine and Hygiene*, Vol. 60, No. 4, p. 567, © 1999, The American Society of Tropical Medicine and Hygiene.

Figure 5–17   *Source:* Reprinted with permission from M.E. Bavia et al., Geographic Information Systems and the Environmental Risk of Schistosomiasis in Bahia, Brazil, *American Jour-*

nal of Tropical Medicine and Hygiene, Vol. 60, No. 4, p. 568, © 1999, The American Society of Tropical Medicine and Hygiene.

Figure 5–18 Source: Reprinted with permission from K.M. Becker et al., Geographic Epidemiology of Gonorrhea in Baltimore, Maryland, Using a Geographic Information System, American Journal of Epidemiology, Vol. 147, No. 7, p. 713, © 1998, Oxford University Press, Inc.

Figure 5–19 Source: Reprinted with permission from K.M. Becker et al., Geographic Epidemiology of Gonorrhea in Baltimore, Maryland, Using a Geographic Information System, American Journal of Epidemiology, Vol. 147, No. 7, p. 713, © 1998, Oxford University Press, Inc.

Figure 5–20 Source: Reprinted with permission from K.M. Becker et al., Geographic Epidemiology of Gonorrhea in Baltimore, Maryland, Using a Geographic Information System, American Journal of Epidemiology, Vol. 147, No. 7, p. 714, © 1998, Oxford University Press, Inc.

Figure 5–21 Source: Reprinted with permission from K.M. Becker et al., Geographic Epidemiology of Gonorrhea in Baltimore, Maryland, Using a Geographic Information System, American Journal of Epidemiology, Vol. 147, No. 7, p. 713, © 1998, Oxford University Press, Inc.

Figure 5–22 Source: Reprinted with permission from F. Tanser and D. Wilkinson, Spatial Implications of the Tuberculosis DOTS Strategy in Rural South Africa: A Novel Application of Geographic Information System and Global Positioning System Technologies, Tropical Medicine and International Health, Vol. 4, No. 10, p. 636, © 1999, Blackwell Science Ltd.

Figure 5–23 Source: Reprinted with permission from F. Tanser and D. Wilkinson, Spatial Implications of the Tuberculosis DOTS Strategy in Rural South Africa: A Novel Application of Geographic Information System and Global Positioning System Technologies, Tropical Medicine and International Health, Vol. 4, No. 10, p. 636, © 1999, Blackwell Science Ltd.

Table 5–3 Source: Reprinted with permission from F. Tanser and D. Wilkinson, Spatial Implica-

tions of the Tuberculosis DOTS Strategy in Rural South Africa: A Novel Application of Geographic Information System and Global Positioning System Technologies, Tropical Medicine and International Health, Vol. 4, No. 10, p. 637, © 1999, Blackwell Science Ltd.

Figure 5–24 Source: Data from J.K. Devasundaram, An Automated Geographic Information System for Local Health Departments, Journal of Public Health Management and Practice, Vol. 5, No. 2, p. 71, © 1999, Aspen Publishers, Inc. and Epidemiology and Disease Control Program, Department of Health and Mental Hygiene, Baltimore, Maryland.

Table 5–4 Source: Data from J.K. Devasundaram, An Automated Geographic Information System for Local Health Departments, Journal of Public Health Management and Practice, Vol. 5, No. 2, p. 71, © 1999, Aspen Publishers, Inc.

CHAPTER 6

Figure 6–1 Source: Reprinted with permission from M. Braddock et al., Using a Geographic Information System to Understand Child Pedestrian Injury, American Journal of Public Health, Vol. 84, No. 7, p. 1159, © 1994, American Public Health Association.

Figure 6–2 Source: Reprinted with permission from M. Braddock et al., Using a Geographic Information System to Understand Child Pedestrian Injury, American Journal of Public Health, Vol. 84, No. 7, p. 1159, © 1994, American Public Health Association.

Figure 6–3 Source: Reprinted with permission from M. Braddock et al., Using a Geographic Information System to Understand Child Pedestrian Injury, American Journal of Public Health, Vol. 84, No. 7, p. 1159, © 1994, American Public Health Association.

Figure 6–4 Source: Data from P. Van Zuyle, Automobile Accidents to Teenagers Requiring Emergency Medical Transport, Ventura County, California, 1996, Journal of Public Health Management and Practice, Vol. 5, No. 2, p. 26, © 1999, Aspen Publishers, Inc. and Ventura County EMS and Center for Health Outcomes Research & Evaluation, 1998 Ventura County Public Health, Ventura County, California.

Figure 6–5   *Source:* Data from M.Y. Rogers, Getting Started with Geographic Information Systems (GIS): A Local Health Department Perspective, *Journal of Public Health Management and Practice*, Vol. 5, No. 4, p. 29, © 1999, Aspen Publishers, Inc. and DeKalb County Department of Public Safety and Office of Assessment, Surveillance, and Epidemiology, Population Based Services, DeKalb County Board of Health, DeKalb County, Georgia.

Figure 6–6   *Source:* Data from M.Y. Rogers, Getting Started with Geographic Information Systems (GIS): A Local Health Department Perspective, *Journal of Public Health Management and Practice*, Vol. 5, No. 4, p. 30, © 1999, Aspen Publishers, Inc. and DeKalb County Medical Examiners Office and Office of Assessment, Surveillance and Epidemiology, Population Based Services, DeKalb County Board of Health, DeKalb County, Georgia.

Figure 6–7   *Source:* Data from J. Slosek et al., Hospitalizations for All Injuries, Average Annual Rates per 1,000 Adults Ages 25-44 by ZIP Code, Boston, Massachusetts, 1994-1996, *Journal of Public Health Management and Practice*, Vol. 5, No. 2, p. 30, © 1999, Aspen Publishers, Inc. and Codman Research Group, Inc. and Massachusetts Health Data Consortium and Office of Research, Health Assessment and Data Systems, Boston Public Health Commission, Boston, Massachusetts.

Table 6–1   *Source:* Data from C. Peek-SAA et al., GIS Mapping of Earthquake-Related Deaths and Hospital Admissions from the 1994 Northridge, California, Earthquake, *Annals of Epidemiology*, Vol. 10, No. 1, pp. 5-13, © 2000, Elsevier Science.

Figure 6–8   *Source:* Reprinted from *Annals of Epidemiology*, Vol. 10, No. 1, C. SAA-Peek, et al., GIS Mapping of Earthquake-Related Deaths and Hospital Admissions from the 1994 Northridge, California, Earthquake, p. 8, Copyright © (2000), with permission from Excerpta Medica.

Table 6–2   *Source:* Reprinted from *Annals of Epidemiology*, Vol. 10, No. 1, C. SAA-Peek, et al., GIS Mapping of Earthquake-Related Deaths and Hospital Admissions from the 1994 Northridge, California, Earthquake, p. 9, Copyright © (2000), with permission from Excerpta Medica.

Table 6–3   *Source:* Reprinted from *Annals of Epidemiology*, Vol. 10, No. 1, C. SAA-Peek, et al., GIS Mapping of Earthquake-Related Deaths and Hospital Admissions from the 1994 Northridge, California, Earthquake, p. 9, Copyright © (2000), with permission from Excerpta Medica.

Figure 6–9   *Source:* Reprinted from *Annals of Epidemiology*, Vol. 10, No. 1, C. SAA-Peek, et al., GIS Mapping of Earthquake-Related Deaths and Hospital Admissions from the 1994 Northridge, California, Earthquake, p. 10, Copyright © (2000), with permission from Excerpta Medica.

Figure 6–10   *Source:* Reprinted from *Annals of Epidemiology*, Vol. 10, No. 1, C. SAA-Peek, et al., GIS Mapping of Earthquake-Related Deaths and Hospital Admissions from the 1994 Northridge, California, Earthquake, p. 11, Copyright © (2000), with permission from Excerpta Medica.

Figure 6–11   *Source:* Reprinted from G. Lapidus et al., Using a Geographic Information System to Guide a Community-Based Smoke Detector Campaign, *Geographic Information Systems in Public Health: Proceedings from the Third National Conference*, ed., R.C. Williams et al., Agency for Toxic Substances and Disease Registry, United States Department of Health and Human Services, August 1998, p. 105.

Figure 6–12   *Source:* Reprinted from G. Lapidus et al., Using a Geographic Information System to Guide a Community-Based Smoke Detector Campaign, *Geographic Information Systems in Public Health: Proceedings from the Third National Conference*, ed., R.C. Williams et al., Agency for Toxic Substances and Disease Registry, United States Department of Health and Human Services, August 1998, p. 106.

Figure 6–13   *Source:* Reprinted from G. Lapidus et al., Using a Geographic Information System to Guide a Community-Based Smoke Detector Campaign, *Geographic Information Systems in Public Health: Proceedings from the Third National Conference*, ed., R.C. Williams et al., Agency for Toxic Substances and Disease Registry, United States Department of Health and Human Services, August 1998, p. 107.

Figure 6–14   *Source:* Reprinted from G. Lapidus et al., Using a Geographic Information System to Guide a Community-Based Smoke Detector

Campaign, *Geographic Information Systems in Public Health: Proceedings from the Third National Conference*, eds., R.C. Williams et al., Agency for Toxic Substances and Disease Registry, United States Department of Health and Human Services, August 1998, p. 107.

Figure 6–15   *Source:* Data from J. Cai and Q.B. Welch, Age-Adjusted Homicide Rates by ZIP Codes, Kansas City, Missouri, 1991-1995, *Journal of Public Health Management and Practice*, Vol. 5, No. 2, p. 28, Aspen Publishers, Inc. and Kansas City Health Department.

CHAPTER 7

Figure 7–1   *Source:* Data from M.Y. Rogers, Using Marketing Information to Focus Smoking Cessation Programs in Specific Census Block Groups along the Buford Highway Corridor, DeKalb County, Georgia, 1996, *Public Health Management and Practice*, Vol. 5, No. 2, © 1999, p. 56, Aspen Publishers, Inc. and Population Based Services, DeKalb County Board of Health, Georgia and Georgia Department of Human Services, Division of Public Health for information licensed through Claritas, Inc.

Table 7–1   *Source:* Reprinted with permission from D. Luke, E. Esmundo, and Y. Bloom, Smoke Signs: Patterns of Tobacco Billboard Advertising in a Metropolitan Region, *Tobacco Control,* No. 9, pp. 16-23, © 2000, BMJ Publishing Group.

Figure 7–2   *Source:* Reprinted with permission from D. Luke, E. Esmundo, and Y. Bloom, Smoke Signs: Patterns of Tobacco Billboard Advertising in a Metropolitan Region, *Tobacco Control*, No. 9, pp. 16-23, © 2000, BMJ Publishing Group.

Table 7–2   *Source:* Reprinted with permission from D. Luke, E. Esmundo, and Y. Bloom, Smoke Signs: Patterns of Tobacco Billboard Advertising in a Metropolitan Region, *Tobacco Control*, No. 9, pp. 16-23, © 2000, BMJ Publishing Group.

Figure 7–3   *Source:* Reprinted with permission from D. Luke, E. Esmundo, and Y. Bloom, Smoke Signs: Patterns of Tobacco Billboard Advertising in a Metropolitan Region, *Tobacco Con-*

trol, No. 9, pp. 16-23, © 2000, BMJ Publishing Group.

Table 7–3   *Source:* Reprinted with permission from D. Luke, E. Esmundo, and Y. Bloom, Smoke Signs: Patterns of Tobacco Billboard Advertising in a Metropolitan Region, *Tobacco Control*, No. 9, pp. 16-23, © 2000, BMJ Publishing Group.

Table 7–4   *Source:* Reprinted with permission from D. Luke, E. Esmundo, and Y. Bloom, Smoke Signs: Patterns of Tobacco Billboard Advertising in a Metropolitan Region, *Tobacco Control*, No. 9, pp. 16-23, © 2000, BMJ Publishing Group.

Figure 7–4   *Source:* Reprinted with permission from D. Luke, E. Esmundo, and Y. Bloom, Smoke Signs: Patterns of Tobacco Billboard Advertising in a Metropolitan Region, *Tobacco Control*, No. 9, pp. 16-23, © 2000, BMJ Publishing Group.

Figure 7–5   *Source:* Reprinted with permission from D. Luke, E. Esmundo, and Y. Bloom, Smoke Signs: Patterns of Tobacco Billboard Advertising in a Metropolitan Region, *Tobacco Control*, No. 9, pp. 16-23, © 2000, BMJ Publishing Group.

Table 7–5   *Source:* Reprinted with permission from D. Luke, E. Esmundo, and Y. Bloom, Smoke Signs: Patterns of Tobacco Billboard Advertising in a Metropolitan Region, *Tobacco Control*, No. 9, pp. 16-23, © 2000, BMJ Publishing Group.

Figure 7–6   *Source:* Reprinted with permission from M. Kulldorff et al., Breast Cancer Clusters in the Northeast United States: A Geographic Analysis, *American Journal of Epidemiology*, Vol. 146, No. 2, p. 164, © 1997, Oxford University Press, Inc.

Figure 7–7   *Source:* Reprinted with permission from M. Kulldorff et al., Breast Cancer Clusters in the Northeast United States: A Geographic Analysis, *American Journal of Epidemiology*, Vol. 146, No. 2, p. 165, © 1997, Oxford University Press, Inc.

Figure 7–8   *Source:* Reprinted with permission from M. Kulldorff et al., Breast Cancer Clusters in the Northeast United States: A Geographic Analysis, *American Journal of Epidemiology*, Vol. 146, No. 2, p. 166, © 1997, Oxford University Press, Inc.

Table 7–6   *Source:* Reprinted with permission from M. Kulldorff et al., Breast Cancer Clusters in the Northeast United States: A Geographic Analysis, *American Journal of Epidemiology*, Vol. 146, No. 2, p. 167, © 1997, Oxford University Press, Inc.

Figure 7–9   *Source:* Reprinted with permission from M. Kulldorff et al., Breast Cancer Clusters in the Northeast United States: A Geographic Analysis, *American Journal of Epidemiology*, Vol. 146, No. 2, p. 168, © 1997, Oxford University Press, Inc.

Table 7–7   Courtesy of Silent Spring Institute Inc., Breast Cancer on Cape Cod, Newton, Massachusetts. http://www.silentspring.org/Projects/Capestudy/Capebrca.html., 1997, Updated 27 February 2001. Accessed 18 March 2001.

Figure 7–10   *Source:* S.J. Melly et al., Exploratory Data Analysis in a Study of Breast Cancer and the Environment, *Geographic Information Systems in Public Health: Proceedings from the Third National Conference*, ed., R.C. Williams et al., Agency for Toxic Substances and Disease Registry, United States Department of Health and Human Services, August 1998, pp. 461-467.

Figure 7–11   *Source:* S.J. Melly et al., Exploratory Data Analysis in a Study of Breast Cancer and the Environment, *Geographic Information Systems in Public Health: Proceedings from the Third National Conference*, ed., R.C. Williams et al., Agency for Toxic Substances and Disease Registry, United States Department of Health and Human Services, August 1998, pp. 461-467.

Figure 7–12   *Source:* S.J. Melly et al., Exploratory Data Analysis in a Study of Breast Cancer and the Environment, *Geographic Information Systems in Public Health: Proceedings from the Third National Conference*, ed., R.C. Williams et al., Agency for Toxic Substances and Disease Registry, United States Department of Health and Human Services, August 1998, pp. 461-467.

Figure 7–13   *Source:* S.J. Melly et al., Exploratory Data Analysis in a Study of Breast Cancer and the Environment, *Geographic Information Systems in Public Health: Proceedings from the Third National Conference*, ed., R.C. Williams et al., Agency for Toxic Substances and Dis-ease Registry, United States Department of Health and Human Services, August 1998, pp. 461-467.

Figure 7–14   *Source:* Reprinted from S.J. Melly, Y.T. Joyce and J.G. Brody, Characterizing the Environmental Features of a Region for a Community-Level Health Study of Breast Cancer, *Geographic Information Systems in Public Health: Proceedings from the Third National Conference*, R.C. Williams et al., ed., Agency for Toxic Substances and Disease Registry, United States Department of Health and Human Services, August 1998, pp. 589-592.

Figure 7–15   *Source:* Reprinted from S.J. Melly, Y.T. Joyce and J.G. Brody, Characterizing the Environmental Features of a Region for a Community-Level Health Study of Breast Cancer, *Geographic Information Systems in Public Health: Proceedings from the Third National Conference*, R.C. Williams et al., ed., Agency for Toxic Substances and Disease Registry, United States Department of Health and Human Services, August 1998, pp. 589-592.

Figure 7–16   *Source:* Reprinted from S.J. Melly, Y.T. Joyce and J.G. Brody, Characterizing the Environmental Features of a Region for a Community-Level Health Study of Breast Cancer, *Geographic Information Systems in Public Health: Proceedings from the Third National Conference*, R.C. Williams et al., ed., Agency for Toxic Substances and Disease Registry, United States Department of Health and Human Services, August 1998, pp. 589-592.

Figure 7–17   *Source:* Reprinted from S.J. Melly, Y.T. Joyce and J.G. Brody, Characterizing the Environmental Features of a Region for a Community-Level Health Study of Breast Cancer, *Geographic Information Systems in Public Health: Proceedings from the Third National Conference*, R.C. Williams et al., ed., Agency for Toxic Substances and Disease Registry, United States Department of Health and Human Services, August 1998, pp. 589-592.

Figure 7–18   *Source:* Reprinted with permission from E. White and T. Aldrich, Geographic Studies of Pediatric Cancer near Hazardous Waste Sites, *Archives of Environmental Health*, Vol. 54, No. 6, p. 391, © November/December 1999, Heldref Publications.

and Suffolk Counties, Long Island, New York, *Archives of Environmental Health*, New York State Industrial Directory, Vol. 51, No. 4, p. 259, © (July/August 1996), Heldref Publications.

Figure 7–23   *Source:* Reprinted with permission from E.L. Lewis-Michl et al., Breast Cancer Risk and Residence Near Industry or Traffic in Nassau and Suffolk Counties, Long Island, New York, *Archives of Environmental Health*, New York State Industrial Directory, Vol. 51, No. 4, p. 260, © (July/August 1996), Heldref Publications.

Table 7–16   *Source:* Reprinted with permission from E.L. Lewis-Michl et al., Breast Cancer Risk and Residence Near Industry or Traffic in Nassau and Suffolk Counties, Long Island, New York, *Archives of Environmental Health*, Vol. 51, No. 4, p. 261, © (July/August 1996), Heldref Publications.

Table 7–17   *Source:* Reprinted with permission from E.L. Lewis-Michl et al., Breast Cancer Risk and Residence Near Industry or Traffic in Nassau and Suffolk Counties, Long Island, New York, *Archives of Environmental Health*, Vol. 51, No. 4, p. 262, © (July/August 1996), Heldref Publications.

Table 7–18   *Source:* Reprinted with permission from E.L. Lewis-Michl et al., Breast Cancer Risk and Residence Near Industry or Traffic in Nassau and Suffolk Counties, Long Island, New York, *Archives of Environmental Health*, Vol. 51, No. 4, p. 262, © (July/August 1996), Heldref Publications.

Figure 7–24   *Source:* Reprinted from M.L. Casper et al., *Women and Heart Disease: An Atlas of Racial and Ethnic Disparities in Mortality*, Office for Social Environment and Health Research, West Virginia University, Morgantown, West Virginia, National Center for Chronic Disease Prevention and Health Promotion, Centers for Disease Control and Prevention, December 1999, p. 73, http://www.cdc.gov/nccdphp/cvd/womensatlas/. Last update 31 January 2001. Accessed February 18, 2001.

Figure 7–25   *Source:* Reprinted from M.L. Casper et al., *Women and Heart Disease: An Atlas of Racial and Ethnic Disparities in Mortality*, Office for Social Environment and Health Research, West Virginia University, Morgan-

town, West Virginia, National Center for Chronic Disease Prevention and Health Promotion, Centers for Disease Control and Prevention, December 1999, p. 75, http://www.cdc.gov/nccdphp/cvd/womensatlas/. Last update 31 January 2001. Accessed February 18, 2001.

Figure 7–26   *Source:* Reprinted from M.L. Casper et al., *Women and Heart Disease: An Atlas of Racial and Ethnic Disparities in Mortality*, Office for Social Environment and Health Research, West Virginia University, Morgantown, West Virginia, National Center for Chronic Disease Prevention and Health Promotion, Centers for Disease Control and Prevention, December 1999, p. 77, http://www.cdc.gov/nccdphp/cvd/womensatlas/. Last update 31 January 2001. Accessed February 18, 2001.

Figure 7–27   *Source:* Reprinted from M.L. Casper et al., *Women and Heart Disease: An Atlas of Racial and Ethnic Disparities in Mortality*, Office for Social Environment and Health Research, West Virginia University, Morgantown, West Virginia, National Center for Chronic Disease Prevention and Health Promotion, Centers for Disease Control and Prevention, December 1999, p. 79, http://www.cdc.gov/nccdphp/cvd/womensatlas/. Last update 31 January 2001. Accessed February 18, 2001.

Figure 7–28   *Source:* Reprinted from M.L. Casper et al., *Women and Heart Disease: An Atlas of Racial and Ethnic Disparities in Mortality*, Office for Social Environment and Health Research, West Virginia University, Morgantown, West Virginia, National Center for Chronic Disease Prevention and Health Promotion, Centers for Disease Control and Prevention, December 1999, p. 81, http://www.cdc.gov/nccdphp/cvd/womensatlas/. Last update 31 January 2001. Accessed February 18, 2001.

Figure 7–29   *Source:* Reprinted from M.L. Casper et al., *Women and Heart Disease: An Atlas of Racial and Ethnic Disparities in Mortality*, Office for Social Environment and Health Research, West Virginia University, Morgantown, West Virginia, National Center for Chronic Disease Prevention and Health Promotion, Centers for Disease Control and Prevention, December 1999, p. 83, http://www.cdc.gov/nccdphp/cvd/womensatlas/. Last update 31 January 2001. Accessed February 18, 2001.

Figure 7–30   *Source:* Reprinted from M.L. Casper et al., *Women and Heart Disease: An Atlas of Racial and Ethnic Disparities in Mortality*, Office for Social Environment and Health Research, West Virginia University, Morgantown, West Virginia, National Center for Chronic Disease Prevention and Health Promotion, Centers for Disease Control and Prevention, December 1999, p. 164, http://www.cdc.gov/nccdphp/cvd/womensatlas/. Last update 31 January 2001. Accessed February 18, 2001.

Figure 7–31   *Source:* Reprinted from M.L. Casper et al., *Women and Heart Disease: An Atlas of Racial and Ethnic Disparities in Mortality*, Office for Social Environment and Health Research, West Virginia University, Morgantown, West Virginia, National Center for Chronic Disease Prevention and Health Promotion, Centers for Disease Control and Prevention, December 1999, p. 164-165, http://www.cdc.gov/nccdphp/cvd/womensatlas/. Last update 31 January 2001. Accessed February 18, 2001.

Figure 7–32   *Source:* Reprinted from M.L. Casper et al., *Women and Heart Disease: An Atlas of Racial and Ethnic Disparities in Mortality*, Office for Social Environment and Health Research, West Virginia University, Morgantown, West Virginia, National Center for Chronic Disease Prevention and Health Promotion, Centers for Disease Control and Prevention, December 1999, p. 164-165, http://www.cdc.gov/nccdphp/cvd/womensatlas/. Last update 31 January 2001. Accessed February 18, 2001.

Figure 7–33   *Source:* Reprinted from M.L. Casper et al., *Women and Heart Disease: An Atlas of Racial and Ethnic Disparities in Mortality*, Office for Social Environment and Health Research, West Virginia University, Morgantown, West Virginia, National Center for Chronic Disease Prevention and Health Promotion, Centers for Disease Control and Prevention, December 1999, p. 165, http://www.cdc.gov/nccdphp/cvd/womensatlas/.

Last update 31 January 2001. Accessed February 18, 2001.

Figure 7–34   *Source:* Reprinted from M.L. Casper et al., *Women and Heart Disease: An Atlas of Racial and Ethnic Disparities in Mortality*, Office for Social Environment and Health Research, West Virginia University, Morgantown, West Virginia, National Center for Chronic Disease Prevention and Health Promotion, Centers for Disease Control and Prevention, December 1999, p. 165, http://www.cdc.gov/nccdphp/cvd/womensatlas/. Last update 31 January 2001. Accessed February 18, 2001.

Figure 7–35   *Source:* Reprinted from M.L. Casper et al., *Women and Heart Disease: An Atlas of Racial and Ethnic Disparities in Mortality*, Office for Social Environment and Health Research, West Virginia University, Morgantown, West Virginia, National Center for Chronic Disease Prevention and Health Promotion, Centers for Disease Control and Prevention, December 1999, p. 165, http://www.cdc.gov/nccdphp/cvd/womensatlas/. Last update 31 January 2001. Accessed February 18, 2001.

Table 7–19   *Source:* Reprinted from http://gis.cdc.gov/cvd from Atlas produced by the Centers for Disease Control, Center for Chronic Disease Prevention and Health Promotion and West Virginia University at www.cdc.gov/nccdphp/cvd/womensatlas/index.htm.

CHAPTER 8

Table 8–1   *Source:* Data from A. Melnick, Clackamas County Department of Human Services Community Health Mapping Engine (CHiME) Geographic Information Systems Project, *Journal of Public Health Management and Practice*, Vol. 5, No. 2, pp. 64-69, 1999 and C.V. Lee and J.L. Irving, Sources of Data for Community Health Planning, *Journal of Public Health Management and Practice*, Vol. 5, No. 4, pp. 7-22, 1999 and A. Melnick, Geographic Information Systems for Public Health, in *Public Health Administration Principles for Population-Based Management*, L.P. Novick and G.P. Mays, ed., © 2001, Aspen Publishers, Inc.

Figure 8–1   *Source:* Reprinted from N.M. Casey, J. Cazzolli and C.W. Keck, Active Patients Attending the North Hill Child Health Clinic, Akron, Ohio, 1997, *Journal of Public Health Management and Practice*, Vol. 5, No. 2, p. 52, © 1999, Aspen Publishers, Inc.

Figure 8–2   *Source:* Reprinted from G.F. White and K.C. Cerny, Client Demographics (Age and Gender) at Low-Income Clinics in Austin/Travis County, Texas, 1995-1996, *Journal of Public Health Management and Practice*, Vol. 5, No. 2, © 1999, p. 48, Aspen Publishers, Inc.

Figure 8–3   *Source:* Reprinted from J.L. Wilson and A. Branigan, Location of East Carolina University School of Medicine Telemedicine Sites in Relation to Primary Care Health Professional Shortage Areas for North Carolina's Health Service Area VI, 1997, *Journal of Public Health Management and Practice*, Vol. 5, No. 2, © 1999, p. 46, Aspen Publishers, Inc. and Division of Health Sciences, East Carolina University and HPSA data from the Federal Register, 62(104), May 30, 1997.

Table 8–2   *Source:* Reprinted with D. Berry and T.W., Ranking Priorities for a State Family Service Integration Initiative by Census Tract in Northern New Castle County, Delaware, 1997, *Journal of Public Health Management and Practice*, Vol. 5, No. 2, © 1999, p. 58, Aspen Publishers, Inc.

Table 8–3   *Source:* Reprinted with D. Berry and T.W., Ranking Priorities for a State Family Service Integration Initiative by Census Tract in Northern New Castle County, Delaware, 1997, *Journal of Public Health Management and Practice*, Vol. 5, No. 2, © 1999, p. 58, Aspen Publishers, Inc.

Figure 8–4   *Source:* Data from D. Berry and T.W., Ranking Priorities for a State Family Service Integration Initiative by Census Tract in Northern New Castle County, Delaware, 1997, *Journal of Public Health Management and Practice*, Vol. 5, No. 2, © 1999, p. 59, Aspen Publishers, Inc. and Delaware Health Statistics Center, 1997, Delaware Health & Social Services.

Table 8–4   *Source:* Data from D. Solet et al., VISTA/PH Software for Community Health Assessment, *Journal of Public Health Management and Practice*, Vol. 5, No. 2, © 1999, p. 62, Aspen Publishers, Inc. and Washington State Department of Health, Washington State Department of Social and Health Services and the 1990 U.S. Census.

Table 8–5   *Source:* Reprinted from A. Melnick et al., Clackamas County Department of Human Services Community Health Mapping Engine (CHiME) Geographic Information Systems Project, *Journal of Public Health Management and Practice*, Vol. 5, No. 2, © 1999, p. 67, Aspen Publishers, Inc.

Figure 8–5   *Source:* Data from A. Melnick et al., Clackamas County Department of Human Services Community Health Mapping Engine (CHiME) Geographic Information Systems Project, *Journal of Public Health Management and Practice*, Vol. 5, No. 2, © 1999, p. 65, Aspen Publishers, Inc. and Clackamas County Sheriffs Department and Clackamas County Information Services.

Figure 8–6   *Source:* Reprinted from A. Melnick et al., GIS in Community Health Assessment and Improvement, *Geographic Information Systems in Public Health: Proceedings from the Third National Conference,* R.C. Williams, ed., Agency for Toxic Substances and Disease Registry, United States Department of Health and Human Services, August 1998, pp. 597-600.

Figure 8–7   *Source:* Reprinted from A. Melnick et al., GIS in Community Health Assessment and Improvement, *Geographic Information Systems in Public Health: Proceedings from the Third National Conference,* R.C. Williams, ed., Agency for Toxic Substances and Disease Registry, United States Department of Health and Human Services, August 1998, pp. 597-600.

Table 8–6   *Source.* Reprinted from A. Melnick et al., Clackamas County Department of Human Services Community Health Mapping Engine (CHiME) Geographic Information Systems Project, *Journal of Public Health Management and Practice*, Vol. 5, No. 2, © 1999, p. 68, Aspen Publishers, Inc.

Table 8–7   Courtesy of J.L. McKnight and J.P. Kretzmann, Mapping Community Capacity, The Asset-Based Community Development Institute, Institute for Policy Research, 1990, Revised 1996, Northwestern University, Evanston, Illinois.

Table 8–8   Courtesy of J.L. McKnight and J.P. Kretzmann, Mapping Community Capacity, The Asset-Based Community Development Institute, Institute for Policy Research, 1990, Revised 1996, Northwestern University, Evanston, Illinois.

Figure 8–8   *Source:* Reprinted from D. Morrison et al., Improving Delivery of Health and Community Services to Welfare Recipients, Columbia, South Carolina, 1997, *Journal of Public Health Management and Practice*, Vol. 5, No. 2, © 1999, p. 50, Aspen Publishers, Inc.

Figure 8–9   *Source:* Reprinted from C.L. Hanchette, GIS and Decision Making for Public Health Agencies: Childhood Lead Poisoning and Welfare Reform, *Journal of Public Health Management and Practice*, Vol. 5, No. 4, © 1999, p. 46, Aspen Publishers, Inc.

Figure 8–10   *Source:* Reprinted from L. Dean, Revitalizing Communities with Geographic Information Systems (GIS): HUD's Community 2020 Software, *Journal of Public Health Management and Practice*, Vol. 5, No. 4, © 1999, p. 50, Aspen Publishers, Inc.

CHAPTER 10

Table 10–1   *Source:* Data from S.E. Thrall, Geographic Information System (GIS) Hardware and Software, *Journal of Public Health Management and Practice*, Vol. 5, No. 2, © 1999, p. 82-90, Aspen Publishers, Inc.

Table 10–2   *Source:* Data from S.E. Thrall, Geographic Information System (GIS) Hardware and Software, *Journal of Public Health Management and Practice*, Vol. 5, No. 2, © 1999, p. 87, Aspen Publishers, Inc.

Figure 10–1   *Source:* Reprinted from A.G. Dean, Epi Info and Epi Map: Current Status and Plans for Epi Info 2000, *Journal of Public Management and Practice*, Vol. 5, No. 4, © 1999, p. 56, Aspen Publishers, Inc.

Table 10–3   *Source:* Reprinted from T.W. Foresman, Spatial Analysis and Mapping on the Internet, *Journal of Public Health Management and Practice*, Vol. 5, No. 4, p. 59, © 1999, Aspen Publishers, Inc.

Figure 10–2   *Source:* Reprinted from T.W. Foresman, Spatial Analysis and Mapping on the Internet, *Journal of Public Health Management and Practice*, Vol. 5, No. 4, p. 60, © 1999, Aspen Publishers, Inc.

Figure 10–3   *Source:* Reprinted from T.W. Foresman, Spatial Analysis and Mapping on the Internet, *Journal of Public Health Management and Practice*, Vol. 5, No. 4, p. 60, © 1999, Aspen Publishers, Inc.

Figure 10–4   *Source:* Reprinted from T.W. Foresman, Spatial Analysis and Mapping on the Internet, *Journal of Public Health Management and Practice*, Vol. 5, No. 4, p. 61, © 1999, Aspen Publishers, Inc.

Figure 10–5   *Source:* Reprinted from T.W. Foresman, Spatial Analysis and Mapping on the Internet, *Journal of Public Health Management and Practice*, Vol. 5, No. 4, p. 62, © 1999, Aspen Publishers, Inc.

CHAPTER 11

Table 11–1   *Source:* Reprinted from G.I. Thrall, The Future of GIS in Public Health Management and Practice, *Journal of Public Health Management and Practice*, Vol. 5, No. 4, p. 77, © 1999, Aspen Publishers, Inc.

Table 11–2   *Source:* Reprinted from Centers for Disease Control and Prevention, Population-Based Prevalence of Perinatal Exposure to Cocaine—Georgia 1994, *Morbidity and Mortality Weekly Report*, Vol. 45, No. 41, October 18, 1996, p. 889, United States Department of Health and Human Services.

Figure 11–1   *Source:* Reprinted from M.D. Brantley, R.W. Rochat, C.D. Ferre et al., Population-Based Prevalence of Cocaine in Newborn Infants—Georgia 1994, *Geographic Information Systems in Public Health: Proceedings from the Third National Conference*, R.C. Williams, et al., ed., Agency for Toxic Substances and Disease Registry, United States Department of Health and Human Services, August 1998, p. 516.

Figure 11–2   *Source:* Reprinted from M.D. Brantley, R.W. Rochat, C.D. Ferre et al., Population-Based Prevalence of Cocaine in Newborn Infants—Georgia 1994, *Geographic Information Systems in Public Health: Proceedings from the*

Third National Conference, R.C. Williams, et al., ed., Agency for Toxic Substances and Disease Registry, United States Department of Health and Human Services, August 1998, p. 517.

Figure 11–3   *Source:* Reprinted from M.D. Brantley, R.W. Rochat, C.D. Ferre et al., Population-Based Prevalence of Cocaine in Newborn Infants—Georgia 1994, *Geographic Information Systems in Public Health: Proceedings from the Third National Conference*, R.C. Williams, et al., ed., Agency for Toxic Substances and Disease Registry, United States Department of Health and Human Services, August 1998, p. 517.

Figure 11–4   *Source:* Reprinted from M.D. Brantley, R.W. Rochat, C.D. Ferre et al., Population-Based Prevalence of Cocaine in Newborn Infants—Georgia 1994, *Geographic Information Systems in Public Health: Proceedings from the Third National Conference*, R.C. Williams, et al., ed., Agency for Toxic Substances and Disease Registry, United States Department of Health and Human Services, August 1998, p. 518.

Figure 11–5   *Source:* Reprinted from M.D. Brantley, R.W. Rochat, C.D. Ferre et al., Population-Based Prevalence of Cocaine in Newborn Infants—Georgia 1994, *Geographic Information Systems in Public Health: Proceedings from the Third National Conference*, R.C. Williams, et al., ed., Agency for Toxic Substances and Disease Registry, United States Department of Health and Human Services, August 1998, p. 519.

Figure 11–6   *Source:* Reprinted from M.D. Brantley, R.W. Rochat, C.D. Ferre et al., Population-Based Prevalence of Cocaine in Newborn Infants—Georgia 1994, *Geographic Information Systems in Public Health: Proceedings from the Third National Conference*, R.C. Williams, et al., ed., Agency for Toxic Substances and Disease Registry, United States Department of Health and Human Services, August 1998, p. 519.

Figure 11–7   *Source:* Reprinted from M.D. Brantley, R.W. Rochat, C.D. Ferre et al., Population-Based Prevalence of Cocaine in Newborn Infants—Georgia 1994, *Geographic Information Systems in Public Health: Proceedings from the Third National Conference*, R.C. Williams,

et al., ed., Agency for Toxic Substances and Disease Registry, United States Department of Health and Human Services, August 1998, p. 521.

Figure 11–8   *Source:* Reprinted from M.D. Brantley, R.W. Rochat, C.D. Ferre et al., Population-Based Prevalence of Cocaine in Newborn Infants—Georgia 1994, *Geographic Information Systems in Public Health: Proceedings from the Third National Conference*, R.C. Williams, et al., ed., Agency for Toxic Substances and Disease Registry, United States Department of Health and Human Services, August 1998, p. 521.

Figure 11–9   *Source:* Reprinted from M.D. Brantley, R.W. Rochat, C.D. Ferre et al., Population-Based Prevalence of Cocaine in Newborn Infants—Georgia 1994, *Geographic Information Systems in Public Health: Proceedings from the Third National Conference*, R.C. Williams, et al., ed., Agency for Toxic Substances and Disease Registry, United States Department of Health and Human Services, August 1998, p. 522.

Table 11–3   *Source:* Adapted from G.I. Thrall, The Future of GIS in Public Health Management and Practice, *Journal of Public Health Management and Practice*, Vol. 5, No. 4, p. 79, © 1999, Aspen Publishers, Inc.

Table 11–4   *Source:* Data from American Public Health Association, *Healthy Communities 2000: Model Standards, Washington, D.C.: American Public Health Association*, 1991 and National Association of County and City Health Officials, *1992-1993, National Profile of Local Health Departments, National Surveillance Series*, Washington, D.C., National Association of County and City Health Officials, 1995.

Figure 11–10   *Source:* Reprinted from T.B. Richards et al., Toward a GIS Sampling Frame for Surveys of Local Health Departments and Local Boards of Health, *Journal of Public Health Management and Practice*, Vol. 5, No. 4, p. 66, © 1999, Aspen Publishers, Inc.

Figure 11–11   *Source:* Reprinted from T.B. Richards et al., Toward a GIS Sampling Frame for Surveys of Local Health Departments and Local Boards of Health, *Journal of Public Health Management and Practice*, Vol. 5, No. 4, p. 68, © 1999, Aspen Publishers, Inc.

Index